Textbook of Clinical Psychology

Second Edition

临床心理学教程（第2版）

主　编　王　伟　方建群

副主编　朱荔芳　周　莉

编　者　（按姓氏笔画排序）

马现仓（西安交通大学医学院）　　　　吴　颢（广州医科大学）

王　伟（浙江大学）　　　　　　　　　邹　涛（贵州医科大学附属医院）

方建群（宁夏医科大学）　　　　　　　辛秀红（宁夏医科大学）

朱　屹（海南医学院第一附属医院）　　张　兰（兰州大学第二医院）

朱荔芳（济宁医学院）　　　　　　　　张雪琴（广州医科大学）

朱菊红（兰州大学第二医院）　　　　　周　莉（大连医科大学）

刘　伟（江苏大学医学院）　　　　　　段熙明（济宁医学院）

苏朝霞（海南医学院第一附属医院）　　祝绮莎（浙江大学）

李　平（齐齐哈尔医学院）　　　　　　顾思梦（江苏大学医学院）

杨世昌（新乡医学院）　　　　　　　　徐国庆（大连医科大学）

学术秘书　祝绮莎（兼）

人民卫生出版社

图书在版编目（CIP）数据

临床心理学教程 = Textbook of Clinical Psychology：英语 / 王伟，方建群主编. —2 版. —北京：人民卫生出版社，2017
　　ISBN 978-7-117-25493-9

　Ⅰ．①临…　Ⅱ．①王…②方…　Ⅲ．①医学心理学－英文
Ⅳ．①R395.1

中国版本图书馆 CIP 数据核字（2017）第 286615 号

| 人卫智网 | www.ipmph.com | 医学教育、学术、考试、健康，购书智慧智能综合服务平台 |
| 人卫官网 | www.pmph.com | 人卫官方资讯发布平台 |

Textbook of Clinical Psychology
临床心理学教程
第 2 版

主　　编：王　伟　方建群
出版发行：人民卫生出版社（中继线 010-59780011）
地　　址：北京市朝阳区潘家园南里 19 号
邮　　编：100021
E - mail：pmph @ pmph.com
购书热线：010-59787592　010-59787584　010-65264830
印　　刷：三河市尚艺印装有限公司
经　　销：新华书店
开　　本：889 × 1194　1/16　印张：20
字　　数：620 千字
版　　次：2010 年 7 月第 1 版　　2017 年 12 月第 2 版
　　　　　2017 年 12 月第 2 版第 1 次印刷（总第 2 次印刷）
标准书号：ISBN 978-7-117-25493-9/R · 25494
定　　价：66.00 元

打击盗版举报电话：010-59787491　E-mail：WQ @ pmph.com
（凡属印装质量问题请与本社市场营销中心联系退换）

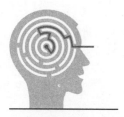

Preface

This textbook is designed for international students majoring in medicine, health and social sciences. Topics in the textbook include the basic psychological processes from peripheral to central nervous systems, clinically common psychological/psychiatric disorders, and the frequently seen consultation-liaison situations. Clinical psychology also covers the discipline of observation and probing inquiry, which is a basic science of behavior, and clinical science of mental disorders and emotional responses to physiological change, somatic illness, and life events. Therefore, we hope the information in this textbook provides a comprehensive scale for the education purpose of clinical psychology.

All contributors to this textbook have been working in fields of medical education and clinical practice for many years. I am indeed grateful to these dear colleagues of mine who have devoted much of their efforts to the textbook. It is their rich experience and kind help that make this textbook possible.

Many thanks,

Prof. Dr. Wei Wang (王伟); Hangzhou, China; Summer, 2017

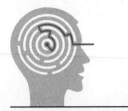

Contents

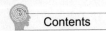

Contents

Chapter 1

Psychological Processes: Early Stages

How do we perceive the world? Why do we forget? How can we understand the processes of learning? How are people motivated to take a certain action? Why some people act aggressively and other people show obedience. Psychological ideas are popular in everyday life. We all use the principles of psychology everyday and probably do not even realize it. When we face a troublesome situation, and talk to ourselves in our minds, "calm down," or "give up," we are utilizing cognitive approaches to change our behaviors and emotions. In a word, psychology covers a great range from our daily lives to a variety of professional fields. It investigates our mental processes and behaviors, and provides meaningful explanations of our experiences.

Psychology is the science involving the scientific study of mental processes and behavior. This definition includes three elements. First, psychological study is a serious and scientific work, and relies on a systematic and scientific method to conduct observations and experiments. The conclusions must depend on the scientific evidence that is based on careful observation and rigorous analysis. Second, psychology explores the mental processes such as memory, emotion, volition, reasoning, imagination, creativity, dreaming and so on; in other words, all the different things that we can do with our minds. As to the mental processes, psychologists share many interests with neurobiologists, especially in the field of cognitive science. Both fields are related to the study of mental processes. Third, behavior is one of the important areas of study in psychology. The term behavior in psychology means any activity of an individual or animal that can be observed and measured. The behaviors usually refer to talking, running, smoking, crying, and even eye blinking. They also refer to some complex behaviors such as making a decision to get married, break up with boyfriend, or give up a job. People behave in certain ways, which are closely linked to their mental processes. The behaviors are determined by multiple causes. Both heredity and environment jointly influence people's behaviors. Psychologists often explore mental processes through observing and studying these behaviors.

1. Sensation and perception

How does the world out there get in? How do we construct our representations of the external world? To represent the world in our mind, we must detect physical energy from the environment and encode it as neural signals, a process traditionally called sensation. Moreover, we must select, organize, and interpret our sensations, a process traditionally called perception.

In our everyday life, sensation and perception blend into one continuous process. What if you were blind and unable to see the faces of your family members? What if you were unable to feel your stomach growl, smell the dinner, or taste the food? Human life would be very difficult without the ability to sense and perceive external and internal stimuli. Thanks to the nose, ears, eyes, tongue, and skin, we can enjoy delicious food, fragrant flowers and plants, a comfortable shower, beautiful sky and sea, and we can have plenty of experiences about our environment and ourselves.

1

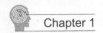

Psychologists are interested in sensation and perception as inputs to and outputs from the brain. Broadly speaking, the study of sensation and perception is one of how an individual knows what is going on around him or her, and then gives explanations about the information. The scientific study of sensation and perception began with the works of Gustav Fechner (1860—1912), a German psychologist and physicist, who examined how the physical properties of stimuli relate to people's experience, and developed the means to quantify the relationship between physical stimuli in the external world and perceptual experience. The early stages of psychological process include initial information processing of sensation, perception, memory and learning. The late stages include thinking, consciousness, motivation and emotion.

1.1　Sensation

1.1.1　The assessment of sense

We live in a world full of information including energies and substances. Sensory systems enable organisms to obtain the information they need to function and survive. A stimulus is any passing source of physical energy that produces a response in a sense organ. Stimuli vary in both type and intensity. Different types of stimuli activate different sense organs. For instance, light stimuli can activate the sense of sight and allow us to see the colors of a tree in autumn. However, all types of sensory receptors have limits. For example, how strong must the information be for it to be detected by the sensory receptor? Commonsense tells us that the intensity of stimuli affects the sensation magnitude. For instance, the louder a sound is, the more it affects the auditory system; the brighter a light is, the more it affects the visual system.

The ability of sensory receptors to perceive the intensity of stimuli is called sensitivity of sensation. Absolute threshold and difference threshold are the measures to assess the sensitivity of sensation by psychologists.

(1) Absolute thresholds

We exist in a sea of energy. At this moment, radio waves and x-rays, ultraviolet and infrared light, sound waves of very high and very low frequencies, are striking us. But to all of them we are blind and deaf. So what stimuli can we detect? At what levels of intensity? The answer to these questions requires an understanding of the concept of absolute thresholds.

An absolute threshold is the smallest intensity of a stimulus that must be present for it to be detected. In other words, the absolute threshold is the point where something becomes noticeable to our senses.

For example, the weakest amount of light that can be reliably discriminated from darkness is an absolute threshold for light detection. Other examples include the softest sound we can hear, and the slightest touch we can feel. The absolute threshold for stimulation is the smallest, weakest stimulus energy that the organism can detect, and it is concerned with the point between not being able to hear a sound, or see a light, and being just barely able to detect it. Therefore the stimuli reaching a receptor must be intense enough to produce a noticeable effect. The absolute threshold is a basic way to assess the sensitivity of a sensory process.

The sensitivity of the sensory process is different in a variety of organisms. Compared to humans, a police dog has a remarkable sense of smell; an eagle has a superior sense of sight; and a dolphin has a superior sense of hearing. We humans cannot sense all the odors around us, or taste every individual spice used in a dish. These and many other examples help to provide evidence that the threshold in humans to detect stimuli is different from other animals.

(2) Difference thresholds

How do we recognize and assess the changes of stimulus once a stimulus becomes detectable to us? How do we notice when it becomes louder or smaller? Psychologists have discussed this comparison problem in terms of difference threshold. The difference threshold is the smallest amount of change that we need to recognize that a change has occurred, in other words, a measure of the smallest increase or decrease in a physical stimulus. The difference threshold is another way to assess the sensitivity of a sensory process. It is the smallest change in stimulation for us to recognize it, or the smallest physical difference between two stimuli that can still be recognized as a difference, a just noticeable difference.

1) Webber's Law. Webber's Law states that a just noticeable difference is a constant proportion of the intensity of an initial stimulus. Over 100 years ago, German scientist Ernst Weber (1795—1878) carried out a famous experiment, and found that the noticeable difference in our sensory process depends on a proportion of change rather than a real amount of change. This finding, named after its original observer, is known as Webber's Law. According to Webber's Law, if the original stimulus is strong, the magnitude of the second stimulus needs to be increased much more for us to notice the difference. For example, if we hold a three-pound weight and one pound was added. Most of us can notice this difference. However, if we hold a fifty-pound weight and one pound was added, we may not notice the change that has occurred due to the addition of this extra weight.

The difference threshold is not the same for all types of sensation. When we are listening to music, we are sensitive to notice the changes such as sounds becoming louder or smaller, or a tone slightly becoming higher or lower. However, it needs a big change between the two stimuli for us to notice the difference in taste during listening to music.

2) Sensory adaptation. You may have such an experience: when you are studying in a noisy classroom, you will notice the noise right away, yet after a while the noise fades into the background. If you enter a stinky bathroom, the smell may be awful for the first few minutes, yet after a little while you do not notice it anymore. Sensory adaptation is the decrease in sensitivity to an unchanging stimulus. The smells do not disappear, but people just become less sensitive to them.

Sensory systems are more sensitive to the change in stimulus input than to a steady input. In most cases, some sensory receptors show reduced sensitivity to a stimulus that remains unchanged for an extended period of time. Sensory adaptation refers to the sensory receptors becoming less sensitive to unchanging stimulus. In addition, for some sensory systems, sensory adaptation may take place in the central nervous system rather than in the sensory receptor. After a period of unchanging stimulation, the brain may just start ignoring it.

Although the sensory adaptation reduces our sensitivity, it offers an important benefit: It enables us to focus our attention on informative changes in our environment without being distracted by the uninformative changes, constant stimulation. Our sense receptors are alert to novelty. We can perceive the world not exactly as it is, but as it is useful for us to perceive it.

1.1.2   Basic senses

Any form of energy and substance that is able to excite a sensory receptor cell can be defined as "stimulus" including sound, light, heat, cold, odor, color, touch, and pressure. The nature of sense organs partially results from their adaptation to the environment. For instance, dogs have a sharp sense of smell whereas their sight is not better than humans, while cats' sight is exclusively sharp in the night that facilitates them to catch grey. Human sense organs have evolved an efficient system for making sense of our world. What happen in the sensing processes? How do our senses work? We need to know the basic physiological processes of sensation, or the common biological properties of the senses.

The different sensory organs detect and receive various forms of energy. It is also called the proximal stimulus. A proximal stimulus triggers a response in specialized receptors, which then transduces that stimulus

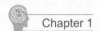

energy into a neural impulse that is carried to the brain. For the sense of vision, the proximal stimulus is a light wave, and the receptor cells are rods and cones in the retina. For the sense of hearing, the proximal stimulus is a sound wave, and the receptor cells are hair cells on the basilar membrane. Many of sensory receptors are found on or near the outside surface of our bodies like the eyes, ears, and skin. They usually detect external stimuli. Other sensory receptors are simply specialized endings of sensory neurons.

Transduction is the way in which sensory stimuli are converted to neural impulses. Sense organs operate through sensory receptor cells that receive and detect external information such as energy and substances, and convert these stimuli into neural impulses that can be transmitted to the brain. The sensory process generally contains the followings steps: sensory receptors detect stimuli, and convert the information into the electrochemical energy (neural impulse) that is meaningful to the nervous system. A variety of stimulations are detected by sensory receptors. The receptors convert the sensory information into a neural signal, and then the intensity and the quality of stimuli are further coded in order to keep the precision during conveying information. By the time it reaches the central nervous system, the information related to the stimulations is still quite precise.

For the five primary senses (vision, hearing, smell, touch, and taste), the basic sensory process works in a similar manner: receiving the proximal stimulus, followed by transduction. We will take a brief look at each.

(1) Vision

Compared to most of animals, humans rely heavily on their sense of vision to perceive the world. We are surrounded by a wide range of electromagnetic waves including light, cosmic rays, x-rays, ultraviolet waves, and so on. The proximal stimulus that the sense of vision responds to is the light wave, and the human eye detects only a narrow band of the electromagnetic spectrum (wavelengths, 350-750 nm).

1) Parts of the visual system. The visual system consists of the eyes, several parts of the brain, and pathways connecting them. The eyes primarily include the cornea, which gathers and focuses the entering light; the pupil, which is a hole allowing light to pass; the lens, which causes light to bend; the retina, upon which the refracted light is focused. In the process leading to vision, light enters the eye through the cornea, and then passes through the pupil and the lens. The amount of light entering the eye is regulated by the size of the pupil. The lens performs the process of focusing the light on the retina by changing its shape. After the optical process of focusing the image on the retina, transduction occurs. Light energy is converted into neural impulses, conveyed to the brain where the visual sensation occurs.

2) Color vision. The human vision system can see an extensive range of colors. Color vision enables human to distinguish and identify lights and objects on the basis of their spectral properties. The hue, saturation, and brightness are three separate components for the experience of color. The hue refers to the wavelength or such as colors red, green, and blue; the brightness refers to the intensity of the hues; and the saturation indicates the purity or richness of the hues. Humans can distinguish only about 150 hues but, through gradations of saturation and brightness, humans can perceive about 300,000 colors.

3) Theories of color vision. Theories of color vision attempt to explain how human sense the colors. There are two main theories of color vision: the trichromatic theory and the opponent-process theory.

The trichromatic theory of color vision is one of the earliest theories. It proposes that the eye contains three kinds of color receptors that are most responsive to the three primary colors: red, green, and blue, and color vision depends on the activity of three different receptor mechanisms. The three-receptor mechanisms are stimulated to different degrees by the light of a particular wavelength. The pattern of activity in the three mechanisms results in the perception of a certain color. According to this theory, perception of color is influenced by the relative strength with which each of the three kinds of cones is activated. If we see a blue

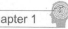

sky, the blue cones are primarily triggered, and the others show less activity. The trichromatic theory of color vision makes clear some of the processes involved in color vision, but it does not explain all aspects of color vision.

The opponent-process theory further describes events later in the visual system. According to this theory, there are some color combinations that we never see, such as reddish-green, yellowish-blue, or black-white. Activation of one member of the pair inhibits activity in the other. The color perception is controlled by the activity of two opponent systems, and no two members of a pair can be seen at the same location. This theory also helps to explain some types of color vision deficiency. For example, people with dichromatic deficiencies will confuse either red and green, or blue and yellow.

In fact, both theories are needed to explain the process of color vision. The trichromatic theory explains that the receptors respond with different patterns to different wavelengths, while the opponent-process theory reflects that neurons integrate the inhibitory and excitatory signals from the receptors. Trichromatic theory describes what is happening at the very beginning of the visual system, in the receptors of the retina. The existence of three different kinds of cone receptors is why it takes a minimum of three wavelengths to match any wavelength in the spectrum. Opponent-process theory describes what is going on later in the visual system. Opponent cells are responsible for perceptual experiences such as afterimages and simultaneous contrast.

(2) Audition

The proximal stimulus that the sense of hearing (audition) responds to is the sound wave. Audition is the sense that detects vibratory changes of sound waves in the air. The amplitude of the sound waves largely determines the loudness of a sound. The frequency of the sound wave, for which the unit of measure is Hertz (Hz), is the primary determinant of pitch, which refers to how high or low the tone appears. Human ears can hear sound waves with frequencies from about 20 to 20,000 Hz.

1) Parts of the audition system. The ear can be divided into three areas: outer ear, middle ear, and inner ear. The outer ear is the external part that helps to collect sound waves. It consists of the pinna, auditory canal, and eardrum. The middle ear refers to the three tiny bones (malleus, incus and stapes) and the surrounding structures. The sound waves are converted into mechanical energy in the middle ear. The cochlea is the primary component of the inner ear. The sound waves (mechanical energies) are translated into nerve signals to be sent to the brain.

In the process leading to audition, the sounds enter into the auditory canal of the outer ear, which funnels the sound waves. The sound waves then strike the eardrum and cause it to vibrate. This vibration of sound waves makes the three ossicles vibrate in sequence. The sound waves are magnified in their passage, through the middle ear to the oval window of the inner ear. In the inner ear, the sound waves cause the fluid inside the cochlea to move. In the cochlea is a structure called the basilar membrane, which is attached to hair cells. The hair cells act as sensory receptors for hearing. Vibrations of the fluid cause the basilar membrane to move up and down. An electrical charge is produced in the hair cells by bending of the hair cells, and then neurotransmitter release onto auditory neurons, which convey the information to the auditory cortex of the brain.

2) Theories of hearing. As mentioned above, human ears can hear sounds from about 20 to 20,000 Hz. Some animals can hear sounds above 20,000 Hz, and other animals probably detect sounds below 20 Hz. How can we tell the difference between different sounds? Researchers developed many theories to explain how different sound-wave patterns are coded into neural messages. We here introduce the two traditional theories of hearing.

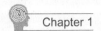

(a) Place theory of hearing. This theory holds that humans differentiate different types of sounds according to the location (place) on the basilar membrane that the waves vibrate. In other words, the hair cells at different places vibrate for different pitches; the brain identifies pitch by the place where the vibration is the strongest. This theory is true for sounds above 4,000 Hz. For example, a 6,000 Hz sound causes one area of the basilar membrane to vibrate, and the 18,000 Hz sound causes another area to vibrate.

The problem with this theory is that it cannot explain sounds below 4,000 Hz (low sounds). It is difficult for us to differentiate between different types of sounds because very low sounds cause the entire basilar membrane to vibrate.

(b) Frequency theory of hearing. Frequency theory proposes that the frequency of vibration on the basilar membrane as a whole is translated into an equivalent frequency of nerve signals. This theory describes the particular sound we hear by the frequency of vibrations on the basilar membrane. It emphasizes that the basilar membrane reproduces the vibrations according to frequency as a whole, and all hair cells fire. It explains how humans differentiate the sounds of less than 1,000 Hz. However, the frequency theory cannot explain how humans differentiate the sounds between 1,000 Hz and 4,000 Hz. Later, researchers modified the frequency theory and proposed that the hair cells on the basilar membrane fire in groups as well as in sequences, then send a rapid series of impulses to the brain. The particular pattern of firing makes humans to differentiate the sounds ranging from 1,000 Hz to 4,000 Hz.

(3) Other senses

1) Olfaction. The human sense of smell (olfaction) can recognize thousands of different smells, and detect odors even in infinitesimal quantities. Smell affects many psychological experiences of life such as attraction, memories, and emotions.

The proximal stimulus of olfaction is an odor particle and the receptors cells are located in the olfactory epithelium at the top of the nasal cavity. The olfactory system is the primary sensory system involved in detecting chemical substances in the air. Scented air contains some chemical substances, which are capable of stimulating the olfactory receptors, and such air may reach the receptor surface by being inhaled through the nose. From there messages are carried directly to the olfactory bulb in the brain, where they are sent to the brain's temporal lobe, and the awareness of smell occurs.

2) Gustation. For the sense of taste (gustation), the proximal stimulus is a substance dissolved in saliva, and the receptors cells are microvilli in the taste buds of the tongue. The taste buds are concentrated along the edges and back surface of the tongue. There are about 10,000 taste buds on the tongue. Each food contains many chemicals substances, which are able to activate a range of taste receptors, thereby providing the unique experience of taste.

The taste buds are sensitive to the five primary taste qualities: sweet, sour, salty, bitter, and umami. Each type of receptor responds intensely to particular types of substances. For example, sweet receptor cells respond primarily to sugars; sour receptor cells respond primarily to acids. All other tastes derive from combinations of these five taste qualities. When something enters the mouth, its chemicals are dissolved by the saliva, and then enter the taste bud. Only substances dissolved in water (or saliva, which is mostly water) can be tasted. Each taste bud contains a cluster of taste receptor cells; the adjacent neurons are activated, and send a nerve impulse to the brain. Then, we have an experience of the sense of taste.

3) The somatosensory system. Skin senses - pressure, touch, temperature and pain, play an important role in survival. The skin is the largest sense organ, and contains numerous nerve receptors, which locate in the epidermis and dermis of the skin. There are three major types of receptors in the skin: mechanoreceptors, thermoreceptors, and pain receptors. The nerve fibers from these receptors travel to the brain, and then we

have an experience of the cutaneous sensations.

The mechanoreceptors detect information such as pressure, vibrations, and texture. When you touch a piece of canvas, an enormous amount of information about the texture of the canvas is transferred to your brain through your fingers because your fingers are full of the sensitive mechanoreceptors.

The thermoreceptors perceive sensations related to the temperature of objects. Human are very sensitive to temperature and able to detect a change of less than one degree centigrade. Thermoreceptors are found all over the body, and including cold and hot receptors. Humans perceive different kinds of temperatures primarily by whether hot or cold receptors are activated.

The pain receptors are found in the skin, muscles, bones, blood vessels, and some organs throughout the body. They can detect pain that is caused by mechanical stimuli such as cutting or scraping, thermal stimuli such as a burn or chemical stimuli such as poison from an insect sting. Pain is a complex sensation that involves more than the simple transmission of pain information from the skin to the brain. The nociception such as pain senses can send the early warning signals to the brain in order to keep the body safe from serious injury or damage. For example, a broken piece of glass or hot water can cause a feeling of sharp pain in your skin, and it can urge you to quickly move away from these harmful stimuli.

Although some theories try to explain the mechanisms of the cutaneous sensations, the direct relationships between the various types of receptors and the cutaneous sensations are not completely understood now.

1.2　Perception

We can sense the sights and sounds, tastes and smells, touch and movement. How do we see not just shapes and colors, but a smile face? How do we hear not just a mix of pitches and rhythms, but a beautiful music? The mind can organize sensations into perceptions.

Perception is a constructive process by which we go beyond the stimuli that are presented to us and attempt to construct a meaningful situation. It involves the selection, organization, and interpretation of sensory information.

1.2.1　Selectivity of perception

Though we are exposed to numerous stimuli, we tend to select only a few at a given time, this is perceptual selectivity. We remember very little of what we do not attend to. During the perceptual process, sensory information is firstly selected, and then sent to the brain. We will not perceive a large amount of information or stimuli if we do not choose to attend to it. For example, at a big dinner party, although we may hear a number of conversations around us, we can easily hear and talk with one friend on a topic of interest, because we select to focus on talking with this friend and ignore the noisy surroundings.

Perceptual selectivity is influenced by some factors. The differences of perceptual selectivity may arise due to the several aspects: the perceiver, the target, and the situation.

Some factors associated with the perceiver are: personality, motives, needs, and expectations. For example, a hungry and thirsty individual must pay more attention to the food and drink while an individual with the need for power will focus on developing affiliation, and on achievement. Some factors associated with the target are novelty, intensity, background, sounds, and size. For example, a novel object, with bright colors increases its probability of being perceived; a larger object is more likely to be noticed than a smaller object; and the stimuli that differ most from the background receive maximum attention. In addition, perceptual selectivity is associated with the situation, such as time and place at the given point. Too many events occur simultaneously in the environment around us. There are several ways in which the brain interprets such complex flow of information and creates perceptual experiences beyond initial sensations.

1.2.2 Organization of perception

After selection, we then employ some principles to make sense of what we are experiencing, in other words, we need to organize the sensory information. Psychologists describe several principles of perceptual organization that people use to make sense of what they see. These principles include figure and ground, and grouping.

(1) Figure and ground

In the perceptual process, the first task is to perceive an object as distinct from its surroundings. The object is called the figure, and its surroundings are called the ground. The figure-ground relationship is the most fundamental principle of perceptual organization, and it is also the most elementary form of the perceptual process. It means when we view the world, certain objects seem to stand out from their background. The object perceived as figure is dependent on our interest, and the ground is usually meaningless, behind the figures. For example, when we look for a friend in a crowded scene, or listen to a presentation in a noisy classroom, we can automatically pick out certain people or sounds as figures and relegate others to the background.

Sometimes, the figure-ground organization can be ambiguous. Please see the following picture (Figure 1-1), it is difficult for you to perceive the figure as both a vase and two faces at the same time. When we look at this figure for a few moments, a vase or two faces alternates to be a figure. The phenomenon demonstrates that the perceptual organization into figure or ground depends on our mind, not the stimulus.

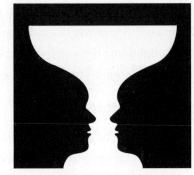

Figure 1-1 Figure-Ground stimulus can be seen as a pair of faces or a vase

(2) Grouping

Having discriminated figure from ground, we must organize the figure into a meaningful form. Gestalt psychologists have studied perceptual organization extensively. The German word "Gestalt" is roughly translated to "whole" or "configuration". Gestalt psychologists believe that the perceived whole is more than the sum of its parts, and the brain automatically imposes a kind of order to sensory perception. Humans have innate organizing tendencies in the brain, facilitating interpretation of the information completely without repetition.

According to Gestalt, "principles stimuli or sensory information can be grouped and seen as a whole by humans" perception. That is, the brain sees things in the world that are not really "there." We may fill in the missing information when we perceive something, and group various objects together so as to see whole objects, or hear meaningful sounds. Please see the Figure 1-2, it is a different perceptual experience when we see one dot, or the eleven dots together; we group eleven dots together by saying "a triangle." Without this tendency to group our perceptions, those same dots would be seen as "dot, dot, dot…" Generally, the Gestalt principles of grouping include the following: similarity, proximity, continuity, and closure.

1) Similarity. The Gestalt principle of similarity refers to how people tend to group things together based upon how similar the objects are. Objects that are of a similar color, size, or shape are frequently grouped together. In the Figure 1-3, we distinguish the cross because the dots with similar shape are seen as a group. The dots and squares are respectively grouped according to similar shape. It is the principle of similarity at work.

2) Proximity. The Gestalt principle of proximity refers to how elements that are closer together are more likely to be perceived as belonging together. When objects are close to one another, we tend to perceive them

as a group rather than separate parts. In the Figure 1-4, we tend to perceive three columns of two arrowheads, rather than six different arrowheads. It is the principle of proximity at work.

3) Continuity. The Gestalt principle of continuity refers to our tendency to perceive interrupted lines and patterns as being continuous by filling in the gaps. We are inclined to group things together so as to continue a pattern or direction. In the Figure 1-5, we tend to perceive a letter X with two continuous curves crossing rather than four separate parts.

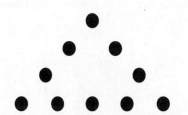

Figure 1-2   The dots are more likely to be perceived as a triangle

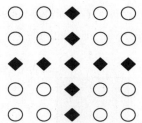

Figure 1-3   The diamonds and circles are respectively perceived as a cross and the squares according to similar shape

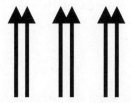

Figure 1-4   The six arrowheads are more likely to be perceived as three columns according to the principle of proximity

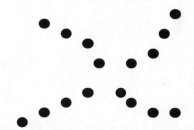

Figure 1-5   The dots are more likely to be perceived as two smooth lines which cross according to the principle of continuity

4) Closure. The Gestalt principle of closure refers to our tendency to complete figures with gaps in them, favoring the more enclosed or complete figures. We tend to perceive a whole object while overlooking some missing or incomplete sensory information. In the Figure 1-6, we perceive a circle and a rectangle at first glance in spite of the gaps.

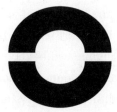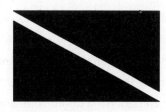

Figure 1-6   The tow semicircles and the two triangles are respectively perceived as a circle and a rectangle according to the principle of closure

(3) Perceptual constancy

When we walk away from a tall building, the image on your retina becomes smaller and smaller. While we get closer, the building should get bigger and bigger. In fact, this does not happen, but instead we still perceive the same height of the building. So we have a tendency to perceive objects as unchanging even though the raw sensory information has changed. A major function of the perceptual system is to achieve perceptual constancy. Perceptual constancy is a phenomenon in which physical objects are perceived as unvarying

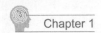

and consistent despite changes in their appearance or in the physical environment. It enables us to perceive fundamental characteristics of the world around us. We will discuss three typical perceptual constancies: shape, size and lightness.

(4) Shape constancy

Shape constancy refers to our ability to perceive that shape remains the same no matter the angle from which it is viewed. When a door opens, it casts a changing shape on our retinal, yet we manage to perceive the door as having s constant door like shape (Figure 1-7). Shape constancy help us to perceive objects as the same shape from a variety of orientations.

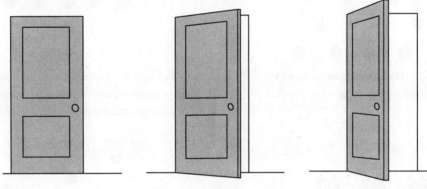

Figure 1-7　Door constancy

(5) Size constancy

Size constancy refers to how we perceive objects as maintaining the same size no matter how far away they are, even when the distance changes and makes them appear larger or smaller. As we walk towards a tall building from a long distance, we generally do not see it as increasing in size. Due to our ability to maintain constancy in our perceptions, we see that the building remains the same height no matter how far away it is. Size constancy enables us to perceive fundamental characteristics of our surroundings though a huge amount of information continuously rushes to our sensory organs. Size constancy of perception depends on a number of factors including the familiarity with the objects concerned, and the availability of distance cues.

(6) Lightness constancy

Lightness constancy refers to our ability to perceive that the lightness of an object remains the same, or changes very little, even when illumination varies. A deep blue shirt remains blue both in sunlight as in shadow, even though it reflects more light when it is directly illuminated by the sun. Color constancy refers to how we see objects as having the same color whether they are outdoors or indoors because the eyes adapt quickly to different lighting conditions. Without color and brightness constancy, our perceptual system would be constantly re-interpreting color and brightness. If this were the case, we would see the continuous changes in the color of our clothes and other things unless we keep not moving. Brightness and color constancy depend on the intensities of light reflected from the objects, and the amount of light an object reflects relative to its surroundings. Although all the examples of constancy that we have described are visual, constancies also occur in the other senses.

1.2.3　Depth perception

The images on retina are flat and two-dimensional. But the world around us is three-dimensional, how do we perceive it that way? Depth perception is the ability to perceive the distance and to perceive the world in

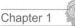

three-dimensions.

How do we transform two-dimensional retina images into three-dimensional perceptions? In fact, we can perceive distance and depth through two different cues: cues from the interaction of both eyes-binocular cues, or from each eye separately -monocular cues.

(1) Binocular cues

Binocular cues refer to distance and depth cues in which both eyes are needed to perceive. It includes two important elements: retinal disparity and convergence.

The retinal disparity is the difference of the images of an object on the retinas of the two eyes; because the two eyes are apart, and their retinas receive slightly different images. An object appears in different places on the two retinas, the distance between these two images also contributes to providing cues regarding the distance of the object, the greater the disparity, the closer the object.

Convergence is a necessary visual neuromuscular response of the eyes in order to focus on objects. The closer the object is, the more the eye muscles tense to turn the eyes inward. Information sent from the eye muscles to the brain helps to determine the distance of the eyes to the object.

(2) Monocular cues

Monocular cues are cues, which can be seen using only one eye. Several different types of monocular cues help us to estimate the distance of objects, including relative size, interposition, relative height and relative motion in the visual field.

The relative size provides a cue to their relative distance. The smaller an object is, the more distant it appears. In the Figure 1-8, we perceive a larger image as closer to us, especially if the two images are of the same object. In face of the two objects with same size, the more distant the object is, the smaller it looks like.

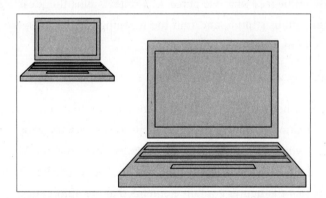

Figure 1-8   Depth cues and the perception of relative size

Interposition. A monocular cue for perceiving distance; nearby objects partially block our view of more distant objects. Due to interposition, an object covering part of another object is perceived as closer. Please see the Figure 1-9.

Relative height also provides a monocular cue for distance. The higher an object is, the farther away it is. Objects that are closer to the bottom of our visual field are seen as closer to us, while higher means farther away. In the Figure 1-10, the tree at the bottom is perceived closer to us while the other higher tree is perceived as farther away.

Relative motion also provides a powerful distance cue. When we move, objects at different distances change their relative positions in our visual image; the faster an object moves, the closer it is; while the slower it moves, the farther away it is. The light or shadows of objects can give clues to their distance. Nearby objects reflect more light, yet dimmer objects are perceived to be more distant than they actually are.

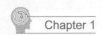

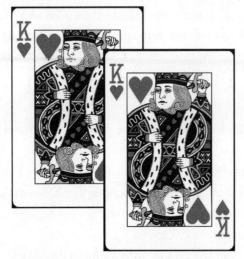

Figure 1-9　Overlap provides a depth cue

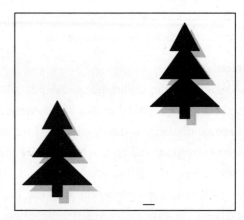

Figure 1-10　Relative height provides a depth cue for distance

Monocular cues are cues, which can be seen using only one eye. Binocular cues are used when looking at objects with both eyes, and depend on the interaction of both eyes. The accuracy of our perception of distance and depth generally depends on the interaction of a number of these cues.

1.2.4　Interpretation of perception

The perception is affected by our learned assumptions and beliefs as well as by sensory input comes from the perceptual set. Our experiences, assumptions, and expectations give us a perceptual set, or mental predisposition, that greatly influences what we perceive. Contexts plus the ideas we have stored in memory help us to interpret the ambiguous stimuli, and find the meaning in what we perceive. Therefore, this helps explain why some people "see" monsters that others do not.

1.2.5　Perceptual illusions

Perceptual illusions occur when we use a variety of sensory cues to create perceptual experiences that do not actually exist. The presentation of multiple stimuli elicits a tendency to group some of them together and others apart, a phenomenon which can create visual illusions. For example, the Müller-Lyer illusions are often cited as visual illusions (Figure 1-11). The lengths of the two lines appear to be different but they are the same. This phenomenon suggests that the figures contain elements that are automatically recognized as perspective cues and which inappropriately trigger the size constancy mechanism. Visual illusions depend primarily on our own perceptual processes and occur because the stimulus contains misleading cues.

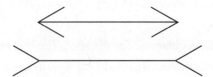

Figure 1-11　Müller-Lyer: the two horizontal lines are of equal length, but the lower one appears longer

Visual illusions are often applied to build particular effects of art. For example, a two-dimensional surface can convey a 3-dimensional picture through many monocular depth cues. Media advertising is directed toward the goal of influencing your perception about products.

2. Memory and learning

2.1   Memory

When we talk about memory, we may recall many interesting experiences: we can remember much information and knowledge when we take exams; we can easily pick up many telephone numbers, and we may remember some unique moments, such as receiving the letter of admission to university three years ago. We may wonder how we remember so much information. Memory plays an important role in comprehension, learning, social relationships, and in many aspects of people's life. Our daily activities such as eating, learning, working, and social life depend on our memory. Without the ability of memory, we would not live a normal life. Memory is the capacity of mind to receive, store, retain, and later retrieve information, and it is a process of recovering information about past events or knowledge.

2.1.1   Types of memory

Memory can be classified into multiple systems, each based on a different perspective.

(1) Episodic and semantic memory

Tulving (1972) distinguished two forms of memory: episodic memory and semantic memory. Episodic memory is concerned with personal experiences such as specific episodes in one's life. Episodic memory is connected with factual information such as a specific event that happened at a precise time and place. Episodic memory represents our memory of life events and experiences in a serial form. It is from this memory that we can reconstruct the actual events that took place at a given point in our lives. Episodic memory always stores information rich with personal meaning, and is concerned with personal experiences. If we were asked to recount something we did at a cocktail party yesterday, we would depend on episodic memory to recall the events. Similarly, episodic memory can help us to describe a family vacations, exciting games, or the circumstances when we won a lottery. Episodic memory contains the personal, autobiographical details of our lives.

Semantic memory refers to our general knowledge of the world such as names, the meaning of words, concepts, chemical equations, and our mathematical ability. It is a form of memory creating a structured record of the concepts and skills that we have acquired. Semantic memory helps people understand thousands of facts, for example, that SOS means save our ship; that cats have four legs; that 3 multiplied by 5 is 15; and that Shakespeare was an English playwright and poet. Semantic memories are usually not associated with the specific time and place of learning. The knowledge or concepts learnt using semantic memory transcend the original context in which it was learned. For example, when people want to remember that Shakespeare was an English playwright and poet, they do not have to recall the time and place where they previously learned this fact. From this aspect, semantic memory is different from episodic memory because the latter is closely related to time and place.

Psychologists notice that brain-damaged patients who have great difficulties remembering their own recent personal experiences can often access their permanent knowledge quite readily. This finding suggested that episodic memory and semantic memory represent independent capacities, and may have a different anatomic and functional basis in the brain. The positron emission tomography scan study by Wheeler and colleagues, have shown that there is more activity in the right prefrontal cortex when participants are trying to retrieve episodic memories. As they said, "the manner in which information is registered in the episodic and semantic systems is highly similar. The major distinction between episodic and semantic memory is no longer best

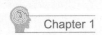

described in terms of the type of information they work with. The distinction is now made in terms of the nature of subjective experience that accompanies the operations of the system at encoding and retrieval". Lepage's study indicated that episodic retrieval leads to greater activation in the frontal lobes, particularly in the prefrontal cortex. Although there are differences between episodic memory and semantic memory, there are some associations between them. Tulving proposed that episodic memory grew out of semantic memory, and besides its own features, it also shares many of features of semantic memory. Episodic memory developed later than semantic memory and therefore is more vulnerable to damage.

(2) Declarative and procedural memory

Declarative memory is the conscious, intentional recollection of facts, concepts, events, and previous experiences. The declarative memory includes names, faces, dates, vocabulary, stories, mathematical formulas, the rules of games and the like. In general, declarative memory comprises episodic memory and semantic memory.

Procedural memory involves motor skills and behavioral habits, for example, when people brush their teeth, write their names, or scratch their eyes, they easily do this because they previously stored these activities and can recall them automatically. Procedural memory is associated knowledge about the sequence of events, and the relationships between events. It is stored due to extensive practice, conditioning, or habit. Procedural memory allows an individual to change his or her performance in some way without knowledge of having learned anything. Procedural memories are accessed and used without the need for conscious control or attention. It is hard to share your procedural knowledge with others. You may have noticed that even you are good rider or drivers themselves, they may not have been very good at communicating the content of compiled good-driving procedures.

(3) Implicit and explicit memory

According to levels of awareness during the memory process, psychologists differentiate implicit memory from explicit memory.

Implicit memory refers to unconscious retention of information, and involves retaining and using prior experiences without realizing it at the time. Many behaviors that people perform reflect past learning and experiences, even when they are not consciously attempting to retrieve those memories. Scientists noticed that people can be influenced by the previous information even though they have scarcely paid any attention to it. People's thoughts and behaviors can be affected by such unconscious retention of information. Implicit memory can be best demonstrated when the performance on a task produces a specific response in the absence of conscious recollection. This type of memory is usually presented through activation of the sensory and motor systems when performing a particular task. The hallmark of all implicit memory tests is that people are not required to remember intentionally, and the retention of past experience or skills can automatically facilitate current performance or improvement. Psychologists propose two subtypes of implicit memory: priming and skill learning.

Priming is when the previous experience with a stimulus facilitates the recognition of that stimulus in later processing. In other words, it is an activation of particular associations in memory, and often unconsciously. Priming is often concerned with perceptual identification of words and objects. For example, we might meet a seldom word when we were reading, which is not the part of our normal working vocabulary base, and one day we heard this word from our friend in a talk. A day later we found that we were using this word in conversation although we could not intentionally remember it. The earlier exposure to this word primed us to retrieve it automatically in the right situation without intentional efforts.

Skill learning is another form of implicit memories. It refers to using previously learned skills or automatic movements without trying to retrieve them. Skill learning relies on associating certain stimuli with a subsequent response. In other words, people learn and retain prior experiences of certain movements or motor skills unconsciously, and subsequently use them without any awareness. For example, when we tie our shoes, ride a bicycle, or brush our teeth, we easily do this because we previously stored these activities and can perform them with ease, and we need not consciously retrieve our experiences about learning these skills. Implicit memory facilitates people automatically take movements or improve motor skills without any conscious recollection. These memories can be accessed only by performing the specific task or through activation of other reflex and motor systems.

Explicit memory refers to the intentional recollection of information and past experiences at the level of awareness. If someone asked you to recall everything you did at the party yesterday, you must consciously recall several episodes. Graf and Schacter's study indicates that explicit memory is revealed when performance on a task requires conscious recollection of previous experiences. People often make an associations between current information and previous related experiences in order to form and store explicit memories. Therefore, explicit memories can be remembered and recalled, and rely on previous experiences and knowledge. How does one examine and assess the explicit memory? Since we have made associations with previous experiences in forming and storing explicit memories, free recall (without cues), cued recall, and recognition are all options for explicit memory testing.

Some studies exhibit that patients with amnesia have poor explicit memories but their implicit memory remains intact. It proposes that explicit memory and implicit memory are distinct forms of memory. Studies also provide evidence that implicit and explicit memory have distinct functional neuroanatomy. Squire's brain-scanning study in normal individuals supports the idea that explicit memory is accompanied by increased neural activity in certain regions, whereas implicit memory is accompanied by a decrease in neural activity in critical regions. A possible explanation for this finding is that there may be separate systems for implicit and explicit memory, and these two types of memories have different functional regions in the brain. However, explicit memories have associations with implicit memories, for example, activities such as riding a bicycle initially required intentional study, which belongs to explicit memory and becomes implicit memory once this task is thoroughly learned.

2.1.2 Processes of memory

Suppose that you are reading a novel, and impressed by the legendary character in the book. That evening, you and your friends talk about the novel. You may say the name of the character in the book, and share feelings with your friends. Obviously, you remember the name of this character and other contents of the book. It is your memory that makes it possible for you to enjoy the book and the talking. When you notice the existence of memory, you must be interested in what memory is, and how memory works. In other words, how memories are formed, how memories are retained, and how memories are recalled. The cognitive perspective plays a very important role in the study of memory. Researchers use the information-processing metaphor to understand the memory process, and view memory as an active, organizing process rather than a passive recording process. Today, the most widely used model of memory is the information-processing model proposed by Atkinson and Shiffrin in 1960s. They propose that the human memory involves a sequence of three stages: sensory memory, short-term memory, and long-term memory. This model describes how information is encoded, stored, and how it is retrieved from memory. This model provides an important framework for memory theories, but it also has some limitations.

Like the way that computers work human memory allows us to store information for later use. This memory process can be broken into three parts: encoding, storage, and retrieval.

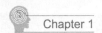

(1) Encoding

In order to form new memories, information must be translated into a form that can be stored in memory. In other words, information input must be selected, identified, labeled, and elaborated upon. This process is called encoding. For a computer this means transferring data into 1's and 0's, binary code, which can be identified and processed by the computer. For the mind, it means we transform sensory input like sound waves or visual stimuli into specific form (a kind of code) that can be placed in the memory. The sensory organs sense all information around us, but only the information with meanings is actually put into memory. The encoding process is an active process in the brain, and requires selective attention to the material to be encoded. A lot of factors may affect selective attention for encoding.

When encoding involves physical aspects of the stimulus, this process is not deep, while encoding involves specific meaning the encoding process occurs at a deeper level. There are several different types of encoding process: structural encoding, phonemic encoding, and semantic encoding.

Structural encoding emphasizes on the structural characteristics of the stimulus, and focuses on what we look at, and belongs to the visual encoding process. For example, the color of an apple or a word made up of several letters. Structural encoding is usually processed at a shallow level. The phonemic encoding is a kind of acoustic encoding, and especially emphasizes on the sounds of the words, and belongs to an intermediate level. For example, the words need to be sounded out in order to get verbal information into memory such as rhyming words. The semantic encoding emphasizes on the meaning of the stimulus especially the meaning of words. Semantic encoding requires a deeper level of processing than structural or phonemic encoding and usually results in better memory. For example, we can endow a group of words with meanings in order to easily get meaning information into memory.

Numerous studies have shown that emotionally rich events in one's life are encoded and remembered more often and with more clarity and detail. In addition, other aspects are related to the encoding process, such as the information relevant to personal experiences, added richness to the material by visual imagery, and associations with other information.

(2) Storage

After the encoding of information, the next stage is storing the information. It refers to maintaining information in memory over a period of time. This process simply means holding onto the information, and similar to a computer physically writing the 1 and 0 onto the hard drive. It also implies that some physiological change must occur for the memory to be stored. The theory developed by Atkinson and Shiffrin (1968) was widely accepted, and it suggested three stages of memory storage: sensory memory, short-term memory, and long-term memory. During the stage of sensory memory, if we do not process input information further, it will disappear. During the stage of short-term memory, we can hold a small amount of information for a short period of time. In order to store the information for a longer period of time, we would need to store it in our long-term memory.

(3) Retrieval

Retrieval involves the process of searching for memory information that we previously encoded and stored, and bringing it into mind. The information is returned to a form similar to what we stored. Furthermore, if we encoded something in the form of vision, it can be retrieved visually while it is difficult to retrieve it acoustically. The more ways the information is encoded, the more ways it can be retrieved. Recall and recognition are the two main ways of retrieving material from memory.

Recall means that information is retrieved directly from memory. It includes free recall, which no hints are given, and cued recall, which facilitated by giving retrieval cues. Recognition occurs when an item is identified as one we have learned or seen before. It includes yes-no recognition and forced-choice recognition. For example, when we take an examination, we are asked to give answers to several types of examination questions. If we are asked to write a paragraph from memory with or without cues, it belongs to recall; if we are asked to answer "yes" or "no" from a list comprised of a target and other irrelevant items, a multiple-choice test it belongs to recognition. In other words, we have to recognize a target from a list of irrelevant items through our stored memory.

Mostly, memory retrieval is not a random process. The proper cues often help with the retrieval process. An effective retrieval cue is usually consistent with the original encoding of the information. Two types of cues are often discussed: context cues and state cues. Context cues are related to a specific situation such as weather, location, hearing a certain song, and seeing a particular food. Memory retrieval can be triggered by replication of a certain condition in which the memory was encoded. For example, a boy can recall that he has to wear the heavy coat to school when he sees his brother's coat in the bedroom, because environmental conditions brings it to mind. State cues refer to memory retrieval that can be facilitated when a specific emotional state is presented again, which is the same as the process of encoding.

2.1.3   The information-processing model of memory

Atkinson and Shiffrin (1968) proposed a widely accepted model of memory which is also known as the information-processing model in Figure 1-12. A large number of external events or stimuli firstly enter the sensory memory (sensory register) through the immediate recording of sensory information. Some important or novel information will be encoded and enter short-term memory (working memory). This information activated memory that holds a few items briefly. Through encoding such as automatic processing and rehearsal, the meaningful information is stored in long-term memory for a long time. When used, this information can be retrieved and carry out tasks.

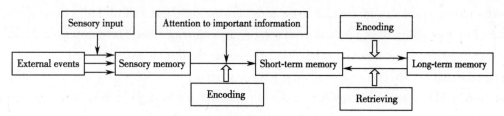

Figure 1-12   Atkinson-Shiffrin model of memory

In this model, memory is conceptualized as consisting of three distinct stages of memory store: sensory memory, short-term memory, and long-term memory. Each stage concerns several aspects: Memory capacity which refers to the amount of information that is maintained; the duration which refers to the length of time information is maintained; what the reason is for forgetting (storage failure versus retrieval failure).

(1) Sensory memory

Sensory memory is also called sensory registers. It is a temporary storage of information, and just maintains a copy of what is seen or heard originally in the sensory areas of the brain for a very brief period of time. The capacity of sensory memory is large, and contains most of the details from sensory input. Huge amounts of information come streaming in from the senses at every moment of our life. Most of information, including all sensory inputs such as visual, auditory, and touch information, is not needed after it is noticed. If we do not process this information further, it disappears. Thus, the sensory registers hold information for very brief periods of time before transferring it to short-term memory. The duration of storage of sensory memory lasts for only a few seconds, and is about 1/10 of a second for visual information. As new visual information

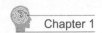

enters the sensory registers, old information is almost immediately replaced and disappears. Auditory information fades more slowly than visual information, and usually lasts 2 seconds.

For a large amount of information in sensory memory, we select some and hold it for further processing. Otherwise, we quickly forget it. The decay theory is proposed to explain the forgetting of sensory memories. The underlying assumption of the decay theory is that forgetting is caused by the disappearance of the biological memory trace over time. Biological memory trace refers to the physiological or physical changes underlying a memory. This theory states that if information is not used or rehearsed, with the disappearance of memory trace, the memory no longer exists in the memory system.

(2) Short-term memory

Some information in sensory memory captures our attention and enters short-term memory (STM), which can hold a limited amount of information in awareness for a brief period. STM is also called working memory and focuses more on the processing of briefly stored information. Working memory is now commonly used to refer to a broader system that can keep information available for short periods until it is used to solve problems, or respond to environmental demands. If something stands out from the information around it, it easily captures our attention, and enters the STM. Any distinctive information is easier to remember than that which is similar, usual, or mundane. In addition, if something is attached to other information, especially if we are interested in it, it easily draws our attention, and becomes easier to remember. The capacity of STM is limited. There are generally seven units of independent information at most, plus or minus two units. Information can be encoded for temporary storage according to the sounds, the visual form, or in terms of its meaning. It depends on the nature of the material to be remembered and what we are trying to do with this information. Researchers conclude that STM has a greater capacity for material encoded with visual images than for information encoded with sounds. A method called chunking can help to increase the capacity of STM. Chunking refers to a process in which the brain organizes information into manageable and meaningful units, thereby allowing for more information to be stored. For example, it is difficult for us to remember a list of single letters, but if we group them into a word it will be easier to remember. The duration of storage of STM lasts for less than 30 seconds without rehearsal. We can increase the duration of short-term memories through maintaining rehearsal, but the memories will disappear very rapidly when we stop repeating the information.

Information in STM disappears rapidly unless it is rehearsed or practiced immediately. Two theories have been proposed to explain storage failure of STM. One is the decay theory, which means that information is lost because memory trace disappears from STM over time. The other is the displacement theory because of the limited capacity of STM. This means that the new information will push out part of the old information. In other words, when the capacity of STM is met, the addition of new information entering STM will push out the previously stored information. For example, some one was telling you several phone numbers and almost instantly you forget the first two numbers after he finished. In addition, if information is interrupted by an accidental interference, it will not have enough time to rehearse and disappear from STM. For example, a friend is telling you his phone number, but another student is asking you a question at the same time, the result is that you forget the phone number.

(3) Long-term memory

Information from STM is transferred into long-term memory (LTM) after a few seconds. The capacity of LTM is virtually unlimited. The duration of storage is up to a lifetime.

1) Encoding process of LTM

Most of the information in LTM seems to be encoded in terms of meaning. For example, when we try to remember the anatomic structures of the blood vessel in the brain, we extract the meaning of the

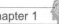

anatomic structures of the blood vessel and link it to much material that is already in our LTM, which is meaningful and familiar for us. The meaningful connections can facilitate information storage in LTM for a long time. Researchers have argued that we have enough space to memorize everything we "know" in our LTM. Obviously, we only use a small fraction of this storage space. Although long-term memory has a preferred encoding for meaning of material, other aspects sometimes are encoded in LTM. For example, some information is encoding with tastes and smells.

2) Storage process of LTM

What information tends to be stored in LTM? Firstly, information that has some significance attached to it is typically stored in LTM. We may remember the day that we took a big entry exam, as well as how hot the weather was. The temperature really does not play an important role, but is attached to the memory of taking a big exam, and was stored in our LTM. Secondly, the memories that we attach to emotional experiences will deem important for transferring to our LTM. Imagine how difficult it would be to forget the day we graduated from the university, or received the first kiss from our girlfriend or boyfriend. Finally, the repeated exposure to a stimulus or the rehearsal of a piece of information can promote information to transfer from STM to LTM, and store in LTM. There are different kinds of rehearsals: maintenance rehearsal and elaborative rehearsal. Maintenance rehearsal refers to a simple recitation or repetition. For example, when we want to remember a group of phone numbers, just repeat them again and again. Elaborative rehearsal refers to when we can link the new information to familiar material in STM, and then store it in LTM. For example, in order to remember a complex English article, we can create a series of connections between the new information and the article, such as familiar pictures or stories, and store them in LTM.

3) Retrieval process of LTM

Information stored in LTM can be used to carry out tasks at hand by the process of retrieval. There are two types of retrieval from LTM: recall and recognition. In recall, the information is reproduced from memory. As on a fill-in-the blank test, we have to search for an answer from our memory. In recognition, information is provided as a cue to access the memory. As on a multiple-choice test, we can choose an answer from a list of materials to access the memory.

Our memory can benefit from the organizational structures of LTM. The more we organize the material (including encode and stored), the easier it is to retrieve. Suppose being at a supermarket and going shopping with a long inventory list, organizing what to buy by dividing the list into several groups such as food, stationery, and cleaning products will make it easier to remember. There are usually several principles for organizing material or information in LTM. Clustering is a common principle for the organization of material. It means that some related pieces of information are usually remembered together, which is like chunking in STM. For example, it is easier to remember a group of English words with approximately the same meanings than separate words. Another organizational principle is conceptual hierarchies. This refers to the classification scheme that is used to organize memory materials. It is effective to use this principle when we study science such as biology and chemistry, and need to remember a variety of knowledge from different domains. In addition, the schema principle is also useful in the organization of material. A schema is a set of beliefs or expectations about something based on an individual's past experience, and it serves as a standard for comparison with a new experience during the encoding process of LTM. A schema can help not only in dealing with the tasks at hand, but also in facilitate the retrieval processes. If schemas are related to the objects abstracted from our prior experience, we tend to recall the objects that fit our schemas.

Although most of the information in LTM remains there permanently, it is impossible for us to retrieve it whenever we need to. Retrieval failure is the main cause of forgetting in LTM. If we cannot find the proper retrieval cue, or use the wrong cues, it will result in retrieval failure.

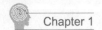

2.1.4 Biological aspects of memory

Physiological mechanisms of memory. The studies of memory from the physiological perspective support that memory has a physiological basis. Memory is a complicated phenomenon. Researchers still do not know exactly how it works at the physiological level. Several physiological theories were proposed to explain the process of memory called the biological or physical approach. Psychologists have made a lot of efforts to identify the mechanisms responsible for memory at the neuroanatomical level. Some scientists propose that certain structures or regions of the brain are associated with memory, such as the cerebral cortex, cerebellum, hippocampus and amygdala. Implicit memory (priming) is associated with hemodynamic decreases in left fusiform gyrus, bilateral frontal and occipital brain regions, while explicit memory was associated with bilateral parietal and temporal and left frontal increases. Retrieval intention did not change these patterns but was associated with activity in right prefrontal cortex. Employing advanced medical techniques in memory studies, such as positron emission tomography and functional magnetic resonance imaging, studies brain regions associated with different forms of memory have been identified in individuals without brain damage directly. For example, working memory are associated primarily with the bilateral prefrontal and parietal regions; semantic memory with the left prefrontal and temporal regions; episodic memory encoding with the left prefrontal and medial temporal regions while retrieval with the right prefrontal, posterior midline and medial temporal regions. The frontal lobe and basal ganglia are important in some forms of declarative memory that require reasoning about the contents of memory.

Some researchers argue that there may be specific neural networks in the brain for specific memories. Some studies proposed that nerve impulses continuously travel through the synapses; information is passed from neuron to neuron, and forms a pattern of junctions. This impulse pattern affects protein and other chemical molecules at the synaptic connections of neurons. The current consensus in this field is that memories are related to specific neural networks in the brain by which plastic neurochemical and neuroanatomical changes occur at connections between neurons, the synapses. In a study of the patients with Alzheimer's disease and they showed a depletion of acetylcholine and glutamate, and scientists suggested that memory storage may occur in biochemical changes at the synapse. The way the brain codes, stores, and retrieves information remains a mystery. We will have a long way to go in exploring the physiological mechanisms of memory.

2.1.5 Forgetting

(1) Ebbinghaus' forgetting curve

You may leave keys in your office when you stand in front of the door of your department, and you may forget to return a phone call to your friend. Forgetting is quite common in our daily life. Forgetting refers to the inability to recall previously learned information, and typically involves a failure in memory retrieval. For Ebbinghaus' forgetting curve please see Figure 1-13.

German psychologist Hermann Ebbinghaus (1850—1909) was the first researcher to conduct scientific studies on forgetting. He devised lists of nonsense syllables as stimulus materials in order to simplify memory tasks and allow for the manipulation and measurement of memory. Each nonsense syllable has a neutral meaning, and is all homogeneous. Therefore, they cannot be associated with each other. Ebbinghaus measured the number of repetitions required to learn the nonsense syllables. He used this new method to measure forgetting, and revealed a relationship between forgetting and time, which is called the Ebbinghaus forgetting curve. The forgetting curve shows that forgetting is most rapid in the first few hours after learning, but the rate of forgetting slows as time goes on. This property of memory suggests that we must rehearse as soon as possible if we want to retain more information in our memory. Ebbinghaus' experimental method revealed some basic properties of memory, and continues to influence our understanding of memory today.

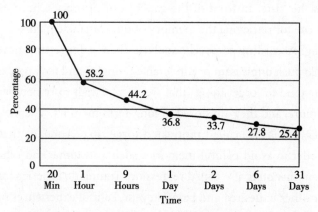

Figure 1-13   Ebbinghaus' forgetting curve. Forgetting is most rapid in the first few hours after learning, but the rate of forgetting slows as time goes on

(2) Causes of forgetting

Everyone forgets things. If information initially did not get encoded into memory, it belongs to encoding failure. The information will disappear from memory if we do not use it. It is no longer in storage. Sometimes the information is in our memory but for various reasons we cannot get access to it, and it belongs to retrieval failure. There are some main causes to explain forgetting, including ineffective encoding, decay, interference, retrieval failure, motivated forgetting, and physical injury or trauma.

1) Ineffective encoding. Processing information at a deeper level makes it harder to forget. We go upstairs and downstairs daily, perhaps, most of us cannot answer the questions about the number of stairs that make up the staircase the third floor where we live. We often take a walk on the campus avenue, if we are asked how many trees on both sides of this avenue, we also possibly cannot answer. This is because this information is not encoded from the very beginning, and has not been stored in the long-term memory.

In an experiment, the subjects were required to draw the portrait from a one-cent coin. Although they use this kind of coin daily, nearly nobody can complete the task. The reason is that very few people consciously know the coin in detail; in other words, they have not encoded this information at a deeper level.

2) Decay. Decay theory believes that information in memory eventually disappears if it is not used; in other words, memory fades as time goes on. As discussed previously, decay explains forgetting of sensory and STM. In LTM, if the information such as events has been stored, forgetting does not seem to depend on how much time has passed. For example, people might easily remember their first day in university but completely forget what they read in the newspaper last Monday.

3) Interference. Interference theory can provide a better explanation of why people lose LTM. There are two types of interference: proactive interference and retroactive interference. Forgetting occurs when newly learned information makes people forget old information, which is known as retroactive interference; when old information makes people forget newly learned information, it is called proactive interference. For example, if we want to remember ten telephone numbers one by one at a given time, wanting to remembering the last three phone numbers will disrupt recollection of the prior learned phone numbers (e.g., the first number), while earlier learned phone numbers will disrupt current remembering.

4) Retrieval failure. Forgetting may also result from failure to retrieve information in memory. Failing to remember something does not mean the information is gone forever though. Sometimes, memory is there but for various reasons we cannot access it. Sometimes proper cues are not available or wrong cues will lead

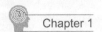

to retrieval failure. On the contrary, proper cues will facilitate us to retrieve information. For example, we may not be able to remember the name of one classmate in fifth-grade. However, his name might suddenly become available if we come across his sister in front of the gate of our primary school. His sister and the primary school will act as a context cue for retrieving the memory of our classmate name.

5) Motivated forgetting. According to psychoanalytic theory, forgetting never means that memories disappear forever but people push unpleasant or intolerable thoughts and feelings deep into their unconscious. Freud believes that we may tend to forget things that we do not wish to remember. In fact, those memories have not disappeared any more, and they are stored in long-term memory. The idea that people forget things they do not want to remember is also called motivated forgetting. It means that we purposefully push a memory out of reach in order to avoid painful memories such as trauma, and other threatening or anxiety-provoking events. This phenomenon is also called repression. Traumatic experiences include experiences such as a violent attack, rape, or other undesired and painful event. Painful experiences of this sort are pushed into the unconscious mind. Individuals intentionally forget them in order to avoid provoking severe anxiety or anguish. Many psychologists argued that repression theory is limited in that most of the information we forget does not relate to anxious or traumatic events.

6) Physical injury or trauma. Forgetting might occur after physical injury or trauma. Many studies support that brain lesions affect memory, especially which different combinations of damaged structures result in different memory impairments. There are generally two types of forgetting: anterograde amnesia and retrograde amnesia. Anterograde amnesia refers to when an individual is not able to remember events that occur after an injury or traumatic event. Retrograde amnesia refers to when an individual is not able to remember events that occurred before an injury or traumatic event.

For more detailed information about memory disorders please see Chapter 11.

2.2   Learning

Learning is a relatively permanent change in behavior and behavior potentials, due to the experience of the interaction with the environment. For example, learning things in school, finding a street in a strange city, learning to predict a potential risk, learning how to express appreciation, worry and other feelings at the appropriate time, and learning civilized behaviors.

2.2.1   Characteristics of learning

Firstly, learning is a change in behavior and behavior potentials. A mastery of new skills means that learning has taken place. When you are able to ride a bike, play a piano, or sing a song, it results in the improvement of your performance. The behavior potentials refer to the acquiring of certain attitudes, thoughts, knowledge, or emotions that can promote individuals to change their performance. For instance, after you experienced life in a needy area, your attitudes toward people in poverty may change. You may become frugal, and decide not to spend too much money on clothes. When you read a health book and understand how important a healthy habit is, you may stop smoking today, and do your best not to eat fatty foods. You improve your life style in that you learned health knowledge, or you might have an experience of suffering certain serious disease.

Secondly, learning is a relatively permanent change. It means that the change in behavior is relatively stable over time and across different occasions. When you learned to ride a bike in childhood, you can still do it well even if you have not touched a bike in many years. You may also hold a certain attitude for many years, even throughout your life.

Lastly, the occurrence of learning includes an interaction with the environment. Behavioral changes are

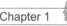

based on the accumulation of human's experiences, and it is the result of experience. Humans have evolved and learned much more about diverse aspects of the environment. The accumulation of experiences is actually the process of learning. The learning process includes several parts: receiving or acquiring information from environment, making responses, and keeping or retaining certain behavior that adapt to the environment. All of these processes only occur in the interaction with the environment.

Learning is concerned with several aspects including the physical, cognitive, emotional and social development in individuals" lives. It also includes academic studies and occupational training. The biological function of learning is to facilitate individuals to survive. Learning makes individuals do things more easily and become more adaptive to their environment.

2.2.2　Types of learning

Learning can be broadly classified into two types: associative learning and observational learning. Associative learning is concerned with certain events occurring together during the learning process. It usually involves an individual making an association between a particular situation, and a particular response. Associative learning can further be subdivided into two types: classical conditioning and operant conditioning.

(1) Classical conditioning

Classical conditioning focuses on the pairing of two stimuli that will lead to new behavior under certain conditions. Classical conditioning is also called Pavlovian conditioning because the general process was first described through Pavlov's experiments, in which a previously neutral stimulus is associated with an unconditioned stimulus through repeated pairing, and the individual begins to produce a response that anticipates for the unconditioned stimulus. This response is not naturally occurring and comes about through the pairing of neutral stimulus and unconditioned stimulus.

(2) Operant conditioning

Operant conditioning emphasizes that a response or behavior is influenced, or changed, by the following consequences. For example, an individual learns to increase certain behaviors that are followed by reinforcing stimuli, and to suppress other behaviors because they are followed by punishing stimuli. Consequently, an individual learns certain responses by operating on the environment to gain something desired or avoid something unpleasant. "Operant" refers to the idea that individuals can perform actions that may change the environment around them. Through operant conditioning, individuals learn to produce some behaviors that are followed by rewards and to reduce those behaviors that are followed by punishing stimuli. Since it is a process of controlling behavior by manipulating its consequences, operant conditioning is also called instrumental learning. Psychologist Edward Lee Thorndike was the first researcher to study operant behavior systematically. Skinner's work was based on Thorndike's and proposed the concept of operant conditioning.

(3) Observational learning

Among higher animals, especially humans, learning occurs not only through personal experience and the making of associations, but also through observation and imitation. Observational learning is another important type of learning. The process of observational learning was demonstrated by American psychologist Albert Bandura's experiments in which children tend to imitate what a model both does and says, and especially to imitate those they perceive to be like them, successful, or admirable.

Today, psychologists generally agree that there are different types of learning processes and that learning may vary greatly across species.

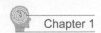

2.2.3 Study of classical conditioning

(1) Pavlov's experiments

Classical conditioning, also called Pavlovian conditioning or conditional reflexes, was first studied and described by Russian physiologist Ivan Pavlov (1849—1936) (Figure 1-14). Dogs usually salivate when they begin to bring in food. In the experiment, Pavlov noticed that dogs started to salivate at the sound of the experimenter's food steps before actually eating food in his laboratory. He became curious about this phenomenon. On the basis of this fact, he found an interesting phenomenon after further observation and studies, and identified that if he used the appropriate sequence of events, a dog would learn a new reflex.

A reflex is a relationship between a specific environmental event, and a stimulus, and a fixed response evoked by this stimulus, in other words, a specific response is always evoked by a certain stimulus. All individuals, including humans, are born with a limited set of reflexes that respond to specific set of environmental stimuli. These reflexes facilitate individuals to have a better chance of survival and reproduction. Let us see the typical procedure of classical conditioning in Pavlov's famous experiment.

Firstly, the experimenters performed a minor operation on a dog to relocate its salivary duct on the outside, in order that drops of saliva could be more easily exported and measured. Dogs have innate responses to certain stimulus. Such a response is called an unconditioned stimulus (UCS). The UCS is usually a biologically significant event, and can reliably elicit an unlearned response (innate response), which is called the unconditioned response (UCR). An example is when a puff of air (UCS) is blown into the eye; the eye will blink in response (UCR). This process is also known as a reflex. Such reflexes are in-born, and serve basic survival value. A UCR is usually a physiological response that can be elicited by the UCS. In this experiment, the food is a UCS and salivation is the UCR, in that a dog does not have to learn to salivate when food is placed in their mouths.

Secondly, the classical conditioning procedure also requires a conditioned stimulus (CS), which is a neutral stimulus that originally has no meaning to the dog, and it does not elicit an automatic response. In this experiment, the sound of a bell was the CS, which originally had no meaning to the dog; the food is the UCS. Then, the CS is paired with the UCS, and presented to a dog frequently. Each presentation of the sound of the bell is followed closely by the presentation of the food.

Thirdly, after a sufficient number of pairings of the CS followed by the UCS, the dog is able to learn the association between the sound of the bell and food.

Lastly, the experimenter only presents the sound of the bell (CS) to the dog. Over a period of time, the dog begins to salivate when exposed to the sound of the bell alone. The salivation is caused by the CS alone. The dog salivates immediately after hearing the bell because the connection between food and bell has been made. The dog begins to produce a behavioral response to the CS. This means that Pavlovian conditioning has occurred, and a new reflex has developed. Pavlov called it a conditioned reflex (CR).

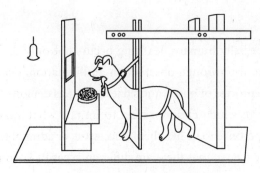

Figure 1-14 Pavlov's experiments

An individual develops a conditional reflex, which is actually a new ability in response to a neutral stimulus. It depends on previously existing unconditional response, then making a connection between the UCS and the CS through repetitive pairings of the UCS and the CS. Classical conditioning is a form of associative learning. An individual is able to develop a new behavior through conducting a conditional reflex. Generally, the development of classical conditioning can be illustrated as following (Figure 1-15):

An unconditioned stimulus can elicit unconditioned response, while a conditioned stimulus (neutral stimulus) cannot elicit any response before conditioning. After conditioning, the unconditioned stimulus is paired with the neutral stimulus; the conditioned stimulus can elicit the same response as the unconditioned stimulus.

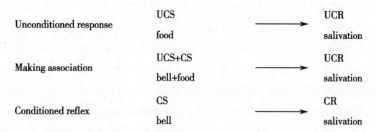

Figure 1-15   The development of classical conditioning

(2) Principles of classical conditioning

Acquisition is the initial stage in classical conditioning in which an association between a CS and a UCS takes place, and a pairing of the UCS and the CS comes to elicit a conditioned response. In classical conditioning, acquisition training involves repeatedly presenting an individual with a pairing of the CS and the US. Some factors will affect the acquisition process in classical conditioning.

For one thing, the selection of a proper CS and a UCS will play an important role in the acquisition of the CR. The strength of a UCS may affect the quality and the magnitude of possible conditioning, while the salience of the CS is also very important in determining the frequency of acquisition of the CR. For example, if we select flour with no flavor to be as a UCS, and a picture of a landscape to be a CS, both the amount and the rate of acquisition may decrease. However, if we choose bread and meat as a UCS, and the sound of a bell to be a CS, and then pair these two types of stimulus; imagine what will happen in a dog? Likewise, the interval between the two stimuli is also an important factor for acquisition. In most cases, the CS needs to be presented before the UCS. This kind of pairing will be most productive for conditioning to occur. When the UCS is presented before the CS, acquisition is usually difficult to obtain. Psychologists also found that the conditioning occurs more rapidly when the food follows the bell within half a second.

1) Extinction. Extinction refers to a learned or conditioned response being reduced or eventually disappearing after repeatedly presenting the CS in the absence of the UCS. When the pairing of the two stimuli are discontinued for several trials, in other words, a CS is no longer followed by the UCS the individual ceases to produce the conditioned response, and the CS loses the capacity to cause the CR. The association between these two stimuli is considered to have extinguished. In Pavlov's experiment, if a dog is repeatedly presented with the bell but not followed with the food, the dog would not salivate when presented with the bell after a long period of time. The dog has forgotten the association between the bell and the food, and it means that the learned response has been extinguished.

2) Spontaneous Recovery. After extinction of a conditioned response, the response reappears after a rest period, usually in a weakened form. It is possible that a CR, having been extinguished, may suddenly reappear even though there has been no reconditioning with the UCS. This means that the extinction does not entirely

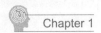

eliminate the association. There are usually two results. First, when an individual is retrained with a previous conditioned response after extinction, the acquisition will occur more rapidly than the original training because some residual association must remain. Second, it is possible that a CR may suddenly reappear even after extinction, and no reconditioning with the UCS. The dog has not completely forgotten the association between the bell and the food. If the experimenter waits a day, the dog may have a spontaneous recovery of the conditioned response and salivate again to the sound of the bell.

Both the extinction and the spontaneous recovery may have biological functions, such as facilitating an individual to become adaptive to the environment. The environment always changes over time; extinction or spontaneous recovery may be indications of the way in which an individual tracks these changes.

3) Generalization. Generalization happens most often when the new stimulus resembles the original conditioned stimulus. It is the tendency in which other stimuli similar to the original CS are also able to elicit the same response as the unconditioned stimulus. The strength or degree of this response is usually weaker than the original. The stimuli that can produce generalization are usually close to the original CS in size, shape, color, or sound but exhibit a small difference. For example, in Pavlov's experiment, a dog heard a sound of a whistle with the similar rhythm, instead of the sound of bell, the dog would still salivate.

As a result of generalization, we are able to learn certain responses through associating different stimuli with the response, without having to actually experience every stimulus event. Generalization does not mean that an individual fails to distinguish between the CS and similar stimuli; it demonstrates the fact that similar stimuli in the environment will usually have similar consequences.

4) Discrimination. In contrast to generalization, discrimination is a learned ability in which an individual can distinguish between a CS and other similar stimuli. Those similar stimuli do not put forth a signal as an unconditioned stimulus to elicit a CR. If a dog is presented with another stimulus such as a bell with a different tone, without following food, the dog would learn not to salivate to the similar stimuli.

(3) Application of classical conditioning

Behaviorists extended the study of Pavlov's classical conditioning, and use it to explain all behaviors, both as animals and humans. Today, the classical conditioning principles provide important insight into emotional learning and drug addiction. Watson's study demonstrated that emotion could be acquired through learning.

In 1920, Watson performed a famous experiment involving an eleven-month-old infant, known as Little Albert. This study demonstrated how emotions are learned under the basis of classical conditioning. At the beginning of the study, Albert was unafraid of the white rat and played freely with the animal. Nothing seemed to disturb or frighten him. Then, experimenters frightened him by making a terrible noise behind him when he was playing with the rat. Albert was startled and began to cry. Thereafter, whenever Little Albert reached for the rat, experimenters presented the terrible noise. After a period of time, as long as a rat was brought close to him, he would cry and avoided the animal. This is an example of typical classical conditioning. The white rat is a neutral stimulus, the terrible noise is an unconditioned stimulus, and Albert's fear of the terrible noise is the unconditioned response. After pairing the noise and rat several times, Albert showed fear of the white rat, the rat became a conditioned stimulus, and Albert's fear became a conditioned reflex. Further observations and studies showed that generalization had taken place, in which Albert's fear could be elicited by showing him any furry object such as hair, or a furry coat that was white.

Watson's experiment showed that emotions, such as fear, could be acquired through the direct experience of learning (classical conditioning). Psychologists use these learning principles to establish new conditioned reflexes in order to control or reduce the maladaptive emotions. For example, we can help a person who is afraid of dogs to conduct a new conditioned reflex through making use of his preference of strawberries. The person is enjoying the strawberries, then, we show a dog to him. Classical conditioning helps associate the dog with good feelings of strawberries. Finally, he is not afraid of dog.

One important area for the application of conditioning principles is the regulation of physiological systems in general, endocrine responses, and the disease-fighting immune system. A few studies supported that endocrine responses, such as insulin secretion, blood-glucose modification, cortisol and growth-hormone release, can be learned in humans. There has been considerable evidence that immunological responses can be modified by classical conditioning. Rodger's study shown that conditioned alteration to an allergic skin test response can be altered by classical conditioning in humans. The significance of this phenomenon can be extended in clinical treatment settings, such as chronic autoimmune conditions (e.g., chronic urticarial, autoimmune thyroid diseases, and lupus erythematosus). In clinical practice, principles of classical conditioning are often used to treat drug addiction. A drug addiction is a strong desire to take a drug for someone to feel good. Simply, classical conditioning consists of pairing a particular feeling with specific event, again and again, until an association is established between them. So, when an individual wants to quit snorting cocaine, psychologists try to make him feel awful instead of feeling nice whenever snorting cocaine. Through pairing snorting cocaine with a terrible stimulus such as a severe electric shock, the individual will establish an association between snorting cocaine and an awful feeling. Finally, snorting cocaine can elicit awful feeling, and the cocaine addiction can be cured.

Extensive research in nonhuman mammals has shown that the amygdala is a critical structure involved in the acquisition, storage and expression of conditioned fear. More recent work demonstrates that the amygdala plays a similar role in humans.

2.2.4 Study of operant conditioning

(1) Thorndike's law of effect

In the late 19th century, American psychologist Edward Thorndike (1874—1949) proposed the law of effect, which states that behaviors followed by favorable consequences will tend to be repeated, and behaviors followed by unfavorable consequences will tend to be avoided. Operant conditioning was first systematically studied by Thorndike about 100 years ago. In his famous experiment, a cat was placed in a cage with a latch on the door, and a piece of fish placed outside the cage, Thorndike noticed that the cat tried to reach the fish by extending its paws, and repeated this behavior again and again, yet still failing to reach the fish. Then the cat began to move the latch of the door several times, and successfully opened the door and got the fish. Ultimately, the cat developed an efficient series of movements for moving the latch. From this Thorndike came to believe that learning occurred through trial and error. Individuals take a set of random responses, many of them are wrong or ineffective, only those that followed by desirable outcomes are retained. In other words, the individuals finally learn those responses through trial and error. Through this experiment, Thorndike proposed the theory of the law of effect, which emphasized that behaviors followed by pleasant consequences are more likely to be repeated, while behaviors followed by unfavorable outcomes are unlikely reoccur.

Skinner's experiments extend Thorndike's idea, especially with the idea concerning how rewarded behavior is likely to occur again. Around 1930, using Thorndike's law of effect as a starting point, Skinner developed a device called an operant box, or the Skinner box, to study operant conditioning.

(2) Principles in operant conditioning

The Skinner box (Figure 1-16) is a soundproof and light-resistant chamber that contains a bar that an animal (rat or pigeon) can press or manipulate in order to gain a reward, such as food, or to avoid a painful stimulus, such as an electric shock. The bar is connected to devices that record the animal's response. It is an

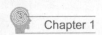

experimental apparatus that Skinner designed to modify animal behavior within an operant conditioning paradigm. In Skinner's experiment, a rat is placed in a box, like the one mentioned above. The rat randomly moves about and explores for food. Occasionally, it presses the bar and gets a small food pellet. The rat can gain food as long as it presses the bar, so the rat begins to press the bar again and again. It is the food that increases the frequency of pressing the bar. In his experiment, Skinner further studied shaping procedures and basic principles in operant conditioning, such as reinforcement and punishment.

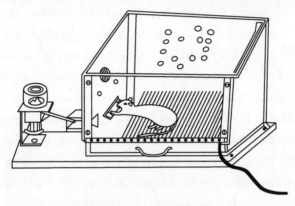

Figure 1-16　Skinner box

1) Reinforcement. In operant conditioning, a reinforcer is any event or stimulus that can increase the frequency of a particular behavior occurring in the future. The increase of certain behaviors may result from the delivery of a pleasant stimulus, or the removal of an unpleasant stimulus. This process is called reinforcement, and the stimulus is called the reinforcer. There are several types of reinforcers as following.

A positive reinforcer is a pleasant stimulus or appetitive event, and the presentation of the stimulus increases the likelihood of that behavior occurs again under the same settings. Positive reinforcement refers to the presentation of a positive reinforcer after a behavior, increasing the frequency of the behavior. In other words, in an attempt to increase the frequency of the behavior occurring in the future, an operant response is followed by the presentation of an appetitive stimulus. In the Skinner box, a food pellet is a positive reinforcer, and its presentation increases the frequency of the behavior; that the rat presses the bar.

A negative reinforcer is an unpleasant stimulus or an aversive event, and the removal of the stimulus increases the likelihood of that behavior occurring again. Again, the rat is placed in the Skinner box, this time with flowing electric current, and the rat suffers a painful electric shock unless it presses the bar. In other words, the electric shock can be avoided if the rat presses the bar, and avoiding the electric shock strengthens the behavior of pressing the bar. The electric shock is a negative reinforcer, and this process is called negative reinforcement, where the withdrawal of negative consequences will increase the likelihood of repeating a desired behavior in similar settings. It is also called avoidance.

Reinforcement theories include three aspects: first, emphasizing the link between individual behavior and specific outcomes; second, focusing on observable behavior and outcomes; and last, experimenter can alter the outcomes to influence behavior in direction, level, and persistence of motivation. In operant conditioning, the terms of "positive" and "negative" do not mean good or bad. Instead, positive means adding a stimulus, and negative means removing a stimulus.

In addition, reinforcer can be divided into primary reinforcer and conditioned reinforcer. A primary reinforcer is an innately reinforcing stimulus, such as one that satisfies a biological need. Food, water, and sex are all primary reinforcers because they satisfy biological desires. A conditioned reinforcer, also known as a secondary reinforcer, is a previously neutral stimulus, and gains its reinforcing power through its association with a primary reinforcer. For example, a good grade is not a primary reinforcer because it does not directly

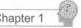

satisfy a boy's biological desires. However, it can be associated with primary reinforcers such as dinner, a kiss from Mom, and a comfortable sleeping bag, which are often rewards. So, the good grade becomes a conditioned reinforcer.

2) Punishment. Punishment refers to administrating negative consequences, or the withdrawing positive consequences, that will reduce the likelihood of repeating certain behaviors in similar settings. In operant conditioning, a punisher is any event that decreases the frequency of a behavior occurring in the future. There are several types of punishers. A positive punisher is an aversive event whose presentation follows a response, which decreases the likelihood of the behavior occurring again. A negative punisher is a pleasant event whose removal decreases the likelihood of that behavior occurring again in the future. For example, for a boy who smokes, he may be punished by having to repeatedly write the same paragraph fifty times as a positive punisher, meanwhile, the removal of desired food or a T-shirt would act as a negative punisher. When either the positive or negative punisher is presented to the boy, the smoking behavior will decrease. Punishment (presenting positive or negative punishers), as an outcome, modifies the behavior of smoking. Both the administration of negative consequences and the withdrawal of positive consequences will reduce the likelihood of repeating the behavior in similar settings.

In addition, there are different types of punishers. Primary punishers are concerned with unpleasant biological experiences, such as pain or freezing temperatures. Secondary punishers refer to unpleasant events that are associated with primary punishers, such as not being promoted or social disapproval. Secondary reinforcers are also called conditioned punishers.

The effects of punishment on behavior are as follows. Punishment is most effective in reducing poor performance. However, arbitrary and capricious punishment will lead to undesirable side effects and poor performance, such as increased aggression and dissatisfaction. In addition, punishment may be offset by positive reinforcement from another source. When we want to modify certain behaviors using punishment, we must realize that the effects of punishment are sometimes limited because it often does not guide one toward more desirable behavior.

3) Shaping. In operant conditioning, shaping is a technique or procedure in which successive approximations to the desired behavior are rewarded. Generally, an experimenter administrates the positive reinforcement to lead to the desired behavior through successive approximations. Behavior is shaped gradually rather than changed all at once.

Shaping can be used to train individuals to perform behaviors that would rarely occur in a natural setting. Usually, shaping is achieved by reinforcing approximations to a desired behavior in a step-by-step fashion. For example, to teach a girl to write her name, you initially give praise for writing the first letter correctly, which is an administration of a positive reinforcer. After the girl has mastered writing the first letter, letter-by-letter you give praise until the entire name is correctly written. This is positive reinforcement through successive approximations.

Experimenters involved with training animals, use the process of shaping to teach the animals to perform tasks. In previous studies, psychologists trained thousands of animals of different species to perform special tasks. However, some studies indicated that not all behaviors could be shaped. Sometimes, it is difficult training some species to perform certain tasks. Operant conditioning, like classical conditioning, operates on environment under biological constraints.

In operant conditioning, generalization is the tendency to respond to other stimuli that are similar, but not identical, to the original stimulus. Extinction, in operant conditioning, is the gradual disappearance of a response when it stops being reinforced. In fact, generalization, discrimination, extinction, and spontaneous recovery work in operant conditioning, just as they do in classical conditioning.

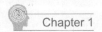

(3) Schedule of reinforcement

A schedule of reinforcement is a prescription that states how and when discriminative stimuli and behavioral consequences will be presented. Schedules of reinforcement are probably the most heavily researched topic within operant conditioning. The schedules explain when and how reinforcements will be delivered. Different schedules of reinforcement produce distinctive effects on operant behavior, and unique rates and patterns of responding depending on the conditions of the schedule selected. In operant conditioning, schedules of reinforcement are the precise rules that are used to present, or remove reinforcers or punishers following certain operant behavior. In other words, to determine when and how the operant behaviors will be reinforced. These rules are important during the learning process. Experimenters can reinforce the strength and rate of a behavior by controlling the amount of time and the number of operant responses. Certain schedules of reinforcement may be more effective in specific situations. Usually, there are two types of reinforcement schedules: continuous reinforcement and intermittent reinforcement.

1) Continuous reinforcement. It means that the desired behavior is reinforced whenever it occurs. Generally, this schedule is best used at the initial stages of operant conditioning in order to create a strong association between the behavior and the reinforcers. However, there are some problems when using this type of reinforcement, and one of them is saturation. For example, in the Skinner box, if an experimenter presents a food pellet every time, the rat may be stuffed and no longer want food. The food will fail to act as a reinforcer if that is the case. So, it is not always best to give reinforcement every single time during the training process.

2) Intermittent reinforcement. It is also known as the partial reinforcement, is when the reinforcer is not administered at each response. For example, in the Skinner box, if every press of the bar is rewarded, the rat is on a continuous reinforcement schedule. Experimenters found that if only some responses are rewarded, behavior can still be maintained effectively, known as intermittent reinforcement. In fact, once the response is firmly associated with the outcome, reinforcement is usually switched to a partial reinforcement schedule. In real life, behavior is not often reinforced each time it occurs. Intermittent reinforcement is much more effective to develop a persistent behavior, because it can economize on time and frequency of the administration of reinforcers. In intermittent reinforcement, behavior is rewarded periodically. When reinforcement depends on a specific number of responses, the schedules are called ratio schedules. In other words, the ratio schedule is the number of responses required per reinforcement. When reinforcement depends on the passage of time the schedules are called interval schedules.

Ratio schedules focus on the direct relationship between the number of responses made by the individual and the amount of reinforcement obtained. The more (faster) the number of responses the individual makes, the more frequently it gets reinforced. So, ratio schedules tend to generate hard work (high rates of response) in individuals.

Interval schedules require a minimum amount of time that must pass between successive reinforced responses. The opportunity for reinforcement is independent of individual's effort, and the individual does not know when reinforcement will be made available. The term interval is in some ways misleading, since it implies that waiting is important. The concept of the interval comes from the fact that laboratory experiments indeed use the various times to schedule the availability of reinforcement. While interval schedules in a sense do imply the passage of time, the important characteristic of these schedules, especially as contrasted with the ratio schedules, is that individual's behavior does not influence the availability of reinforcement. Due to this lack of a relationship, between individual's behavior and the availability of reinforcement, interval schedules produce much lower amounts of behavior per reinforcement when compared to ratio schedules.

In addition, we need to know two other terms to fully understand reinforcement schedules. One is fixed schedules, which requires that reinforcement is always the same. The other is a variable schedule, which means that reinforcement changes randomly. We generally discuss four major schedules of reinforcement that Skinner studied.

(a) Fixed Ratio Schedule. As to the ratio schedule, it requires a certain number of operant responses to acquire the next reinforcement. If each reinforcement requires a fixed number of responses, it is called fixed ratio schedule. For example, in the training of a young boy to form an eating habit using chopsticks instead of his hands, a mother may choose a fixed ratio schedule; the boy will be rewarded after he uses chopsticks three times. Another example of a fixed ratio schedule is an industrial worker whose wages are adjusted according to the unit output produced. Usually, this schedule elicits rapid rates of responding, if the pause is brief after the delivery of the reinforcer. The length of the pause is directly proportional to the number of responses required.

(b) Variable Ratio Schedule. Variable ratio schedule is when the individual is still rewarded after a certain number of responses; however, the number of responses that will be reinforced is unpredictable. Under the conditions of the variable ratio schedule, the number of responses required for reinforcement is uncertain, and this results in high rates of responding. For example, the student does not know when he will be awarded because this schedule uses random reinforcing of a desired behavior. Consequently, he continues to show the behavior in hopes that the next time he will acquire the reward. A familiar example of a variable ratio schedule is seen in lottery games. People know there is a possibility of acquiring a prize by buying lottery tickets, but they cannot predict which time they may win a prize, which encourages them to buy lottery tickets again and again. Therefore, variable schedules typically result in more consistent patterns of behavior than do the fixed schedules.

(c) Fixed Interval Schedule. Fixed interval schedule is when an organism's response is reinforced in a fixed time period. After the first response is rewarded, the successive responses will be reinforced in a specified amount of time. For example, in the Skinner box, the experimenter designs the reinforcement with a fixed interval schedule of 30 seconds. From the first time the rat is rewarded for pressing the bar, the successive reinforcements occurs every 30 seconds. The responses occurring before this time has elapsed are not reinforced. This schedule causes high amounts of responding near the end of the interval, because the individual learns the length of the interval.

(d) Variable Interval Schedule. Variable interval schedule is when an individual's responses are reinforced in a variable time period, from a few seconds to longer periods of time. In other words, the reinforcement for the desired responses from one to the next uses an unpredictable time interval. This schedule produces a slow, steady rate of response, and it tends to be resistant to extinction. For example, in the Skinner box, when the experimenter uses reinforcement with a variable interval schedule, from the first time the rat is rewarded for pressing the bar, each successive reinforcement occurs irregularly; this may be from 15 second to 60 second. In real life, a teacher usually uses a variable interval schedule with a consistent average length when she wants a student to develop a desired behavior. When a student performs a target behavior, such as finishing his homework in time, he will be rewarded about once a week, but on different days of the week, maybe on Monday this time and next on Friday.

(4) Comparison of classical and operant conditioning

There are many similarities and differences between the two types of conditioning.

1) Similarities. Both classical conditioning and operant conditioning are basic forms of associative learning. New behaviors are acquired by associative learning in both patterns. In classical conditioning, we learn to associate two stimuli and change our behaviors; in operant conditioning, we learn to associate a response and its consequence and alter our behavior according to the consequences of previous behavior. Both classical and operant conditioning can be used to increase or decrease the instances of a behavior and that they can both

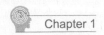

be demonstrated in animals and humans. Some principles of learning can work in both operant conditioning and classical conditioning. Like Kimble (1961) pointed out, the basic principles of learning such as acquisition, generalization, extinction, discrimination, and spontaneous recovery are common to both types of learning. In addition, both types of learning are often affected by some biological factors such as neural mechanisms, fatigue, and use of drugs, etc.

2) Differences. There are significant differences between the two types of learning. First, classical conditioning is based on involuntary reflexive behavior, while operant conditioning is based on voluntary behavior. In classical conditioning, besides a pairing of neutral stimuli and unconditioned stimuli, the precondition is that an organism has an innate reflexive behavior, that is, it occurs as an automatic response to some stimulus. In operant conditioning, an organism performs a specific behavior, and then acquires reinforcement. It involves operant behavior, that is, an organism operates on the environment to produce rewarding or punishing stimuli. It is an experience of active learning whereas the classical conditioning is a process of passive learning. However, this distinction is not as strong as it once was believed to be. Neal Miller (1978) has pointed out that the involuntary responses, such as heart rate and respiration rate, can be modified through operant conditioning; meanwhile many instances of classical conditioning also involve the reinforcement process.

Second, as to the pattern of associative learning, classical conditioning is based on the pattern of stimulus-response. The neutral stimuli will elicit a specific response through pairing the unconditioned stimuli together. Operant conditioning is based on the pattern of response-reinforcement, in which organisms learn particular behaviors follow by certain consequences.

Third, the effectiveness of classical conditioning is usually assessed by size of response, while the effectiveness of operant conditioning is usually assessed by frequency of response. For example, in Pavlov's experiment, the effectiveness is assessed by the amount of salivation of dogs; in Skinner's experiment, the effectiveness is assessed by the frequency of the rat's pressing bar.

(5) Applications of operant conditioning

The principles of operant conditioning are broadly applied in many fields such as education, training in workplace, and clinical treatment.

Shaping of behavior is an example of operant conditioning. In the training of certain behaviors, shaping focuses on, and reinforces, each necessary step leading to the target, and finally an individual acquires a desired behavior. This method is broadly applied in educational activities. Shaping procedures are also applied in the training of animal's performance, such as personal assistants for blind humans. When a dog is trained to behave according to the commands of a blind man, the man offers a command antecedent to the desired behavior; the dog is rewarded as long as it performs the behavior in response to the command. Finally, the dog becomes an assistant for the blind man, and acts according to commands. Reinforcement in time plays an important role during shaping procedures.

Operant conditioning also has made significant contributions in therapeutic settings. The typical example is the application of biofeedback. Biofeedback is a technique in which people are trained to adjust and improve their behaviors by monitoring signals from their own bodies. Biofeedback uses special equipment to help individuals become more aware of their body's reactions, and they learn to control certain internal bodily processes that normally occur involuntarily, such as heart rate, blood pressure, muscle tension, respiration, and skin temperature.

Psychologists use biofeedback to help the tense and anxious patients learn to relax. Clinicians use biofeedback to help patients with many diseases and painful conditions. For example, biofeedback technique is used to help an individual with the tension and anxiety they face in stressful situations. Respiration biofeedback devices monitor the rate and amplitude of respiration. When the individual is tense or anxious, the rate and amplitude of respiration increase; when the individual tries to control his respiration, the signal about his respiration from the biofeedback device may act as a kind of reward for reducing tension and anxiety. This signal can guide or reinforce the individual to control and improve his behaviors during the exercises. Relaxation is a key component in biofeedback treatment of many disorders. Biofeedback techniques tell individuals that their efforts to control their own physiological functions are being successful reinforced, and they learn to relax in the face of anxious situations. Subsequently, they learn to reduce those maladaptive behaviors. Biofeedback techniques are widely used to treat a host of conditions such as tension-type headaches, many other types of pain, insomnia, high blood pressure, digestive disorders, and attention deficit disorder. Operant conditioning techniques and procedures have had many applications across various circumstances and problem areas.

2.2.5   Study of observational learning

(1) Bandura's experiment

Among higher animals, learning does not occur through direct experience alone. In the 1960s, American psychologist Albert Bandura suggested another form of learning especially among humans, observational learning. It refers to when individuals can learn a behavior simply by watching and imitating the behavior of another person. Observational learning, sometimes called modeling, is a type of social learning because it often occurs in social settings. A model is someone who serves as an example.

In Bandura's famous "Bobo doll" experiment, the nursery school children imitated the aggressive behavior of an adult model just through seeing them in a movie. Three groups of nursery school children were exposed to presentations of an adult punching an inflatable clown (Bobo doll). The first group observed the adult's behavior live; the second group watched the same aggressive scenes on video; and the third group watched a cartoon version of the adult's behavior. When the children were later allowed to play in a room with the same inflatable clown, some of them began to imitate the adult's aggressive behaviors they had previously observed. The children were influenced to differing degrees based on the presentation style they viewed, either live, on video or cartoon. Those children who had observed the adult's aggressive behaviors live were more likely to have aggressive behaviors when they were frustrated in their life. This experiment supports Bandura's argument that people learn from observing others. The process of observing and imitating a specific behavior is often called modeling. Many of our behaviors are learned from modeling. Modeling means that we imitate what a model does and says. Parents and teachers are often the models to children. Observational learning often occurs through exposure to events and people in the media. For example, many young people like to copy the clothes or behaviors of television personalities.

(2) Steps to successful modeling

In 1986 Bandura published his famous book, Social Foundations of Thought and Action: A Social Cognitive Theory, in which describing many studies involving observational learning, or modeling. Modeling is the process of observing and imitating a specific behavior. Bandura identified three basic models of observational learning: a live model, which involves an actual individual demonstrating or acting out a behavior; a verbal instructional model, which involves descriptions and explanations of a behavior; and a symbolic model, which involves real or fictional characters displaying behaviors in books, films, television programs, or online media. Especially, people are likely to imitate those they perceive to be like them, successful, or admirable. According to Bandura, four basic steps are necessary for an observer to learn successfully the behavior of a model: attention, retention, reproducing modeled behavior, and motivation.

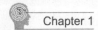

1) Attention. The first step is that an observer pays attention to the model. This process decides what an individual observes and learns from the modeled behavior. Many factors contribute to the quality and the amount of attention. In particular, both the experiences of the observer and the characteristics of the model play important roles. An observer will be attracted by some important characteristics of the modeler such as expertise, appearance, and status. If a modeler is interesting or novel, an observer is more likely to dedicate his attention to learn.

2) Retention. In this process, an observer needs to remember the behaviors and the activities of the model, in other words, he or she needs to deal with learned information including organization, rehearsal and coding. Imagery and language aid in the process of retaining information. The stored information in the form of mental images or verbal descriptions will facilitate observers to recall later, and reproduce the activity with their own behavior. It is also ability for observer to pull up information later and act on. It is important part of observational learning.

3) Reproducing Modeled Behavior. Reproduction refers to the ability to replicate the behavior that the model has just demonstrated. Once observer has paid attention to the model and retained the information, he begins to actually perform the behavior what he observed. The reproduction process involves converting stored information about the model, in the observers mind, into explicit actions. Behavioral reproduction is accomplished by organizing the observer's own responses and experiences in accordance with the modeled pattern. Some simple actions can be learned through directly observing and imitating, but possession of complex behaviors needs a series of procedures such as repeated imitation, guided practice, and appropriate feedback. Continual practice of the learned behavior leads to improvement and skill advancement.

4) Motivation. If a model is successful or observer's behavior is rewarded, the behavior is more likely to recur. Motivation is the key factor during the process of observational learning. An observer will perform the certain behavior only if he or she has some motivation or reason to do so. Since an observer's behavior can be affected by the positive or negative consequences, it is very important for the presence of reinforcement or punishment. In other words, reinforcement and punishment play an important role in motivation. For example, if a model's behaviors are followed by many incentives, an observer will have stronger motivation to imitate the model's behavior. These incentives act as reinforcers; in contrast, negative reinforcers or punishers discourage the continuation of the modeled activity. Bandura noticed that external, environmental reinforcement was not the only factor to influence learning and behavior. He suggested intrinsic reinforcement as a form of internal reward, such as pride, satisfaction, and a sense of accomplishment. He emphasized that internal motivation can promote observational learning or modeling.

(3) Possible mechanism of observational learning

As mentioned above, emotion such as fear is learned on the basis of classical conditioning, and requires personal experience with an aversive event. A recent study demonstrated that fear can be acquired indirectly, merely through observation rather than personal experience of the aversive event.

Scientists conducted a study that participants watched a video: a person watched several colored squares on a computer screen. Once a blue square appeared, the person received an electrical shock; there was no shock while other colored squares appeared. The person in the video responded with fear and anxiety whenever the blue square appeared. In this experiment, when the participants were presented with the blue square that predicted with electric shocks like the person in the video, they would have a response of fear. The fear is learned by observing other's behaviors and responses. The scientists monitored the brain activity of each participant during the experiment. The researchers use functional magnetic resonance brain imaging techniques, and found that certain part of the brain, especially amygdala, responded both when watching others receive a shock and when presented with the blue square that was previously paired with a shock in the video. It seems that there are similar processes in the brain for directly experiencing fear and observing others fear. This study suggests that learned fears, from observation, may work under similar mechanisms as fears learned from direct experiences.

Many studies explored the neurological mechanisms of observational learning. Neurophysiologist Rizzolatti and colleagues discovered the mirror neurons in the neurological experiments of the Macaque monkey. They noticed when a monkey imitated another monkey's activities, the mirror neurons always fired. A mirror neuron is a neuron that fires both when an animal acts and when the animal observes the same action performed by another. Scientists have planned to conduct further studies in human. These mirror neurons may play a fundamental role in both understanding the actions and emotions of other people, and for learning new skills by imitation.

Observational learning is actually a highly complex cognitive process, involving vision, perception, representation, memory and motor control. The recent neuroimaging experiments suggest that the regions in the human brain that contain mirror neurons may be associated with imitation and language.

（周　莉　徐国庆）

Chapter 2

Psychological Processes: Late Stages

You have learned related psychological knowledge in the former lessons, and you have known the terms of sensation, perception, memories, and so on. Then you will learn some more complicated processes.

Thinking may be the most complicated and amazing achievements for human-beings. We think when talking, making schedules, studying, even when you are intending to lie to someone, you need to make up a story that never happened. Language is also another kind of characteristic ability which only belongs to mankind. How do we think? How do we solve problems? How do we create ideas? How did Copernicus come up with his idea? In our daily lives, we are capable of doing things with information that make the most complicated ones simple. These processes—thinking and problem solving—are most impressive when they show originality or creativity.

Consciousness is one of those words that different philosophers and psychologists use in different ways and about which they often debate. For practical purposes, most psychologists define consciousness simply as the experiencing of one's own mental events in a manner that one can report on them to others. Defined this way, consciousness and awareness are synonyms. Consciousness is the awareness of internal and external stimuli. Your consciousness includes your awareness of external events ("The professor just asked me a difficult question about medieval history"), your awareness of your internal sensations ("My heart is racing and I'm beginning to sweat"), the awareness of yours as the unique being having these experiences ("Why me?"), and your awareness of your thoughts about these experiences ("I'm going to make a fool of myself!"). To put it more concisely, consciousness is personal awareness. What aspects of consciousness to researchers study? Topics such as sleep, dreams, hypnosis, and the effects of psychoactive drugs are just a few of the major topics studied by psychologists.

Motivation concerns the forces that direct future behavior, emotion pertains to the feelings we experience throughout our lives. The study of emotions focuses on our internal experiences at any given moment. All of us feel a variety of emotions: happiness at succeeding at a difficult task, sadness over the death of a loved one, anger at being treated unfairly. Because emotions not only play a role in motivating our behavior but also act as a reflection of our underlying motivation, they play an important role in our lives.

1. Thinking and language

1.1 Thinking

Thinking which belongs to a higher mental process is defined as the manipulation of mental representations of information. We can transform representations including words, visual images, sounds or information in any other sensory modality stored in our memory into new and different forms in order to understand the outside world, solve problems, making decisions or reach goals.

1.1.1 Mental images

Mental images are representations of object, event, or scene in the mind of the physical world, when the relevant object, event, or scene is not actually present to the senses. Every sensory modality may produce corresponding mental images. For example, if you are asked to think of one of your old friends, you may "see" the visual image of him or her. Besides the visual representations, our ability to "hear" a tune in our heads also relies on a mental image. When a musician hears a song, he or she can sometimes "see" the song notes in their head.

Mental images have many of the properties of the actual stimuli they represent. It takes longer time to scan mental images of larger objects than of small ones, just as the eye takes longer to scan an actual large object than an actual small one. Research has found that we can manipulate and rotate mental images of objects, just as we are able to manipulate and rotate them in the real world (Figure 2-1).

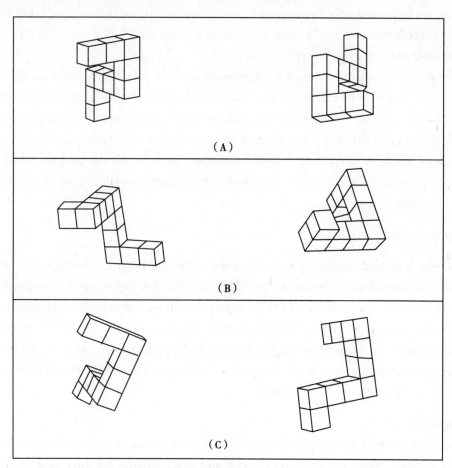

Figure 2-1   Materials used in the experiment of Shepard and Metzler (1971)

(A) One of the two patterns cannot be mentally rotated to match the other, (B) and (C) one of the two patterns can be mentally rotated to match the other.

In the mental rotation experiment, participants were asked to mentally rotate one of each pair of patterns to see if it is the same as the other member of that pair. The results found a linear relationship between the degree of rotation in the mental imagery task and the time it took participants to reach their answers.

The production of mental images can be a way to improve various skills. Experts found that the use of mental imagery can lead to improved performance in sports. Students can form mental images of playing a 5-finger piano exercise, and such mental practice will significantly improve in performance of their playing without mental practice.

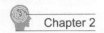

1.1.2　Concepts

Concepts are usually defined as categorizations of objects, events, or people that share common properties. For example, if you are asked to tell what was in your kitchen cabinets, you might answer with a detailed list of items, such as a jar of sugar, six unmatched dinner plates and so forth. Or even you would respond by naming some broader categories, such as "food" and "dishes".

Concepts in our everyday lives are usually ambiguous and difficult to define. For instance, broader concepts such as "table" and "bird" have a set of general, relatively loose characteristic features, rather than unique, clearly defined properties that distinguish an example of the concept. When we consider these more ambiguous concepts, we usually think in terms of examples called prototypes. Prototypes are typical, highly representative examples of a concept that correspond to our mental image or best example of the concept. For instance, although a robin and an ostrich are both examples of birds, the robin is an example that comes to most people's minds far more readily. Consequently, robin is a prototype of the concept "bird". Similarly, when we think of the concept of a table, we're likely to think of a coffee table before we think of a drafting table, making a coffee table closer to our prototype of a table.

Concepts enable us to organize complex phenomena into simpler, more easily usable and cognitive categories. Concepts can help us classify newly encountered objects on the basis of our past experience. Concepts also can influence our behavior. For instance, we would assume that if might be appropriate to pet an animal after determining that it is a dog, whereas we would behave differently after classifying the animal as a wolf. Concepts enable us to think about and understand more readily the complex world in which we live. For example, physicians make diagnoses by drawing on concepts and prototypes of symptoms that they learned about in medical school.

1.1.3　Problem solving

Problem solving is defined as a higher-order mental process that requires moving a given state toward a desired goal state. In psychology, problems can vary from ill-defined to well-defined. Ill-defined problems are those that do not have clear goals, solution paths, or expected solution. For example, how to bring peace to the areas in war. On the contrary, well-defined problems have specific goals, clearly defined solution paths, and clear expected solutions. For example, solving a mathematical equation in an exam. Well-defined problems allow for more initial planning than ill-defined problems. Thus, we can make straightforward judgments about whether a potential solution is appropriate.

(1) Types of problem

1) Arrangement problems. It requires the problem solver to rearrange or recombine elements in a way that will satisfy a certain criterion. Anagram problems and jigsaw puzzles are the examples of arrangement problems. Usually, several different arrangements can be made, but only one or a few of the arrangements will produce a solution. For example, given a set of random letters "I N E A V", and then asked you to rearrange the set to make an English word, "NAIVE".

2) Problems of Inducing Structure. In problems of inducing structure, a person must identify the existing relationships among the elements presented and then construct a new relationship among them. In such a problem, the problem solver must determine not only the relationships among the elements but also the structure and size of the elements involved. For example, given a series of numbers "1 4 2 4 3 4 4 4 5 4 6 4", with the question "What number comes next in the series?" A person must first determine that the solution requires the numbers to be considered in pairs (14-24-34-44-54-64). Only after identifying that part of the problem can let a person determine the solution rule that is the first number of each pair increases by one,

while the second number remains the same.

3) Transformation problems. They consist of an initial state, a goal state, and a method for changing the initial state into the goal state. The Tower of Hanoi problem is an example. In the problem, the initial state is the original configuration, the goal state is to have the three disks on the third peg, and the method is the rules for moving the disks.

In the Tower of Hanoi puzzle, three disks are placed on three posts in the order shown in the Figure 2-2. The goal of the puzzle is to move all three disks to the third post, arranged in the same order, by using as few moves as possible. There are two restrictions: Only one disk can be moved at a time, and no disk can ever cover a smaller one during a move. Psychologists are interested in the Tower of Hanoi puzzle, because the way people go about solving such puzzles helps illuminate how people solve complex, real-life problems.

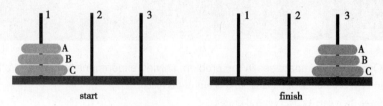

Figure 2-2   The Tower of Hanoi puzzle

(2) Problem solving strategies

1) Trial and error. It is a fundamental method of problem solving. It is characterized by repeated, varied attempts which are continued until success, or until one stops trying. We can solve problems through trial and error. For instances, Thomas Edison invented the light bulb only because he tried thousands of different kinds of materials for a filament before he found one that worked. But the difficulty with trial and error, of course, is that some problems are so complicated that it would take a lifetime to try out endless possibilities. Thus, solving complex problems often involve the use of heuristics.

2) The means-ends analysis. It involves repeated tests for differences between the desired outcome and what currently exists. In a means-ends analysis, each step brings the problem solver closer to a resolution. Although this approach is often effective, if the problem requires indirect steps that temporarily increase the discrepancy between a current state and the solution, means-ends analysis can be counterproductive. For example, sometimes the fastest route to the summit of a mountain requires a mountain climber to backtrack temporarily; a means-ends approach, which implies that the mountain climber should always forge ahead and upward, will be ineffective in such instances.

3) Forming subgoals. It is a commonly used heuristic to divide a problem into intermediate steps, or subgoals, and solve each of those steps. For instance, in the Tower of Hanoi problem, we could choose several obvious subgoals, such as moving the largest disk to the third post. If solving a subgoal is a step toward the ultimate solution to a problem, identifying subgoals is an appropriate strategy. In some cases, however, forming subgoals is not all that helpful and may actually increase the time needed to find a solution. For example, a complicated mathematical problem is so complex that it takes longer to identify the appropriate subdivisions than to solve the problem by other means.

4) Insight. It means a sudden awareness of the relationships among various elements that had previously appeared to be unrelated during the process of solving a problem.

Researchers examined learning and problem-solving processes in chimpanzees. In the studies, they exposed chimps to challenging situations in which boxes and sticks were strewn about, and a bunch of tantalizing bananas hung from the ceiling, out of reach. Initially, the chimps made trial-and-error attempts to get to

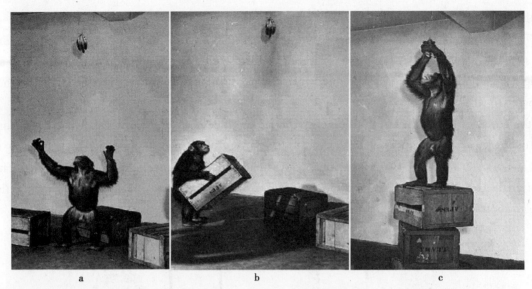

a   b   c

Figure 2-3   One of the chimpanzees in the problem solving experiments made by Wolfgang Kohler

a. The chimpanzee sees a bunch of bananas that is out of his reach.

b. The chimpanzee then carries over several crates.

c. The chimpanzee stacks the crates and stands on them to reach the bananas.

the bananas: They would throw the sticks at the bananas, jump from one of the boxes, or leap wildly from the ground. Frequently, they would seem to give up in frustration, leaving the bananas dangling temptingly overhead. But then, in what seemed like a sudden revelation, they would stop whatever they were doing and stand on a box to reach the bananas with a stick. The researcher called the cognitive process underlying the chimps' new behavior insight.

5) Algorithm. It is a rule that, if applied appropriately, guarantees a solution to a problem. We can use an algorithm even if we cannot understand why it works. For example, you may know that the length of the third side of a right triangle can be found by using specific mathematical formula. However, no algorithm is available for many problems and decision.

(3) Impediments to solutions

1) Functional fixedness. It is the tendency to think of an object only in terms of its typical use. For instance, in the candle problem, you are given a set of tacks, candles, and match each in a small box, and told your goal is to place three candles at eye level on a nearby door, so that wax will not drip on the floor as the candles burn. How would you approach this challenge? Functional fixedness leads most people to see the box with objects inside simply as containers for the objects they hold rather than as a potential part of the solution. They cannot envision another function for the boxes.

The Candle Problem

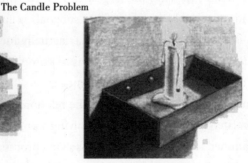

initial state   one solution

Figure 2-4   The difficulty most people experience with the candle problem is caused by Functional fixedness

2) Mental set. It is the tendency for old patterns of problem solving to persist. A classic experiment demonstrated this phenomenon. As you can see in the following Figure 2-5, the object of the task is to use the jars in each row to measure out the designated amount of liquid.

Given jars with these capacities(in ounces):

	A	B	C	Obtain:
1	21	127	3	100
2	14	163	25	99
3	18	43	10	5
4	9	42	6	21
5	20	59	4	31
6	23	49	3	20

Figure 2-5   The object is to use the jars in each row to measure out the designated amount of liquid

The first five rows are all solved in the same way: First fill the largest jar (B) and then from it fill the middle-size jar (A) once and the smallest jar (C) two times. What is left in B is the designated amount (Stated as a formula, the designated amount is B-A-2C.) The demonstration of mental set comes in the sixth row of the problem, a point at which you probably encountered some difficulty. If you are like most people, you tried the formula and were perplexed when it failed. Chances are, in fact, that you missed the simple solution to the problem, which involves merely subtracting C from A. Interestingly, people who were given the problem in row 6 first had no difficulty with it at all.

3) Confirmation bias. It is a tendency to selectively look for information that conforms to the original hypothesis and to overlook information that supports alternative hypotheses or solutions. Even when we find evidence that contradicts a solution we have chosen, we are apt to stick with our original hypothesis. Confirmation bias occurs for several reasons. For one thing, rethinking a problem that appears to be solved already takes extra cognitive effort, and so we are apt to stick with our first solution. For another, we give greater weight to subsequent information that supports our initial position than to information that is not supportive of it.

1.1.4   Reasoning and decision making

We live in a world filled with uncertainty. Should you spend much money to see movies? Are you ready to commit yourself to a long-term relationship? What pen should I bring to my exam? Thus, we must use the processes of reasoning and decision making to deal efficiently with those uncertainties. There are two kinds of reasoning: deductive reasoning and inductive reasoning.

(1) Deductive reasoning

Deductive reasoning is a form of thinking in which one draws a conclusion that is intended to follow logically from some statements or premises. Syllogism that involves the logical rules of deductive reasoning consists of three parts: two premises and a conclusion. An example:

Premise 1: All cats are animals.

Premise 2: Kitty is a cat.

Conclusion: Kitty is an animal.

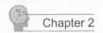

Syllogism shows that we are quite capable of applying deductive reasoning to arrive at conclusions.

However, we will have difficulties to perform some reasoning tasks. In Watson selection task, imagine that you are given the array of four cards with A, D, 4, and 7 printed on them. Your task is to determine which cards you must turn over to test the rule. If a card has a vowel on one side, then it has an even number on the other side. Most participants turn over the A, which is correct, and the 4—which is incorrect. Actually, no matter what character appears on the flip side of the 4, the rule will not be falsified. Instead, you must flip the 7.

Researchers identified that the task tends to be solved correctly by presented in a context of social relations. For example, if the rule used is "If you are drinking alcohol then you must be over 18", and the cards have an age on one side and beverage on the other, e.g., "16", "drinking beer", "25", "drinking coke", most people have no difficulty in selecting the correct cards ("16" and "beer").

(2) Inductive reasoning

Inductive reasoning is the attempt to infer some new conclusions from available evidence and past experience. In inductive reasoning, the conclusion is reached by generalizing or extrapolating from specific cases to general rules. The inferred information is at best an educated guess, not a logical necessity. In real-life circumstances, much of the problem-solving ability relies on inductive reasoning. Scientists reason inductively as they try to infer rules of nature from their observations of specific events in the world. Detectives engage in inductive reasoning when they piece together bits of evidence to make inferences as to who might have committed a crime. However, most psychologists focused on the mistakes of inductive reasoning in their study. As an example, when asked to estimate the percentage of people who die from various causes, most people overestimate causes that have recently been emphasized in the media, such as terrorism, murders, and airplane accidents, and underestimate less-publicized but much more frequent causes, such as heart disease and traffic accidents. Because, the heavily publicized causes are more available to them than are the less-publicized causes. When we reason, we tend to rely too strongly on information that is easily accessible to us rather than on information that is less available.

(3) Decision making

Decision making is regarded as the cognitive process resulting in the selection of a belief or a course of action among several alternative possibilities. Decision-making is the process of identifying and choosing alternatives based on the values and preferences of the decision-maker. The basic principle to make a decision is to judge which option will bring about the biggest gain or which option will bring about the smallest loss. Imagine you were asked how happy you would be to get a ￥1000 raise in your job. If you were expecting no raise at all, you would see this as a great gain, and would be quite happy. But if you were expecting a raise of at least ￥5000, you may feel as if you've lost money and no happy at all. Kahneman (1992) believed reference points are important in decision making. What seems like a gain or a loss will be determined in part by the expectations to which a decision maker refers.

1.2   Language

No other species that uses a language as complex as any human language. People can produce an unlimited number of messages with a limited number of words. Our ability to make sense out of nonsense, if the nonsense follows typical rules of language, illustrates the complexity of both human language and the cognitive processes that underlie its development and use. Language is the communication of information through symbols arranged according to systematic rules. The use of language is an important cognitive ability for people communicating with each other. Not only is language central to communication, it is also closely tied to the very way in which we think about and understand the world.

1.2.1   Basic components of language

(1) Grammar

The basic structure of language rests on grammar, the system of rules that determine how our thoughts can be expressed. Grammar deals with three major components of language: phonology, syntax, and semantics. Despite the complexities of language, most of us acquire the basics of grammar without even being aware that we have learned its rules. Moreover, even though we may have difficulty explicitly stating the rules of grammar, our linguistic abilities are so sophisticated that we can utter an infinite number of different statements.

(2) Phonology

Phonology is the study of the smallest basic units of speech, called phonemes, that affect meaning, and of the way we use those sounds to form words and produce meaning. For instance, a sound in fat and a sound in fate represent two different phonemes in English. Linguists have identified more than 800 different phonemes among all the world's languages. Speakers in certain language use phonemes from as few as 15 to as many as 141. Differences in phonemes are one reason people have difficulty learning other languages. For example, to a Japanese speaker, whose native language does not have an r phoneme, English words such as roar present some difficulty.

(3) Syntax

Syntax refers to the rules that indicate how words and phrases can be combined to form sentences. Every language has intricate rules that guide the order in which words may be strung together to communicate meaning. English speakers have no difficulty recognizing that "Radio down the turn" is not a meaningful sequence, whereas "Turn down the radio" is. To understand the effect of syntax in English, consider the changes in meaning caused by the different word orders in the following three utterances: "John kidnapped the boy", "John, the kidnapped boy", and "The boy kidnapped John".

(4) Semantics

Semantics are the meanings of words and sentences. Semantic rules allow us to use words to convey the subtlest nuances. For instance, we are able to make the distinction between "The truck hit Laura" (which we would be likely to say if we had just seen the vehicle hitting Laura) and "Laura was hit by a truck" (which we would probably say if someone asked why Laura was missing class while she recuperated).

1.2.2   Language comprehension

Comprehension is the process of accessing meanings about spoken and written utterances in a language. Language processes can use context powerfully and efficiently to resolve ambiguities. Suppose a speaker has produced the utterance "I come from the bank." You can probably think of at least two meanings about the word "bank", one having to do with rivers and the other having to do with money. To resolve the ambiguity, you should use surrounding context, such as talking about rivers or money during the conversation. Inference, which will fill up the missing information with logical assumptions based on prior experiences or knowledge can make listeners understand utterances well too. Consider following pair of utterances:

I am heading to the Deli to meet Mary.

She promised to buy me a sandwich for lunch.

Listeners can draw this inference "Deli is a place where you can buy a sandwich" automatically.

1.2.3   Language production

Language production is concerned with what people choose to say, sign and write, as well as the processes

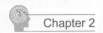

they go through to produce the message. How do speakers produce the right words to communicate the meaning they intend? As a good speaker, one should have accurate expectations about what the listeners are likely to know. The expectations are based on the common knowledge or common ground shared by the language users. The judgment of common ground includes three sources: Community membership, that is language producers often make strong assumptions about what is likely to be mutually known based on shared membership in communities of various sizes; Co-presence for actions, that is language producers often assume that the actions and events they have shared with other conversationalists become part of common ground; perceptual co-presence, that exists when a speaker and a listener share the same perceptual events.

Speech Errors are optimal windows for psychologists to study language production.

Spoonerism that is an exchange of the initial sounds of two or more words in a phrase or sentence is one of speech errors that language producers make. For example, a speaker might exchange initial consonants—"tips of the slung" for "slips of the tongue". Speech errors give researchers insight into the understanding of producing of utterances. In the above example, speakers would never say "tlips of the sung," which would violate the rule of English that "tl" does not occur as an initial sound. Findings suggest that while you are producing utterances, some of your cognitive processes are devoted to detecting and editing potential errors. These processes are reluctant to let you pronounce sounds that are not real English words.

2. States of consciousness

2.1　Consciousness

For more detailed information, please see Chapter 3.

2.1.1　Characteristics of consciousness

Consciousness is the awareness of an individual's perceptions, thoughts, and feelings being experienced at a given moment. The main characteristics of consciousness include the following: subjectivity, uniformity, change, and initiative.

(1) Subjectivity

Subjectivity refers to the idea that consciousness is unique in each individual, and it is a truthful personal experience. Every thought is part of a personal consciousness. The universal fact is not "feeling and thoughts exist", but "I think" and "I feel". We can directly be aware of our own thoughts, feelings and moods, while only understanding other people's awareness of the experience through indirect observation. This subjectivity is also demonstrated when we make a selection in face of the huge amount of information around us, we may choose or neglect some information. In fact, we can only be aware of a small part of our conscious experience in any given moment.

(2) Uniformity

Uniformity refers to the idea that awareness of our experience is a unified whole. The various forms of our awareness have been integrated into a unique and coherent personal experience. For example, when we come to the park, we may see flowers blooming everywhere, smell their fragrance, and touch cool water in a brook. We have a general and unified experience about the park in the moment. Later, when we recall those experiences we can still have a whole experience about the park.

(3) Change

Change refers to the idea that the contents of consciousness are constantly changing rather than keeping static. As William James said, "within each personal consciousness thought is always changing". Consciousness contents vary continually. The same state of consciousness can never occur twice within an individual. For example, when we watch a pianist playing the piano at the same odium again, we can never have exactly the same feelings or thoughts as the first time we watched it.

(4) Initiative

Initiative refers to the idea that consciousness is an active process. As William James said, "human thought appears deal with objects independent of itself, that is, it is cognitive, or possesses the function of knowing". On the one hand, we can be aware of the interaction between ourselves and our environment, which can facilitate us to take action in order to maintain a balance with the environment, in other words, making us becoming more adaptive to the environment. On the other, consciousness provides a continuous personal experience from the past, the current, and the future, which can promote self-understanding, and controls and plans our actions to meet future needs.

2.1.2 Levels of consciousness

According to Freud, consciousness is divided into three levels of awareness: the conscious, the preconscious, and the unconscious levels.

(1) The conscious level

The conscious level of awareness usually contains cognitions and emotions to which one currently is attending. For example, right now, you probably are aware that you are playing chess, which you can notice is the focus of your awareness. Yet your attention is constantly shifting, and what is in your awareness is always changing. It is known that it is nearly impossible to keep one's attention focused on a single thing for an extended period of time. This is why teachers often repeat important points several times in a class because they realize that many students' attention may change and focus on elsewhere at any one time.

(2) The preconscious level

There are many memories and thoughts that are out of the current awareness of our minds; when we process information, it can be brought to consciousness. This is called the preconscious level. The preconscious level of awareness contains cognitions and emotions to which one is currently not attending, but could easily retrieve when necessary. For example, your memory of what you wore at the birthday party yesterday is probably at the preconscious level. You can easily shift your attention to this memory and recall what you wore. Therefore, attention plays an important role during the shift from the preconscious level to the conscious level. A variety of knowledge, experiences, skills, and habits are stored in our minds. Usually, we are not aware of the existence of such information unless we intentionally recall when in use. For example, at this point you may not be aware of some events during last year's Spring Festival, but you can remember if you want to, and then these memories will become clear in your mind.

(3) The unconscious level

The unconscious is a concept of psychoanalytic theory, which was introduced by Freud. The unconscious level of awareness contains certain memories, impulses, desires, and emotions to which it is very difficult or impossible to bring to the level of consciousness. The phenomenon of having something at the "tip of your tongue" is an example of people processing information at the unconscious level. You may feel as if the word or the event exists somewhere in your mind, but you cannot reach it. Furthermore, according to Freud, although

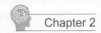

painful or undesired memories have been suppressed in the unconscious mind, they continue to affect people's behavior in an indirect or disguised manner, such as in dreams, irrational behavior, and parapraxis, etc.

In general, we can think of the three levels of awareness as existing on a continuum, with mental content and mental processes currently within awareness at one end of the continuum, and levels of consciousness that could never be brought into awareness at the other end.

2.1.3   Functions of consciousness

Consciousness generally contains two basic functions: monitoring and controlling.

(1) Monitoring

Monitoring refers to that consciousness can make us aware of what is going on in our surroundings, as well as within our own body, through processing the relative information. If our bodies do not provide changed information, we may focus on the things we are interested in with the environment. For example, in certain moment, we may be enjoying a fashion show, or watching the beautiful scenery of the mountains. If we are very hungry, then eating is certainly the first thing that we are aware of rather than other things such as study. Our attention is selective, and the stimuli or events that are important to survival usually have top priority within our consciousness.

(2) Controlling

Controlling refers to the idea that consciousness can guide our actions. We are able to initiate and terminate behavioral and cognitive activities when we are aware of the changes going on in ourselves and our environment. For example, it suddenly begins raining while a group of boys are playing basketball in an open air; consequently they stop playing and come back to the classroom.

Consciousness coordinates our actions with our environment in our daily activities such as making decisions, concentrating on something falling asleep, and so on. Sometimes, decision-making may occur at an unconscious level.

2.1.4   States of consciousness

Consciousness is not static. Subjective experiences constantly move in and out of our awareness as our state of mind and environment change. Psychologists generally divide states of consciousness into two areas: waking consciousness and altered states of consciousness.

(1) Waking consciousness

Most of our lives take place in a waking state of consciousness. Waking consciousness is clear, organized, and the common state of consciousness. In this state, we are aware of time, place and events, which are real, meaningful and familiar to us. For example, we can be aware of our activities and environment: we are having lunch at a dining-room table, and two boys are playing a game in the playground. Usually, there are three types of normal waking consciousness: directed consciousness, flowing consciousness, and daydreaming.

The directed consciousness is orderly and focuses on "one tracked" awareness, centered on a specific stimulus. For example, you are carefully reading an information booklet, or you are learning to sing a folk song, or you are feeling hungry and want to find some food.

The flowing consciousness is a kind of drifting, unfocused awareness. Your awareness or attention randomly moves from one stimulus to another. For example, when you are walking on the beach, you may see a drifting boat, then a swimming boy, and shift to look at a flock of birds. Your awareness randomly shifts from one seascape to another without particular attention.

Daydreaming refers to the state where you involve fantasies without any stimulus. It occurs without any effort. American psychologist Jerome Singer described it in his book "The Inner world of Daydreaming". Daydreaming represents a shift of attention away from some primary physical or mental task we have set for ourselves, or away from directly looking at or listening to something in the external environment, toward an unfolding sequence of private responses made to some internal stimulus. Some psychologists see no positive or practical value in daydreaming. Others suggest that daydreaming allow people to express and deal with desires and emotions free of guilt or anxiety.

(2) Altered states of consciousness

Altered states of consciousness refer to states of mind when mental function is changed or out of the ordinary state. The mental state differs noticeably from normal waking consciousness during altered states of consciousness. Some altered states of consciousness are experienced by everyone such as sleep and dream. Others may occur in special circumstances such as hypnosis, meditation, and drug use. For example, while in a state of hypnosis, an individual may not answer when spoken to, stare straight ahead, and have no facial expression. Others may think the individual is acting confused, odd, or sleepy. Later, the individual may not be able to recall what happened.

2.2   Sleeping and dreaming

We all need to sleep. One's life is about one-third of the time spent sleeping. Sleep is necessary for healthy life and survival, similar to eating, drinking and breathing. Many studies have demonstrated that sleep is essential for survival. Without sleep we could not survive, and it plays a critical role in the sequence of life. Studies found that laboratory rats deprived of all sleep survived only about three weeks while these animals will normally live for several years. Sleep is not unique to humans. All mammals, birds, fish, reptiles, and insects, go through periods of inactivity and unresponsiveness that are remarkably similar to mammalian sleep. Sleep is the way that most animals recharge and rest.

2.2.1   Functions of sleep

If we have not slept for a long time, we will receive signals of decrease in the efficiency and effectiveness from our body, and we will begin to feel sleepy. This suggests that sleep fulfills some very important function, and appears to be necessary. As scientists do not yet know exactly why we sleep, and a number of hypotheses have been proposed to explain the functions of sleep. The main theories include the restoration theory, and the preservation and protection theory.

(1) The restoration theory

The restoration theory emphasizes the restorative functions of sleep. During the day when we are awake, our body and brain are working tirelessly on both our body and the environment, and progressively become tired, even worn out. Sleep is a way of recharging the brain, because the brain has a chance to repair neurons and to exercise important neuronal connections. Animal studies show that sleep can enhance changes in brain connections in early life. Frank and colleagues found that sleep enhances plasticity in the developing visual cortex, and can modify experience-dependent neuronal connections. This finding also suggests that sleep in early life may play a crucial role in brain development. In addition, being awake disrupts homeostasis of the body and sleep is a response to restore an internal balance, including replacing aging or dead cells and repair muscles and other tissues. A study conducted by Gumustekin and colleagues in 2004 shows that sleep deprivation hinders the healing of wounds in rats. Sleep deprivation refers to a general lack of the necessary amount of sleep.

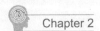

(2) The preservation and protection theory

The preservation and protection theory refers to the idea that sleep is an adaptive response that evolved to preserve energy and to protect us from dangers. During sleep, most of the functions of the body are carried on at the lowest level that is possible in health. Some scientists proposed that sleep could reduce unnecessary activity and energy consumption below the level of rest alone because rest alone is not enough to conserve energy. Other scientists proposed that sleep is an enforcement of rest and sets a limit for activity and energy expenditure. Compatible with findings on sleep deprived rats: deprivation leads to increased metabolism that cannot be compensated by increased food intake. It is easier for some animals to search for food during the day because they do not see well in the dark. Sleep may be the best way for animals to protect themselves when there is little value and considerable danger in the night. Sleeping during the night evolved to be the most efficient way to reduce exposure to danger by lying still and keeping very quiet. In addition, frogs and snakes are not able to go out foraging or migrate, like migratory birds in the winter. So, these animals evolved the ability to hibernate in order to protect them from harm. The preservation and protection theory emphasizes the adaptive function of sleep.

Besides the above-mentioned functions of sleep, many studies suggest that adequate sleep can help people improve memory. By using functional magnetic resonance imaging, Matthew Walker and colleagues studied the activities of different brain regions when the participants were performing certain memory tasks. In this research, they found that certain brain regions were more active in the participants who had slept than those who had not been allowed to sleep. In other words, adequate sleep can better facilitate the participant's performance on the memory task. This study shows that a nights' sleep is beneficial to memory. As Walker and colleagues found, "the brain regions shift dramatically during sleep. When you are asleep, it seems you are shifting memory to more efficient storage regions within the brain. Consequently, when you awaken, memory tasks can be performed both more quickly and accurately and with less stress and anxiety." The exact mechanisms about why sleep can improve memory are not clear. One of the possible explanations is that sleep may provide the brain an opportunity to reorganize data, process newly learned information and organize and archive memories. In addition, in children and young adults, growth hormones are released during deep sleep, which is an important process in development.

2.2.2 Sleep patterns

Most of our physiological and behavioral functions occur on a rhythmic basis. Circadian rhythms are regular changes in mental and physical characteristics that occur in the course of a day. There are patterns of brain wave activity, hormone production, body temperature, and other biological activities linked to the circadian rhythm. When a person falls asleep and wakes up is largely determined by his or her circadian rhythm. Circadian rhythms greatly influence the timing, amount and quality of sleep.

(1) Brain waves and the electroencephalogram

Generally, sleep accounts for nearly one third of our lives. Sleep is a kind of altered state of consciousness. Scientists found that the brain is still active during sleep though our eyes are closed, muscles are relaxed, and we do not respond to sound, light, and other stimuli. The electrical activity of the brain is recorded by using the electroencephalogram (EEG), which is obtained by attaching electrodes to the scalp and then connecting these electrodes to the special devices. The wavy lines of the EEG are what most people know as brain waves.

EEG recordings provide a rough depiction of psychological states. Scientists have recorded various EEG patterns in humans. Normally, an individual has the following EEG patterns: alpha wave, beta wave, theta wave, and delta wave. Alpha wave is the wave with the largest amplitude, regular, between 8 to 12 Hz. It often indicates the states of relaxed wakefulness, and with person's eyes closed. Beta wave refers to the low amplitude, irregular waves, between 13 to 25 Hz. When people are attentive to an external stimulus or are thinking hard about something, the EEG rhythm with alpha wave is replaced by the beta waves. This transformation is known as the EEG arousal and is associated with the act of paying attention to a stimulus. Theta wave is the slow (5 to 8 Hz) and irregular waves; Delta wave is slow (1 to 5 Hz), irregular, and high-amplitude waves. These two types of brain waves usually occur during deep sleep. The EEG can accurately show the brain electrical activity during sleep.

(2) Stages of sleep

The sleep to wakefulness cycle is one that the body does daily, and is also a part of the circadian rhythm. Several brain structures and hormone fluctuations, such as melatonin, regulate our circadian rhythm. Some rhythmic change continues at close to a 24-hour cycle. In the absence of time cues, the cycle period will become somewhat longer than 24 hours.

Analysis of the brain waves of the EEG suggests that human's sleep cycle is very regular pattern during a normal night. There are usually five stages of sleep with different EEG patterns during sleep. A typical sleep cycle (or the duration of the series) is about 1.5 hours long. An individual usually has 4 to 6 sleep cycles occurring in an average night sleep. Sleep ranges from light to deep, and become progressively insensitive to external stimuli.

The records of EEG reveal different patterns of the brain waves. When people are in the state of wakefulness, the EEG presents the following patterns: Awake but non-attentive, EEG presents large, regular alpha waves; when people are in the state of wakefulness and attention, the EEG presents low amplitude, fast, irregular beta waves. Before a person falls asleep, the EEG is typically punctuated by bursts of alpha waves. When an individual falls asleep, the EEG progresses in sequence through initial stage 1 to stage 5. The EEG measures of brain wave activity during sleep reveal different brain-wave patterns of sleep.

Stage 1 is a brief transition stage from semi-wakeful state to light sleep. The stage is sometimes called as "drowsy sleep". It appears at sleep onset, as it is mostly a transition state into Stage 2. People lose some muscle tension and most conscious awareness of the external environment. They are easily aroused by moderate stimuli. The EEG presents alpha waves that are reduced in frequency and amplitude compared to wakefulness. The gaps in alpha rhythm fill with theta and delta waves.

In Stage 2, people's muscular activities decrease, conscious awareness of the external environment disappears, and the brain activities are slow further. The brain waves of the EEG are of higher amplitude and slower than stage 1. The most obvious characteristics in this stage are the occurrence of K complexes and sleep spindles. K complexes are a single large negative wave followed by a single large positive wave. Sleep spindles refer to the bursts of brain waves, and it consists of 12-16 Hz waves that occur for 0.5 to 1.5 seconds. Sleep spindles indicate the onset of the Stage 2 sleep.

Stage 3 is the state of deep sleep, and the brain waves are slowing further. This stage functions primarily as a transition into stage 4. EEG is characterized by much theta waves and the occasional presence of delta waves.

Stage 4 is the deepest form of sleep. In this stage, individuals are only responsive to vigorous stimuli. You must shake a person strongly if you want to awaken him from this stage because brain waves are at their slowest. The EEG pattern is a predominance of delta waves, and accounts for 50% or more of the EEG record during this stage.

From stage 2 to stage 4, sleep progresses deeper and deeper, it is characterized by an increasing percentage of slow, irregular, and high-amplitude delta waves. Usually, stages 3 and 4 together are also called slow-wave sleep. Upon reaching stage 4, sleep begins to become lighter, returns through stages 3 and 2, and stage 5

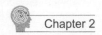

emerges which is also called the rapid eye movement sleep (REM). The REM sleep is also called dream sleep. The brain waves begin to move faster; return to beta wave patterns of alert wakefulness though individuals are still asleep. Muscles are most relaxed, rapid eye movements occur, and dreams occur during this stage.

According to the criteria of sleep stages developed by Rechtschaffen and Kales, the difference between Stages 3 and 4 was that delta waves made up less than 50% of the total wave-patterns in stage 3, while they were more than 50% in stage 4. The newer standard published by the American Academy of Sleep Medicine (2007) eliminated stage 4 sleep and leaves only stage 3 to describe deep sleep, which is known as delta sleep or slow-wave sleep.

In adults, one cycle from stage 1 to REM sleep takes about 90 minutes. In this 90-minute cycle, humans fall into progressively deeper sleep, then, go back through the stages until they enter REM sleep. This cycling repeats several times every night while humans sleep. At the end of stage 4, individuals go back through the stages in reverse, from stage 4 to 3 to 2. When they reach stage 2, instead of waking up, people go into REM sleep (rapid eye movement sleep.) Sleep proceeds in cycles of these stages, the order normally being: stage 1 → stage 2 → stage 3 → stage 4 → stage 3 → stage 2 → REM sleep → stage 1.

(3) Types of sleep

Scientists have observed that there is a considerable amount of eye movement occurring during sleep even though muscles are relaxed, and one is not aware of environmental stimuli. According to the occurrence of eye movement, sleep is also divided into REM sleep and non-rapid eye movement (NREM) sleep.

In 1953, American physiologists Aserinsky and Kleitman reported REM sleep that refers to the observable movements of the eyeball under the eyelid occur during a period of sleep. They found that most people reported vivid dreams when they are awakened during REM sleep. Scientists found that if people are deprived of REM sleep by waking them up during this period, they may get anxious and irritable. Scientists believe that REM sleep is closely related to wakefulness because brain wave activity during REM sleep is dominated by beta waves, which is the pattern similar to brain wave activities of the waking state. REM sleep in the beginning of the night usually last about ten to fifteen minutes, and increases becoming progressively longer, lasting up to 30 minutes in the early hours of the morning. During REM sleep, the sleeper appears to be deeply asleep, and is incapable of moving because of paralysis of body's voluntary muscles. Research suggests that REM sleep has also been thought to be important for memory and learning. REM sleep is more prevalent in infants than adults, and so it may play a role in the development of the brain.

The NREM sleep encompasses four stages from stage 1 to stage 4, which accounts for 75%-80% of total sleep time. NREM sleep alternates with REM sleep during the sleep cycle. Brain wave activity during NREM sleep is marked by high-amplitude, low-frequency waves (delta waves). So the NREM sleep is also called slow-wave sleep. Scientists found that if people are awakened from periods of NREM sleep, they are much less likely to report dreams. The restoration theory of sleep suggests that NREM sleep is important for restoring physiological functions, while REM sleep is essential in restoring mental functions. Studies have shown that the NREM sleep is related to fatigue. If people are deprived of NREM sleep by waking them up during this period of time, they may complain of being physically tired. The more physical exercise an individual does, the more NREM sleep he or she will have.

Human's cycle between REM sleep and NREM sleeping in very regular patterns. Furthermore, sleep patterns change as people age. Newborn babies usually spend about 50% of their sleep time in NREM and 50% in REM sleep, while adults usually spend about 20% of their sleep time in REM and 80% in NREM sleep.

A typical sleep cycle is about 1.5 hours long, and an individual has 4 to 6 sleep cycles occurring every night. The normal sleep required by adults is about 7 to 8 hours per night. The REM sleep lasts longer and longer as the night passes, while NREM sleep becomes shallower as the night goes on. During the first sleep cycle in night, the REM sleep lasts about ten minutes, while in the last sleep cycle individuals may spend about 40 to 60 minutes in REM sleep. (For stages of sleep please see Table 2-1)

Table 2-1 Stages of Sleep

Stage	Behavior	Eye Movement	Type of Brain Wave
Alert wakefulness	Awake, alert, and attention	Eyes open	Beta rhythm
Relaxed wakefulness	Awake, relaxed, not attentive	Eyes closed	Mainly alpha rhythm
NREM sleep			
Stage 1	Drowsy sleep; losing some conscious awareness of the external environment; awaken easily.	The eyes move slowly	Alpha waves reduce in frequency and amplitude; The gaps in alpha rhythm fill with theta and delta waves.
Stage 2	The conscious awareness of the external environment further disappears.	Eye movement stops	The brain waves are of higher amplitude and slower than stage 1; complexes and sleep spindles occur.
Stage 3	Slow-wave sleep; arousal is not easy; bed wetting and sleepwalking often occur in some children.	No eye movement	Much theta waves and the occasional presence of delta waves.
Stage 4	Slow-wave sleep; the deepest forms of sleep.	No eye movement	Predominant delta waves
REM sleep	Deep sleep; heart rate and blood pressure resemble the awake state; limbs are incapable of moving; dreams occurred	Eyes move rapidly under closed lids.	Mostly beta waves; EEG resembles that of an alert awake state.

2.2.3 Dreaming

Dreaming is an interesting phenomenon. It has been seen as a mystery since ancient times, and we all have had the experience of complex and strange dreams.

There are enormous differences among various cultural contexts. In many cultures, dreaming is seen as an important source of information related to the future, and the spiritual world. Dreaming is the most important psychological activity occurring during sleep. When dreaming, the dreamer perceives herself/ himself more as a participant than an observer. The dream environment may be vivid, and without any of limitations of time, place and characters.

Dreaming is actually the perception of sensory images during sleep and mostly occurs during the stage of REM sleep. Although numerous hypotheses have been put forward about the possible functions and the nature of dreams, there is no convincing explanation as to why people experience dreams during sleep. We try to explain why we dream through introducing two influential theories about dreams.

(1) Psychoanalytic perspective

Freud believed that dreams have two levels of contents. One is the manifest content, which reflects the superficial content of the dream itself, and often represents the daily activities and underlying unconscious material. The other is the latent content, which represents the unconscious meanings of the dream, including wishes and desires that are unacceptable by the ethical standards and rules of society. The manifest content results from the latent content, which is disguised by a process called the dream-work. According to Freud, a dream to some extent fulfills the individuals' wishes, and relieves sexual frustration created by repressed desires, allowing them to act on forbidden impulses through disguising their true feelings using symbolic imagery.

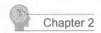

Freud's theory has been popularized through literature and film, and had profound influences on people's life. Till now Freud's terms have been widely used in our everyday life such as slip of the tongue and suppression. Freud developed his theory from the patients with mental abnormality and extended them in general people, which is inevitable to lead to generalization. Some contemporary psychologists have become skeptical about the Freud's dream theory. In particular, the unconscious desire is always interpreted as sexual impulse, which limits the comprehensive understanding of dreams. Moreover, there is no significant evidence to support that dreams can be distinguished by the manifest and latent content. In fact, the contents of dreams have shown regularities across age, gender, and culture, and dreams reflect or express more than they disguise. However, the theory is still widely accepted by Western culture.

(2) Activation-synthesis theory

In 1977, Hobson and McCarley firstly proposed the activation-synthesis hypothesis of dreaming. This theory states that dreams are a random biological process caused by the firing of neurons in the brain, and thus views dreams as the result of random neural activity. According to this theory, when we sleep, all sensory and motor input is blocked and neurons in the cerebral cortex are activated by random neural impulses (activation). Then, the brain tries to reconcile and make sense of this nonsensical activation and by synthesizing the random impulses into what we experience as dreams. There is random firing of neurons in the cerebral cortex during REM sleep. The fore brain then creates a story in an attempt to make sense of the nonsensical sensory information presented to it, resulting in the many types of dreams people have.

Since individuals are relatively insensitive to outside sensory input during sleep, they have to draw on internal information from memory. Several studies suggest that dreams initiate from the information reprocessing in the brain that occurred during the day. For example, we often dream of the previous day's events, which are most likely to come to mind. Studies suggested that the dream images are loaded from memory, and dreaming during REM sleep might have a function in memory processing.

Moreover, the dream process is viewed as a response to a disturbance by some dangers during sleep. For example, the loud noises that might be a warning of dangers in the environment can make a terrible dream for instant awakening. The dreams are also viewed as semi-consciousness, and can facilitate the ability for neural systems to remain partially active in which body could be re-activated instantly.

2.3 Altering consciousness

Have you ever been totally absorbed while reading a book, or watching a movie? This is a state where you are experiencing "losing yourself" in a book or movie. This is actually an altered conscious state where you do not notice what else is going on around you as you focus on a certain point. People with altered states of consciousness usually involve several common characteristics. They may experience distortions in perception, and intense emotions, both positive and negative. Sometimes, altered states are illogical and indescribable. Some states of altered consciousness do not occur naturally, and must be induced in some way. These mainly include hypnotic states, meditative states, and drug-induced states.

2.3.1 Hypnosis

Hypnosis is a trance-like and wakeful state with extreme relaxation and sleepiness, in which the individual responds readily to suggestions. The individual in hypnosis exhibits diminished peripheral awareness, and it is not really like the state of sleep because the individual is alert during the whole period. The history of hypnosis is more than 200 years old, but scientists have not fully explained how it actually happens. Following are some theories proposed to explain hypnosis.

Dissociation theory contends that dissociation of consciousness exists during hypnosis, and some distinct states of consciousness can be present during hypnosis, such that certain actions may become dissociated from the conscious mind. Dissociation of consciousness is the common phenomena in our life. Ernest Hilgard proposed, in his book: Theories of Hypnosis: Current Models and Perspectives, that hypnosis causes participant to divide their consciousness into two parts, which are out of touch with each other. One part responds to the suggestion, and the other part observes but does not participate. In other words, the individual is actually aware of only one line of thought and action at this time, usually concentrating deeply on suggestions, while exclude most of the stimuli around them. For example, hypnosis can make people not react to the undesired signal such as pain as well as change to the desired behavior, because hypnosis separates the part of consciousness that registers pain signal from the part of consciousness that communicates with the outside world.

Social psychological theory maintains that hypnotic behavior is similar to other forms of behavior. Barber and colleagues addressed that the premise of hypnosis that hypnotizable individuals retain control over suggested responses. Hypnotic responses are regarded as goal-directed actions. According to this theory, hypnotized individuals simply behave as they think they are expected to.

Hypnosis and personality (Wang et al, 2011; Zhang et al, 2017)

Hypnosis is also called hypnotherapy. It can be used to create the certain state of mind where the therapist can give suggestions for desired results in order to help the individual. For example, hypnotherapy may be used to reduce stress and anxiety; to decrease the intensity of phobias; to control pain. Hypnosis seems to work best to the individuals with higher suggestibility meanwhile a well-trained therapist. Although hypnosis may have the potential effects to a variety of conditions, it is only typically used as one part of a more comprehensive treatment plan rather than as a stand-alone therapy.

2.3.2　Meditation

Meditation is the practice of focusing attention, and can produce an altered state of consciousness. Meditation can help people to enhance awareness and gain more control of physical and mental processes. Techniques used in meditation usually focus concentration to a single point of reference and away from thoughts and feelings. When the mind is calm and focused in the present, it is neither reacting to the memories from the past nor being preoccupied with the plans for the future. Meditation enables us to keep attention pleasantly on the present moment, and generates a sense of relaxation.

Studies found that meditation has long-term effects on improving physical and mental health, because the practitioners of meditation often present a sense of focus and calm that lasts even after a meditation session has ended. Meditation has been applied to reduce the stress and strain of daily life. By meditating, individuals can acquire a sense of relaxation and learn how to become free of thought, feeling, and emotion. There are a number of ways of practicing meditation. The meditation techniques generally can be grouped into two basic types: concentrative meditation and mindfulness meditation.

Concentrative meditation focuses the attention on the breath, an image, or a sound, in order to ease the mind and acquire a greater awareness and clarity to emerge. This kind of way can help individuals to narrow the focus to a selected field, and help them to control their mind and body. For example, you can try when you focus the attention on the continuous rhythm of inhalation and exhalation; your mind becomes absorbed in the rhythm of the breath. When the mind is calm, your breathing will become slower and deeper, and then, the mind becomes more tranquil and aware. This is the simplest form of concentrative meditation.

Mindfulness meditation refers to an individual simply witnessing whatever goes through the mind, but not becoming involved with these thoughts, memories, worries, or images. This technique can help individuals

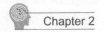

become calmer, and more non-reactive. Compared to the concentrative meditation, which focuses on a selected field, mindfulness meditation helps the individual to become aware of the entire field, is to gain insight as to the true nature of reality.

Meditation is a simple way to improve physical and mental health. More and more doctors are prescribing meditation as an alternative therapy. Meditation can facilitate lowering blood pressure, improve exercise performance in people with angina, promote healing, increase immune system functioning, and bring relief from insomnia and mood fluctuation. However, one should bear in mind that the meditation and related therapeutics including hypnotherapy need stronger evidence-based support. Clinical longitudinal designs aiming to elucidate the long-term effects of these therapies are especially needed.

2.3.3 Altered states with drugs

Psychoactive drugs refer to the chemical substances that can induce an altered state including changes in sensory experience, perception, mood, thinking, and behavior. Psychoactive drugs are usually used for recreational rather than medical purposes, though some have legitimate medical uses. Psychoactive drugs generally include four types: stimulants, depressants, narcotics, and hallucinogens.

Stimulants are drugs that stimulate the central nervous system, which include amphetamines, cocaine, caffeine, and nicotine. Depressants are drugs that slow down the central nervous system, which include sedatives and tranquilizers. Narcotics also called opiates, can relieve pain, which include morphine, heroin, codeine, and demerol. Hallucinogens are drugs that cause sensory and perceptual distortions, which include mescaline and marijuana.

Individuals have variable responses to psychoactive drugs, and many factors can influence how an individual reacts to drugs, including: the amount of the drug, purity of a drug, an individual's expectations to a given drug, an individual's personality and mood, and motivation. In addition, how the drug is administered also influences the user's reactions.

Drug use can be dangerous because heavy or frequent use of drugs can damage body tissues and organs. An overdose of some drugs can be lethal. Especially, when individuals use certain psychoactive drugs, they tend to behave in risky, accident-prone, or unhealthy ways. This is also the most dangerous effect caused by psychoactive drugs.

3. Motivation and emotion

3.1 Motivation

"Why did you do that way? What caused your behavior?" In psychology, the question is "what motivated you to do that?" Motivation is a psychological term that we used to describe and account for why we do things. The term motivation is derived from Latin word "movere", which means, "to move". Motivation is a need or desire that energizes and directs behavior. Arouses, sustains, and directs behavior toward a goal is the physiological and psychological process of motivation.

Motivation is considered a hypothetical state. We cannot directly see or touch people's motivation; we infer it from their observable behavior. The same behavior may be motivated by different reasons, or different behavior may be motivated by the same reasons. For example, some students work hard in order to obtain external rewards such as grades, approval, and some students do so because the study itself gives them a lot pleasure.

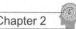

3.1.1 Motivational theories

Motivation has biological, cognitive, and social aspects, and the complexity of the concept has led psychologists to propose a variety of theories. All these theories seek to explain the energy that guides people's behaviors in particular directions.

(1) Instinct theory

An instinct is a complex, innate (unlearned), biological behavior pattern characteristic of a species. William McDougall (1871—1938), one of the early pioneers in social psychology, in his influential book An Introduction to Social Psychology (1908) argued that human beings are motivated by a variety of instincts, including instincts for acquisitiveness, curiosity, pugnacity, gregariousness, and self-assertion. At about the same time, Sigmund Freud (1917) based his theory of personality on unconscious instincts, believing that sex and aggression were especially powerful instincts; and William James claimed that human are motivated by more instincts than any other animal.

In the 1920s, psychologists, influenced by behaviorists John B. Watson, who believed that human behaviors are learned, not innate, rejected instincts as a factor in human motivation.

Instinct theory of motivation presents several difficulties. For one thing, psychologists do not agree on what kind of or how many primary instincts exist. William McDougall suggested that there are eighteen instincts. Some theorists came up with laundry lists of instincts. For example, one sociologist claimed that there are exactly 5759 distinct instincts. Furthermore, the instinct theorists failed to explain the behaviors they labeled as instinct. Think about the following hypothetical dialogue about an alleged "aggressive instinct":

Why does one person have aggression?

Because s/he has an aggressive instinct.

But how do you know he/she has an aggressive instinct?

Because s/he has aggression.

Such circular reasoning neither explains why this person is aggressive towards others nor provides evidence of an aggressive instinct. Each assertion is simply used to support the other. In addiction although it is clear that much animal behavior is based on instincts, because much of the variety and complexity of human behavior is learned, behavior cannot be seen as instinctual.

(2) Drive reduction theory

Following the decline of the instinct theory, the drive reduction theory by Clark Hull (1943) dominated psychology in the 1940s and 1950s. Hull based his theory on the concept of homeostasis — the maintenance of steady internal state. His theory was one of the first systematic attempts to explain motivation and it inspired an enormous amount of research. Drive reduction theory claimed that a lack of some basic biological requirement such as water produces a drive to obtain that requirement.

A drive is an arousal, an internal state that is created by a physiological need. Many basic drives, such as hunger, thirst, sleep, and sex, are related to biological needs of the body or of the species as a whole. These basic drives are called primary drives. But some behaviors fulfills with secondary dives, such as achievement needs.

The goal of drive reduction is the restoration of homeostasis, underlies primary drives. Animal cells and organs will only work optimally when their operating environment is maintained within a certain range. Homeostasis refers to the physiological process by which an organism maintains a fairly steady internal body environment (e.g., body temperature, electrolyte concentration, pH of body fluids, oxygen level, and carbohydrate concentration of tissues). When the body deviates from these optimal levels, automatic reactions restore equilibrium.

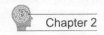

Drives are only reduced when the motivated behaviors are effective in restoring homeostasis and balance, satisfying body's needs. The strength of each drive determines our behavior. We seek to reduce the strongest drive first, then the second strongest and so on.

Drive reduction theory provide a good explanation of how some basic drives motivate behaviors, but the explanation is not complete. A number of social, developmental and psychological factors are involved in all the basic drives, from hunger and thirst, to sleep and sex. Furthermore, the drive reduction ignores higher psychological and social need (e.g., self-esteem and achievement). In addition, drive reduction theory cannot fully explain a behavior in which the goal is not to reduce a drive, but rather to maintain or even increase the level of excitement or arousal. For example, some behaviors seem to be motivated by nothing more than curiosity. Many people pursue thrilling activities such as rapids of a river. In both cases, people appear to be motivated to increase the level of stimulation and activity rather than to reduce the drive.

Modern approaches to human motivation borrow the language of drive reduction theory, but apply it in a more general way. Thus, the term "drive" is used to describe the state of feeling motivated to perform some action. A "need" does not relate to a tissue deficit, but to a feeling that something is missing. Underlying these approaches is the notion that the satisfaction of needs or drives is pleasant, either intrinsically, or because it reduces an unpleasant feeling of need.

(3) Optimum arousal theory

Rather than reduce a physiological need or minimize tension, some motivated behaviors increase arousal. In the 1950s, Hebb and others came up with optimum arousal theory of motivation. According to this theory, each person tries to maintain a certain level of stimulation and activity. In contrast to the drive reduction model, the optimum arousal theory suggests that if our arousal level falls below the optimum, we will try to increase it by seeking novelty or other types of stimulation, and if our stimulation and activity levels become too high, we try to reduce them.

Two psychologists described that optimum arousal might be their formulation, now known as the Yerkes-Dodson law; states that performance is best under conditions of moderate arousal than either low or high arousal (Figure 2-6).

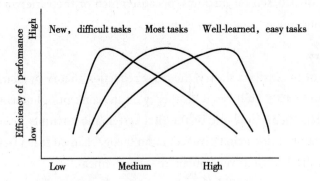

Figure 2-6　Arousal and performance

Moderate arousal often serves us best in tackling life's tasks, but there are times when low or high arousal produces best performance. For well-learned or easy tasks (signing your name, pushing a button on request), optimal arousal may be quite high. In contrast, for new or quite complex tasks (solving an algebraic equation), much lower arousal is preferred. Figure 2-6 shows how arousal might influence easy, moderate, and difficult tasks.

(4) Incentive theory

Not only are we pushed by our need to reduce drives and achieve optimum arousal, we are also pulled by incentives—positive or negative stimuli that lure or repel us.

When a delicious dessert appears on the table after a filling meal, its appeal has little or nothing to do with internal drives or the maintenance of arousal. Rather, if we choose to eat the dessert, such behavior is motivated by the external stimulus of the dessert itself, which acts as an anticipated reward. This reward, in motivational terms, is an incentive. Incentive theory of motivation suggests that motivation stems from the desire to obtain valued external stimuli—whether grades, money, affection, sex, success, approval, or status.

Although the theory explains why we succumb to an incentive (such as a mouthwatering dessert) even though we lack internal cues (such as hunger), it does not provide a comprehensive framework for understanding motivation, because organisms sometimes seek to fulfill the needs even when incentives are not apparent. Consequently, many psychologists believe that the internal drives proposed by drive reduction theory work in tandem with the external incentives to "push" and "pull" behavior, respectively. Whereas a drive is an internal state of tension that "pushes" you toward a goal, an incentive is an external stimulus that "pulls" you toward a goal. Thus, at the same time that we seek to satisfy our underlying hunger needs (the push of drive reduction theory), we are drawn to foods that appear particularly appetizing (the pull of incentive theory). Rather than contradicting each other, drives and incentives may work together in motivating behavior. Incentives often are used by teachers and employers to motivate students and employees.

(5) Cognitive theory

The contemporary view of motivation emphasizes cognitive factor. Cognitive theories of motivation suggest that motivation is a product of people's thoughts, expectation, and goals. For instance, when you are hungry, you do not always eat just to reduce a drive. You make decisions about what and when you will eat. Cognitive theories view individuals as thinking about, planning, and exercising control over their behavior. Cognitive consistency theory, expectancy-value theory, attribution theory, and self-efficiency theory explain the motivation from the cognitive approach.

1) Cognitive consistency theory. According to Leon Festinger (1957), a psychological state known as cognitive dissonance occurs when a person has two inconsistent or incompatible thoughts or cognitions. Because people value consistency in their attitudes and behavior, and cognitive dissonance is an unpleasant or aversive state, they seek to reduce and avoid tension and contradiction. Therefore, the basic premise of cognitive consistency theory is that we are motivated to achieve a psychological state in which our beliefs and behaviors are consistent; we perceive inconsistency between beliefs and behaviors to be unpleasant. Students who think about studying but never get around to it need to achieve consistency between their thoughts and actions. They may achieve consistency by deciding they are too tired to study. You might think of this motive as the need to achieve psychological homeostasis.

2) Expectancy-value theory. Sometimes, people are motivated by the expectation that the probability they could obtain the goals. For instance, the degree to which people are motivated to study for a test is based on their expectations of how well studying will pay off in term of a good grade. Expectancy-value theory developed by Julian Rotter (1954) suggests that the motivation to engage in a given activity is determined by: (a) expectancy (a person's belief that more effort will result in success); (b) instrumentality (person's belief that there is a connection between activity and goal), and (c) valence (the degree to which a person values the results of success). In sum, the equation is: motivation = expectancy x instrumentality x valence.

3) Self-efficiency theory. Self-efficiency also plays a large role in motivation (Bandura, 1997). It refers to a person's self-perceived level of competence and capacity to succeed. Some researchers have showed that self-efficiency is the second most important predictor of a student's academic achievement after ability.

For more details about Cognitive Therapy please see Chapter 3.

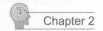

(6) Maslow's hierarchy of needs

For more detailed information, please see chapter 3.

3.1.2 Intrinsic and extrinsic motivations

Intrinsic motivation is the desire to carry out an activity for enjoyment, to show one's ability, or to gain skill. In contrast, extrinsic motivation is the desire to perform an act in order to obtain external rewards such as pay, grades, praise, obligations, and prestige. For example, you might work hard because you find it satisfies your achievement needs (an intrinsic reason) or because you can earn more money (an extrinsic reason). Until the 1970s, most psychologists agreed with B. F. Skinner's commonsense belief that rewards will increase the probability of behavior, but then researcher found that this is not always the case. Some researches with children show that external rewards could undermine the intrinsic motivation. For example, children strongly rewarded for drawing with Magic Markers, later spent less time and showed little interest in drawing, though they were interested in drawing in the first place.

Note that cross-cultural research reveals that the effects of intrinsic motivation might be culturally dependent. A study on the effect of free choice on intrinsic motivation in task performance found that European American students—from more individualistic cultures—showed greater intrinsic motivation after making their own choices than after the choices were made for them by trusted others. In contrast, Asian American students—from more interdependent cultures—showed the opposite tendency, that is, they showed greater intrinsic motivation after the choices were made for them by trusted others than after making their own choices.

In order to avoid taking spontaneous interest and satisfaction out of motivation for others, especially children, you can follow some rules summarized by Greene and Lepper (1974):

(1) if there is no intrinsic interest in an activity to begin with, there is nothing to lose by using extrinsic rewards;

(2) if needed skills are lacking, extrinsic rewards may be necessary to begin;

(3) extrinsic rewards may focus attention on an activity so that real interest can develop—this is especially true for motivating learning in children;

(4) if extrinsic rewards on incentives are to be used, they should be as small as possible, used only when absolutely necessary, and faded out as soon as possible. A good rule of thumb to remember is that the more complex an activity is, the more it is hurt by extrinsic reward.

3.1.3 Motives conflict

Both drive reduction theory and Maslow's hierarchy of needs may make you think that people deal with only one motive at a time. In fact, this is not the way the real world operates. We are frequently confronted by several motives. Psychologists have identified four situations involving multiple motives: approach-approach, avoidance-avoidance, avoidance-approach, and multiple approach- avoidance. In each situation, to satisfy one motive leaves one or more unsatisfied.

(1) Approach-approach conflict

Approach-approach conflict is that you are attracted to two equally desirable goals. Satisfy one motive, however, prevents you from satisfying the second. For example, you are trying to decide whether to spend one-month savings on a TV set or a mobile phone. The desire for each goal is high, but the income will pay for only one; a choice must be made. If either goal can be made a bit more attraction than the other, you will be able to make a choice and resolve the conflict.

(2) Avoidance-avoidance conflict

Avoidance-avoidance conflict refers to a conflict arising from having to choose between two equally unpleasant alternatives. For instance, some children find themselves faced with a choice of doing their homework or going to bed without supper. Avoidance-avoidance conflict is difficult to resolve, and one option must be chosen.

(3) Approach-avoidance conflict

Approach-avoidance conflict means one goal has both good and bad aspects. Suppose a person has some kind of disease, and he will die in three months if he does not have a particular operation, but he only has 30% chance of surviving the operation if he does. It might seem that the avoidance-approach conflict would be easy to resolve -just make a choice and the agony will be over. It sounds simple, but it is often difficult to accomplish. In the above mentioned example, should he have operation or not? How could this dilemma be resolved? In an approach-avoidance situation, only when one motive (attractive or repulsion) becomes stronger than the other will this conflict be resolved.

(4) Multiple approach-avoidance conflict

Multiple approach-avoidance conflict involves a choice among several goals with good and bad features. Suppose you are trying to choose one among a variety of brands of mobile phones, and each brand has good and bad aspects. You are caught in a multiple approach-avoidance situation. Multiple approach-avoidance conflicts are similar to many daily experiences in which we are attracted to and repulsed by a variety of goals. By evaluating the features of the various brands, costs, and dealer reputation, you can resolve the mobile phone problem without much difficulty. When, however, such conflicts occur over interpersonal relationships that may have several positive and negative aspects, such as marriage, they can have serious long-lasting effects.

3.2   Emotion

Emotions add color to our life. Each of us has experienced the strong feelings that accompany very pleasant or very negative experiences. Perhaps it was the joy of being in love, the sorrow over someone's death, or the anguish of inadvertently hurting someone. Everyone has an intuitive sense of what an emotion is, but emotion can be exceedingly difficult to define. Wseten (1996) define emotion as an evaluative response (a positive or negative feeling) that typically includes some combination of physiological arousal, subjective experience, and behavioral or emotional expression.

Before we provide an account that unites arousal, feelings, and actions, we need to make a distinction between emotions and another closely related state, moods. Emotions are distinct from moods in multiple ways. First, emotions typically have a clear cause. They are about something or someone. Moods, on the other hand, are often free-floating and diffuse affective states. The second difference is that emotions are typically brief, lasting only seconds or minutes, but moods endure longer, lasting for hours, even days. A third difference is that emotions typically implicate the multiple aspects described previously, but moods may be salient only at the level of subjective experience. Finally, emotions are often conceptualized as fitting into discrete categories, like joy, fear and anger. Moods, by contrast, are often conceptualized as varying along the dimensions of pleasantness and arousal level. However this last idea is still hotly debated.

3.2.1   Physiology of emotion

(1) Physiological changes of emotion

When we experience certain emotions intensely, such as fear or anger, we may be aware of a number of bodily changes. Many of the physiological changes that take place during emotional arousal result from activation

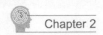

of the sympathetic division of the autonomic nervous system. These physiological changes include: 1) Blood pressure and heart rate increase; 2) Respiration becomes more rapid; 3) The pupils dilate; 4) Perspiration increases while secretion of saliva and mucus decreases; 5) Blood-sugar level increases to provide more energy; 6) The blood clots more quickly in case of wounds; 7) Blood is diverted from the stomach and intestines to the brain and skeletal muscle; 8) The hairs on the skin become erect, causing goose pimples.

All these responses are designed to mobilize your body for action to deal with the source of the emotion. The autonomic nervous system prepares the body for emotional responses through the action of both its sympathetic and parasympathetic divisions. The balance between the divisions depends on the quality and intensity of the arousing stimulation. With quality and intensity of the arousing stimulation, the sympathetic division is more active; with mild, pleasant stimulation, the parasympathetic division is more active. With more intense stimulation of either kind, both divisions are increasingly involved. Physiologically, strong emotions such as fear or anger activate body's emergency reaction system, which swiftly and silently prepares the body for potential danger. The sympathetic nervous system takes charge by directing the release of hormones (epinephrine and norepinephrine) from the adrenal glands, which in turn leads the internal organs to release blood sugar, raise blood pressure, and increase sweating and salivation. As the emotion subsides, the parasympathetic nervous system takes over and returns the body to its normal state.

(2) The neuropsychology of emotion

Derryberry and Tucker (1992) have found that affects are distributed throughout the nervous system and are not located in any particular region. Three areas of the brain, however, are particularly important: the hypothalamus, the limbic system, and the cortex.

Since the 1930s, psychologists have recognized the role of the hypothalamus in emotion. Electrical stimulation of this region can produce attack, defense, or flight reactions, with corresponding emotions of rage or terror. Papez (1937) considered the hypothalamus a crucial component of a circuit involved in the generation of emotion. Papez argued that when the hypothalamus receives emotionally relevant sensory information from the thalamus, it instigates activity in a circuit of neurons higher up in the brain. These neurons, which include the limbic system and the cortex, process the information more deeply to assess its emotional significance. Once the circuit is completed, it feeds back to the hypothalamus, which in turn activates autonomic and endocrine responses. Many aspects of Papez's theory have turned out to be anatomically correct.

Contemporary research places more emphasis on the limbic system. Perhaps the most important limbic structure for emotion is the amygdala. In 1937, Kluver and Bucy discovered that lesioning (destroying) a large temporal region (which later turned out primarily to involve the amygdala) produced a peculiar syndrome in monkeys. The monkeys no longer seemed to understand the emotional significance of objects in their environment, even though they had no trouble recognizing or identifying them. The animals showed no fear of previously feared stimuli and were generally unable to use their emotions to guide behavior. The amygdala plays a crucial role in associating sensory and other information with pleasant and unpleasant feelings. This allows humans and other animals to adjust their behavior based on positive and negative emotional reactions to objects or situations they encounter.

The amygdala is, in many respects, the neuronal hub of emotions because of its connections with both the cortex and the hypothalamus. The emotional reaction to stimulus may pass through two stages, reflecting two somewhat independent processes. One is a quick response based on a cursory reaction to gross stimulus features, involving a circuit running from the thalamus to the amygdala. The second process is slower, based on a more thorough cognitive appraisal, involving a thalamus-to-cortex-to-amygdala circuit. The initial thalamus-to-amygdala process typically occurs faster because it involves fewer synaptic connections. The endocrine and autonomic responses it triggers in turn produce sensations that are processed by the cortex, which must interpret their significance.

The cortex plays several roles with respect to emotions. It allows people to consider the implications of a stimulus for adaptation or wellbeing. It is also involved in interpreting the meaning of peripheral responses, as when a person's experience of shaky knees and a dry throat while speaking in front of a group shows her that she is anxious. In addition, the frontal cortex plays an important part in the social regulation of the face, such as the ability to amplify, minimize, or feign an emotion.

Finally, the right and left hemispheres appear to be specialized, with the right hemisphere dominant in processing emotional cues from others and producing facial displays of emotion. Current research also suggests that pleasant, approach-related emotions are associated with activation of the left frontal cortex, whereas unpleasant, avoidance-related emotions are associated with activation of the right frontal lobe.

3.2.2　Expressing emotion

To describe emotions, we can look at their faces, listen to their voices, and read their bodies. Furthermore, each individual way is capable of carrying a particular message. Emotions occur in the social context of family, friends, and culture. Not only do social stimuli trigger emotions, but also emotions in turn serve social roles in which emotions provide visible cues that help other people know key aspects of our thoughts and desires.

(1) Facial expressions

Facial expressions represent the primary means of communicating emotional states, and so we will examine their role in the experience of emotions. A facial expression results from one or more motions or positions of the muscles of the face. These movements convey the emotional state of the individual to observers. Different facial expressions are associated with different emotions. Terror is marked by eyes that are wide open in a fixed stare or moving to the side away from the dreaded object. The relationship between emotion and facial muscle movements is uniform enough across individuals and cultures that electrodes attached to the face to detect muscle movements allow psychologists to assess directly the valence (positive or negative) and intensity of emotion.

Facial expressions not only indicate a person's emotional state, but they also influence his physiological components. In a classic study, Ekman, and colleagues (1983) gave subjects specific directions to contract their facial muscles in particular ways. For instance, they instructed subjects to raise their eyebrows and pull them together, then raise their upper eyelids, and finally stretch their lips horizontally. The result was an expression of fear, even though the subjects had not been instructed to show a particular emotion. The subjects also showed a rise in heart rate and a decline in body temperature, physiological reactions that were characteristic of fear. This experiment acts as support for a hypothesis called the facial-feedback hypothesis. According to this hypothesis, you feel emotions in part because of the way your muscles in your face are positioned. This means that "wearing" an emotional expression provides muscular feedback to the brain which helps produce an emotion congruent with the expression.

(2) Culture and emotion display rules

Do facial expressions also have different meaning in different cultures? To find out, two investigative teams—one led by Paul Ekman and Wallace Friesen (1975, 1987, 1994), the other by Carroll Izard (1977, 1994) — showed photographs of different expressions to people in different of the world and asked them to guess the emotion. Six facial expressions recognized by people of every culture examined: surprise, fear, anger, disgust, happiness, and sadness. These finding suggest that some emotions are biologically linked not only to distinct autonomic states but also to certain facial movements, which people in all cultures can decode.

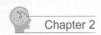

Not all facial expressions, however, are the same from culture to culture. Different cultures have different standards for how emotions should be managed. Some forms of emotional response are unique to each culture. People learn to control the way in which they express emotion, using standards considered appropriate within their culture or subculture, called display rules. Display rules are learned during childhood, and they act to exaggerate, minimize, or mask emotional expressions. According to Ekman (1980), each of us learns a set of display rules for our culture that indicates when, to whom, and how strongly certain emotions can be shown. Display rules are partly a function of habit (individuals do differ in their styles), but they largely reflect "the way things are done" in a particular region, class, or ethnic culture. People are fairly good at using display rules, since we all have a lot of practice. For instance, people who receive an unwanted gift learn to feign a smile, at least in the presence of the gift-giver.

In a study by Ekman (1977) examining cultural differences in display rules, Japanese and North American subjects viewed a film depicting a painful initiation rite. As long as they were unaware that they were being observed, subjects from the two cultures showed the same facial responses. When subjects believed they might be observed, however, their reactions were quite different. The North Americans still showed revulsion, but the Japanese, socialized to show far less emotion, masked their expressions.

Culture affects not only how willing you are to express emotion in specific situations, but also how sensitive you are to the emotional expressions of others. It is almost as if when a culture makes emotions harder to detect, its members develop better abilities to detect them. For example, although China has more restrained display rules than Australia, Chinese children can detect basic emotions more accurately than Australian children can.

(3) Gender and emotional expression

Display rules differ not only by culture but also by gender. Whether men and women actually experience their emotions differently is difficult to ascertain, but consolidating across multiple studies, psychologists have learned that men and women differ more in the expression of emotions—both facially and verbally—than in the subjective experience of emotions. Women probably experience emotions more intensely, are better able to read emotions from other people's face and nonverbal cues, and express emotion more intensely and openly than men. This is true for all emotions except anger, with which males tend to be more comfortable.

When gender differences in reports of subjective experience do emerge, they can often be traced back to differences in gender stereotypes. For instance, Grossman and Wood (1993) found that endorsement of the gender stereotypes was, for women, associated with reporting high-intensity emotions and, for men, associated with reporting low-intensity emotions. This suggests that gender stereotypes color people's reports of their own experiences. Studies by Feldman Barrett (1998) have shown that stereotypes most color reports on emotion when those reports are made at a global level ("How often do you feel sad") or from hindsight ("How anxious were you during last week's interview"). It turns out that gender differences in reported experience vanish when men and women report how they feel in the moment ("How anxious do you feel right now"), presumably because in the moment, people are focused on the specifics of their circumstances and feelings, and less on how those feelings conform to their gender-based beliefs about themselves. These findings suggest that emotions may be a medium through which men and women behave in gender-appropriate ways.

3.2.3　Experiencing emotion

The components of emotion include not only physiological arousal and expressive behavior but also our conscious experience. We can feel angry, afraid, sad, joy and love. The experiences of different emotions include two dimensions-pleasant versus unpleasant, and intensely aroused versus sleepy. For example, anger is unpleasant, but happiness is pleasant; enraged is angrier than angry, delighted is happier than happy.

(1) Types of emotion

Charles Darwin (1872) believed that many emotional behaviors are inborn. He noticed that people of many races and cultures appear to have very similar facial expressions to signal their emotional states. Moreover, blind people show those same expressions, even if they have never had the chance to observe the way others look when they have particular emotional reactions. Darwin believed that all humans are born with a built-in set of emotions, and these emotions would be an essential part of "human nature".

Ekman and Friesen (1971) described the results of experiments that were designed to investigate the possibility of Darwin's thought. They wanted to know whether people who had never seen Caucasian faces could nevertheless identify the emotions underlying their facial expressions. They visited a New Guinea tribe, the Fore, who had rarely if ever seen White people in person, in movies, or on television. Nonetheless, the Fore was able to identify expressions of happiness, anger, sadness, disgust, fear, and surprise. The one difficulty they had was in distinguishing the expression of fear from that of surprise, probably because the two are very similar emotions. Also, it is possible that in the Fore culture the two often go together. Ekman concludes that surprise, happiness, anger, fear, disgust, and sadness are basic emotions, emotions that are innate and shared by all humans.

Other psychologists have also tried to sort through the list of basic emotions, as well as to try to determine how our emotions are related to one another. Robert Plutchik (1984) carried out a comprehensive effort; he believed that emotions are like colors. Every color of the spectrum can be produced by mixing the primary colors. Possibly some emotions are primary, and, if mixed together, they combine to form all other emotions. Plutchik asked people to rate each of a large set of emotions along thirty-four different rating scales. Then, by mathematically combining the ratings, he was able to determine the relationships among the various emotions, as well as which emotions were most fundamental. Eight different fundamental emotions emerged (joy, acceptance, fear, surprise, sadness, disgust, anger, and anticipation). Furthermore, these primary emotions could be consolidated into the two-emotion combinations. For example, combining sadness and surprise gives disappointment. Mixture of primary emotions adjacent to each other combines to produce other emotions. Emotions nearer one another in the circle are more closely related, while those opposite each other are conceptual opposites. For instance, sadness is opposite joy, disgust is opposite acceptance.

Although theorists generate slightly different lists, and the precise number of basic emotions is debated, most classifications include five to nine emotions. All theorists of basic emotions list anger, fear, happiness, sadness, and disgust. Surprise, contempt, interest, shame, guilt, joy, trust, and anticipation sometimes make the roster. There is widespread agreement that humans do have a set of built-in emotions that express the most basic types of reactions.

Perhaps a distinction even more fundamental than differences among the basic emotions is between positive affect (pleasant emotions) and negative affect (unpleasant emotions). Factor analysis of data from several cultures suggests that these two factors underlie people's self-reported emotions. Within these two factors, emotions are substantially correlated. In other words, people who frequently experience one negative emotion, such as guilt, also tend to experience others, such as anxiety and sadness. Positive affect and negative affect are independent dimensions, in that a person can be high along both dimensions at the same time. The distinction between positive and negative affect is congruent with behaviorist research and neuropsychological data establishing the existence of a pleasure-seeking, approach-oriented behavioral system driven by positive affect and an aversive or avoidance-oriented system driven by negative affect.

(2) Functions of emotion

Why do you have emotions? What functions do emotions serve for you? Thinking about these questions,

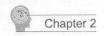

it might help to review your day and imagine how different it would have been if you couldn't experience or understand emotions. Let's examine some of the roles researchers have suggested that emotion plays in your life.

1) Serving as motivation and impacting attention. Emotions serve a motivational function by arousing you to take action with regard to some experienced or imagined event. Emotions then direct and sustain your behaviors toward specific goals. Emotional responses also have an impact on how you focus your attention. We tend to pay more attention to events that fit our current feelings than to events that do not. Consider an experiment by Anderson and Phelps (2001) in which participants were asked to report two words presented in green type among a larger group of words presented in black type. Because of the attentional-blink effect, in which means that when your attention has become focused on one stimulus, you'll have less awareness of another one that comes shortly after, participants typically had some trouble on the second of the two green words: They were able to name the word correctly 61.5 percent of the time. However, when the second word evoked negative emotions, performance rose dramatically to 79.8 percent. That's solid evidence that emotional stimuli command extra attention.

2) Modifying cognitive processes. Emotions serve cognitive functions by influencing what you attend to, the way you perceive yourself and others, and the way you interpret and remember various features of life situations. Bradley and Forgas have demonstrated that emotional states can affect learning, memory, social judgments, and creativity. Your emotional responses play an important role in organizing and categorizing your life experiences. Psychologist Bower proposes that when a person experiences a given emotion in a particular situation, that emotion is stored in memory along with the ongoing events, as part of the same context. Material that is congruent with one's prevailing mood is more likely to be noticed, attended to, and processed more deeply and with greater elaborative associations. Here's an example you might have noticed: People who are in pleasant moods tend to recall more positive events from their lives than do people who are in unpleasant moods.

3) Regulating social interaction. On a social level, emotions serve the broad function of regulating social interaction. The emotions we experience are frequently obvious to observers, as they are communicated through our verbal and nonverbal behaviors. These behaviors can act as a signal to observers, allowing them to better understand what we are experiencing and to predict our future behavior. Imagine what life would be like if you could not understand when people were trying to communicate negative emotions. The emotions you experience have a strong impact on how you function in social settings. Forgas's experiment (1999) found that people in sad moods were more politely on the ways in which they made requests than people in happy or neutral moods. Carlson (1988) also found that when individuals are made to feel good, they are more likely to engage in a variety of helping behaviors.

3.2.4 Theories of emotion

Psychologists have developed a variety of theoretical perspectives to try to explain emotions. Theories of emotion generally attempt to explain the relationship between physiological and psychological aspects of the experience of emotion. Some theorists suggest that specific bodily reactions cause us to experience a particular emotion, such as you are afraid because you feel your heart pounding? In contrast, other theorists suggest that the physiological reaction is the result of the experience of an emotion, for instance, your heart pound because you are afraid.

(1) James-Lange theory

The pioneering psychologist William James (1884) proposed that emotions occur as a result of physiological reactions to events. The Danish physiologist Carl Lange arrived at a similar conclusion at about the same time. Their view can be summarized in James's statement (1890), "We feel sorry because we cry, angry because we strike, afraid because we tremble". James-Lange view of emotion was 180 degrees out of our common sense; common sense tells us that we cry because we are sad, strike because we are angry, tremble because we are afraid.

According to James and Lange, perceiving a stimulus causes autonomic arousal and other bodily actions that lead to the experience of a specific emotion. For example, if you come across someone who begins acting like a mugger, you would first run and then feel afraid, not the other way around. The emotion of fear arises because you sense your bodily state as you are feeling.

In sum, James and Lange proposed that we experience emotions as a result of physiological changes that produce specific sensations. In turn the brain interprets these sensations as particular kinds of emotional experiences. This view that emotions stems from bodily feedback became known as the James-Lange theory. According to the theory, because the perception of autonomic arousal (and perhaps of other bodily changes) constitutes the experience of an emotion, and because different emotions feel different, there must be a distinct pattern of autonomic activity for each emotion. The James-Lange theory therefore holds that autonomic arousal differentiates the emotions (Figure 2-7).

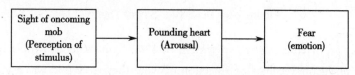

Figure 2-7   James-Lange Theory

(2) Cannon-Bard theory

The James-Lange theory came under severe attack in the 1920s. The attack was led by the physiologist Walter Cannon (1927), who offered three major criticisms: 1) Internal organs are relatively insensitive structures and are not well supplied with nerves, therefore internal changes occur too slowly to be the primary source of emotional feeling; 2) Artificially inducing the bodily changes associated with an emotion—for example, injecting a drug such as epinephrine—does not produce the experience of a true emotion; 3) The bodily changes that occur during varied emotional states are nearly the same, regardless of the emotion felt, for example, anger makes our heart beat faster, but so does the sight of a loved one.

Taking into account the above mentioned critiques, Cannon and Bard suggested an alternative view, in what has come to be known as the Cannon-Bard theory. The theory assumes that both physiological arousal and the emotional experience are produced simultaneously by the same nerve impulse, which Cannon and Bard suggested emanates from the brain's thalamus. According to this theory, after an emotion-inducing stimulus is perceived, the thalamus is the initial site of the emotional response. In turn, the thalamus sends a signal to the autonomic nervous system, thereby producing a visceral response. At the same time, the thalamus communicates a message to the cerebral cortex regarding the nature of the emotion being experienced.

The Cannon-Bard theory focuses on the central mechanism of emotional experience. However, recent research has found that it is the hypothalamus and the limbic system, and not the thalamus, which play a major role in emotional experience (Figure 2-8).

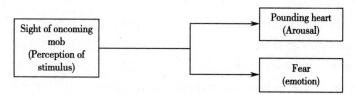

Figure 2-8   Cannon-Bard Theory

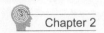

(3) Cognitive perspectives on emotion

Following with the development in the field of cognitive psychology, researchers Schachter and Singer devised a new theory of emotion that took into account the influence of cognitive factors. Schachter and Singer (1962) proposed that the experience of emotion is the joint effect of physiological arousal and cognitive appraisal, with both parts necessary for an emotion to occur. All arousal is assumed to be general and undifferentiated, and arousal is the first step in the emotion sequence. You appraise your physiological arousal in an effort to discover what you are feeling, what emotional label best fits, and what your reaction means in the particular setting in which it is being experienced. This view is known as the Schachter-Singer theory (Figure 2-9).

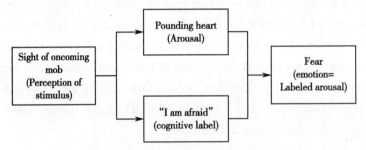

Figure 2-9   Schachter-Singer Theory

Schachter and Singer reported a classic experiment in 1962. The subjects, who believed that they would be taking part in a test of vision, received an injection of what they were told was a vitamin supplement. In reality, they were given epinephrine, a drug that causes an increase in physiological arousal, including higher heart and respiration rates and a reddening of the face. Although one group of subjects was informed of the actual effects of the drug, another was left unaware. Each subject then waited in a room with a "confederate"—that is, someone posing as a participant who in fact cooperates with the investigators in establishing the conditions of the experiment. The experiment consisted of having the confederate act in different ways during the waiting period, and records the effects of his behavior on the participant. In one condition, the confederate acted angry and hostile, complaining that he would refuse to answer the personal questions on a questionnaire that the experimenter had asked him to complete. In the other condition, his behavior was quite the opposite. He behaved euphorically, flying paper airplanes and tossing wads of paper, in general acting in an exuberant manner.

The purpose of the experiment was to determine how the subjects would react emotionally to the confederate's behavior. When they were asked to describe their own emotional state at the end of the experiment, subjects who had been told of the effects of the drugs were relatively unaffected by the behavior of the confederate. They thought their physiological arousal was due to the drug and therefore were not faced with the need to find a reason for their arousal. Hence, they reported experiencing relatively little emotion. On the other hand, subjects who had not been told of the drug's real effects were influenced by the confederate's behavior. Those subjects exposed to the angry confederate reported that they felt angry, while those exposed to the euphoric confederate reported feeling happy. In sum, the results suggest that uninformed subjects turned to the environment and the behavior of others for an explanation of the physiological arousal they were experiencing.

The results of the Schachter-Singer experiment, then, support a cognitive view of emotions, in which emotions are determined jointly by a relatively nonspecific kind of cognitive arousal and the labeling of the arousal based on cues from the environment. Psychologists have had difficulty replicating the Schachter and Singer experiment, but the Schachter-Singer theory lead to some clever experiments in several areas of psychology. In general, research supports the belief that misinterpreted arousal intensifies emotional experiences.

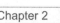

In Schachter and Singer's study, subjects initially became aroused by a shot of epinephrine. In normal life, however, people typically become aroused by their experiences rather than by injection. According to another cognitive psychologist, Richard Lazarus, people's emotions reflect their judgments and appraisals of the situations or stimuli that confront them. Lazarus believes cognitive activity is a precondition for emotion and we cognitively appraise ourselves and our social circumstances. These appraisals, which include values, goals, commitments, beliefs, and expectations, determine our emotions. Lazarus maintains that "emotional experience cannot be understood solely in terms of what happens in the person or in the brain, but grows out of ongoing transactions with the environment that are evaluated" (Lazarus, 1984). This position has become known as the cognitive appraisal theory of emotion.

(4) The opponent-process theory

Richard Solomon (1980) developed a theory of motivation/emotion that views emotions as pairs of opposites, for example, fear-relief or pleasure-pain. The opponent-process theory states that when one emotion is experienced, the other is suppressed. For example, if you are frightened by a wild dog, the emotion of fear is expressed and relief is suppressed. If the fear-causing stimulus continues to be present, after a while the fear decreases and the relief intensifies. For example, if the dog did not move, your fear would decrease and relief that the dog did not attack would increase. If the stimulus is no longer present, then the first emotion disappears and is replaced totally with the second emotion. If the dog turns and runs, you are no longer afraid, but rather feel very relieved.

Solomon and Corbit (1974) analyzed the emotions present when skydivers jump from planes. Beginners experience extreme fear as they jump, which is replaced be great relief when they land. With repeated jumps, the fear decreases and post-jump pleasure increases. This theory attempts to explain a variety of thrill-seeking behaviors. It has also been proposed as a model of drug addiction. The drug originally produces pleasurable feelings, but then a negative emotional experience occurs afterwards. Eventually, the drug user takes drugs not for their pleasurable effects, but to avoid the aversive experience of withdrawal symptoms. The opponent-process theory is an attempt to link emotional states with motivation. Although it is an intriguing idea, some researchers have not found support for the opponent-process theory. Additional research is needed to test the usefulness of the opponent-process theory.

After we have discussed the theoretical perspective of emotion, maybe you want to ask why there are so many theories of emotion and, perhaps even more importantly, which provides the most complete explanation? Actually, we have only scratched the surface. There are almost as many explanatory theories of emotion as there are individual emotions.

Why are theories of emotion so plentiful? The answer is that emotions are such a complex phenomenon that no single theory has been able to fully explain all facets of emotional experience. For each of the four theories there is contradictory evidence of one sort or another, and therefore no theory has proved invariably accurate in its predictions. On the other hand, this abundance of theoretical approaches to emotions simply reflects the fact that psychology is an evolving, developing science. As more evidence is gathered, the specific answer to questions about the nature of emotions will become clear. Furthermore, even as our understanding of emotions continues to grow, there are ongoing efforts to apply our knowledge of emotions to some practical problems.

（周　莉　徐国庆）

Chapter 3

Basic Theories of Psychology and Psychotherapy

Psychology has come a long way since the days of studying bumps on skulls. In the fifth and sixth centuries B.C., the Greeks began to study human behavior and decided that people's lives were dominated not so much by the gods as by their own minds: people were rational. Early philosophers attempted to interpret the world they observed around them in terms of human perceptions—objects were hot or cold, wet or dry, hard or soft—and these qualities influenced people's experience of them. As one psychologist has expressed it, "Modern science began to emerge by combining philosophers' reflections, logic, and mathematics with the observations and inventiveness of practical people" (Hilgard, 1987). The history of psychology is a history of alternative perspectives. As the field of psychology evolved, various schools of thought arose to compete and offer new approaches to the science of behavior. This chapter we will discuss the most important theories of psychotherapy.

1. Historical approaches

The history of psychology is a history of alternative perspectives. As the field of psychology evolved, various schools of thought arose to compete and offer new approaches to the science of behavior.

The first section of this chapter is about four historical approaches. The remaining sections are about contemporary theories, which have strong connections with clinical psychotherapy.

1.1 Structuralism

In 1879 in Leipzig, Germany, Wilhelm Wundt (1832—1920) started his Laboratory of Psychology. Because of his efforts to pursue the study of human behavior in a systematic and scientific manner, Wundt is generally acknowledged for establishing modern psychology as a separate, formal field of study. Although he was trained in physiology—the study of how the body works—Wundt's real interest was in the study of the human mind. Wundt was a structuralist, which means that he was interested in the basic elements of human experiences. In his laboratory, Wundt modeled his research on the mind after research in other natural sciences he had studied. He developed a method of self-observation called introspection to collect information about the mind. In carefully controlled situations, trained participants reported their thoughts, and Wundt tried to map out the basic structure of thought processes. Wundt's experiments were very important historically because he used a systematic procedure to study human behavior. This approach attracted many students who carried on the tradition of systematic research.

1.2 Functionalism

William James (1842—1910) taught the first class in psychology at Harvard University in 1875. James is often called the "father of psychology" in the United States. It took him 12 years to write the first textbook of psychology, "The Principles of Psychology" (1890). James speculated that thinking, feeling, learning, and remembering—all activities of the mind—serve one major function: to help us survive. Rather than focusing on the structure of the mind as Wundt did, James focused on the functions or actions of the conscious mind and the goals or purposes of behaviors. Functionalists studied how animals and people adapt to their environments. Although James was not particularly interested in experimentation, his writings and theories are still influential.

1.3   Inheritable traits

Sir Francis Galton (1822—1911), a nineteenth century English mathematician and scientist, wanted to understand how heredity influences a person's abilities, character, and behavior (Heredity includes all the traits and properties that are passed along biologically from parent to child.). Galton traced the ancestry of various eminent people and found that greatness runs in families. He therefore concluded that genius or eminence is a hereditary trait. This conclusion was like the blind men's ideas about the elephant. Galton did not consider the possibility that the tendency of genius to run in distinguished families might be a result of the exceptional environments and socioeconomic advantages that tend to surround such families. He also raised the question: Would not the world be a better place if we could get rid of the less desirable people? Galton encouraged "good" marriages to supply the world with talented offspring. Later, scientists all over the world recognized the flaws in Galton's theory. A person's heredity and environment interact to influence intelligence.

The data Galton used were based on his study of biographies. Not content to limit his inquiry to indirect accounts, however, he went on to invent procedures for directly testing the abilities and characteristics of a wide range of people. These tests were the primitive ancestors of the modern personality tests and intelligence tests.

Although Galton began his work shortly before psychology emerged as an independent discipline, his theories and techniques quickly became central aspects of the new science. In 1883 he published a book, "Inquiries into Human Faculty", that is regarded as the first study of individual differences. Galton's writings raised the issue of whether behavior is determined by heredity or environment—a subject that remains a focus of controversy today.

1.4   Gestalt psychology

A group of German psychologists, including Max Wertheimer (1880—1943), Wolfgang Köhler (1887—1967), and Kurt Koffka (1886—1941), disagreed with the principles of structuralism and behaviorism. They argued that perception is more than the sum of its parts—it involves a "whole pattern" or, in German, a Gestalt. For example, when people look at a chair, they recognize the chair as a whole rather than noticing its legs, its seat, and its other components. Another example includes the perception of apparent motion. When you see fixed lights flashing in sequence as on traffic lights and neon signs, you perceive motion rather than individual lights flashing on and off. Gestalt psychologists studied how sensations are assembled into perceptual experiences. This approach became the forerunner for cognitive approaches to the study of psychology.

2. Psychoanalysis and psychoanalytic therapy

Sigmund Freud (1856—1939), a physician who practiced in Vienna until 1938, was more interested in the unconscious mind. He believed that our conscious experiences are only the tip of the iceberg, and that beneath the surface are primitive biological urges that are in conflict with the requirements of society and morality.

According to Freud, these unconscious motivations and conflicts are responsible for most human behavior. He thought that they were responsible for many medically unexplainable physical symptoms that troubled his patients.

2.1 Topographical model

Freud believed that the majority of what we experience in our lives, the underlying emotions, beliefs, feelings, and impulses are not available to us at a conscious level. He believed that most of what drives us is buried in our unconsciousness. While buried there, however, they continue to impact us dramatically according to Freud.

The role of the unconscious is only one part of the model. Freud also believed that everything we are aware of is stored in our consciousness. Our consciousness makes up a very small part of who we are. In other words, at any given time, we are only aware of a very small part of what makes up our personality; most of what we are is buried and inaccessible.

The final part is the preconscious or subconscious. This is the part of us that we can access if prompted, but is not in our active consciousness. It is right below the surface, but still buried somewhat unless we search for it. Information such as your telephone number, some childhood memories, or the name of your best childhood friend is stored in the preconscious.

Because the unconscious is so large, and because we are only aware of the very small conscious at any given time, this theory has been likened to an iceberg, where the vast majority is buried beneath water's surface. The water, by the way, would represent everything that we are not aware of, have not experienced, and that has not been integrated into our personalities, referred to as the subconscious.

2.2 Structural model

Freud proposed that the human psyche could be divided into three parts: id, ego and super-ego. Freud discussed this model in the 1920 essay Beyond the Pleasure Principle, and fully elaborated upon it in the ego and the id, in which he developed it as an alternative to his previous topographic schema. The id is the completely unconscious, impulsive, childlike portion of the psyche that operates on the "pleasure principle" and is the source of basic impulses and drives; it seeks immediate pleasure and gratification. The super-ego is the moral component of the psyche, which takes into account no special circumstances in which the morally right thing may not be right for a given situation. The rational ego attempts to exact a balance between the impractical hedonism of the id and the equally impractical moralism of the super-ego; it is the part of the psyche that is usually reflected most directly in a person's actions. When overburdened or threatened by its tasks, it may employ defense mechanisms including denial, repression, undoing, rationalization, and displacement. This concept is usually represented by the "Iceberg Model" (Figure 3-1). This model represents the roles the id, ego, and super ego play in relation to conscious and unconscious thought. Freud compared the relationship between the ego and the id to that between a charioteer and his horses: the horses provide the energy and drive, while the charioteer provides direction.

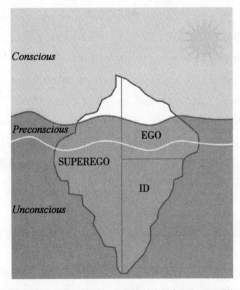

Figure 3-1 An iceberg diagram of topographical model

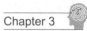

2.3 Psychosexual stages of development

Freud advanced a theory of personality development (for more detailed information of personality please see Chapter 6) that centered on the effects of the sexual pleasure drive on the individual psyche. At particular points in the developmental process, he claimed, a single body part is particularly sensitive to sexual, erotic stimulation. These erogenous zones are the mouth, the anus, and the genital region. Child's libido centers on behavior affecting the primary erogenous zone of his age; he cannot focus on the primary erogenous zone of the next stage without resolving the developmental conflict of the immediate one.

A child at a given stage of development has certain needs and demands, such as the need of the infant to nurse. Frustration occurs when these needs are not met; overindulgence stems from such an ample meeting of these needs that the child is reluctant to progress beyond the stage. Both frustration and overindulgence lock some amount of child's libido permanently into the stage in which they occur; both result in a fixation. If a child progresses normally through the stages, resolving each conflict and moving on, then little libido remains invested in each stage of development. But if he fixates at a particular stage, the method of obtaining satisfaction, which characterized the stage, will dominate and affect his adult personality.

(1) The oral stage. The oral stage begins at birth, when the oral cavity is the primary focus of libidinal energy. The child, of course, preoccupies himself with nursing, with the pleasure of sucking and accepting things into the mouth. The oral character that is frustrated at this stage, whose mother refused to nurse him on demand or who truncated nursing sessions early, is characterized by pessimism, envy, suspicion and sarcasm. The overindulged oral character, whose nursing urges were always and often excessively satisfied, is optimistic, gullible, and is full of admiration for others around him. The stage culminates in the primary conflict of weaning, which both deprives the child of the sensory pleasures of nursing and of the psychological pleasure of being cared for, mothered, and held. The stage lasts approximately one and one-half years.

(2) The anal stage. At one and one-half years, the child enters the anal stage. With the advent of toilet training comes child's obsession with the erogenous zone of the anus and with the retention or expulsion of the feces. This represents a classic conflict between the id, which derives pleasure from expulsion of bodily wastes, and the ego and superego, which represent the practical and societal pressures to control the bodily functions. The child meets the conflict between parent's demands and child's desires and physical capabilities in one of two ways: Either he puts up a fight or he simply refuses to go. The child who wants to fight takes pleasure in excreting maliciously, perhaps just before or just after being placed on the toilet. If the parents are too lenient and the child manages to derive pleasure and success from this expulsion, it will result in the formation of an anal expulsive character. This character is generally messy, disorganized, reckless, careless, and defiant. Conversely, a child may opt to retain feces, thereby spiting his parents while enjoying the pleasurable pressure of the built-up feces on his intestine. If this tactic succeeds and the child is overindulged, he will develop into an anal retentive character. This character is neat, precise, orderly, careful, stingy, withholding, obstinate, meticulous, and passive-aggressive. The resolution of the anal stage, proper toilet training, permanently affects the individual propensities to possession and attitudes towards authority. This stage lasts from one and one-half to two years.

(3) The phallic stage. The phallic stage is the setting for the greatest, most crucial sexual conflict in Freud's model of development. In this stage, child's erogenous zone is the genital region. As the child becomes more interested in his genitals, and in the genitals of others, conflict arises. The conflict, labeled the Oedipus complex (The Electra complex in women), involves child's unconscious desire to possess the opposite-sexed parent and to eliminate the same-sexed one. In the young male, the Oedipus conflict stems from his natural love for his mother, a love that becomes sexual as his libidinal energy transfers from the anal region to his

genitals. Unfortunately for the boy, his father stands in the way of this love. The boy therefore feels aggression and envy towards this rival, his father, and also feels fear that the father will strike back at him. As the boy has noticed that women, his mother in particular, have no penises, he is struck by a great fear that his father will remove his penis, too. The anxiety is aggravated by the threats and discipline he incurs when caught masturbating by his parents. This castration anxiety outstrips his desire for his mother, so he represses the desire. Moreover, although the boy sees that though he cannot possess his mother, because his father does, he can possess her vicariously by identifying with his father and becoming as much like him as possible: this identification indoctrinates the boy into his appropriate sexual role in life. A lasting trace of the Oedipal conflict is the superego, the voice of the father within the boy. By thus resolving his incestuous conundrum, the boy passes into the latency period, a period of libidinal dormancy. Fixation at the phallic stage develops a phallic character, which is reckless, resolute, self-assured, and narcissistic--excessively vain and proud. The failure to resolve the conflict can also cause a person to be afraid or incapable of close love; Freud also postulated that fixation could be a root cause of homosexuality.

(4) Latency period. The resolution of the phallic stage leads to the latency period, which is not a psychosexual stage of development, but a period in which the sexual drive lies dormant. Freud saw latency as a period of unparalleled repression of sexual desires and erogenous impulses. During the latency period, children pour this repressed libidinal energy into asexual pursuits such as school, athletics, and same-sex friendships. But soon puberty strikes, and the genitals once again become a central focus of libidinal energy.

(5) The genital stage. In the genital stage, as child's energy once again focuses on his genitals, interest turns to heterosexual relationships. The less energy the child has left invested in unresolved psychosexual developments, the greater his capacity will be to develop normal relationships with the opposite sex. If, he remains fixated, particularly on the phallic stage, his development will be troubled as he struggles with further repression and defenses.

2.4 Ego-defense mechanisms

In Freud's view, the human is driven towards tension reduction, in order to reduce feelings of anxiety. In Freudian psychoanalytic theory, defense mechanisms are unconscious psychological strategies brought into play by various entities to cope with reality and to maintain self-image. Healthy persons normally use different defenses throughout life. An ego defense mechanism becomes pathological only when its persistent use leads to mal-adaptive behavior such that the physical and mental health or both of the individual is adversely affected. The purpose of ego defense mechanisms is to protect the mind/self/ego from anxiety, social sanctions or to provide a refuge from a situation with which one cannot currently cope.

The following is an explanation of each of the ego defense mechanisms:

(1) Denial. Denial is the act of refusing to acknowledge the presence of the threat or the occurrence of the unpleasant event. Examples of denial would be refusing to acknowledge the death of a person or questioning the qualifications of the doctor who diagnosed the disease. The problem with denial is that it blocks the road to acceptance. You won't be able to get over that event until you first accept it.

(2) Displacement. Displacement is transferring or discharging your emotions on a less threatening object. For example, shouting at your children or having a fight with your neighbor right after your boss shouts at you is an example of displacement. You are angry at your boss but you are shouting at your kids instead. If your displacement ego defense mechanism gets fired, then try to control yourself a bit and then work on identifying your real enemy. Do not attack innocent people just because someone you cannot harm has emotionally hurt you.

(3) Repression. Repression is the complete memory loss of a painful event. In this case, your subconscious

mind does not want you to remember what happened because it may negatively affect your mood.

(4) Projection. Projection is throwing the blame for the unwanted event upon others. For example, saying that you failed an exam because the teacher is a racist.

(5) Rationalization. Rationalization is the act of rationalizing your wrong actions and creating a self-serving explanation for what you did. Saying "I have the right to cheat in the exam because the lessons were not well explained" is a basic example of rationalization.

(6) Suppression. Avoiding thinking about the unwanted event and burying it deep. Suppressed emotions can result in mood swings that come out of nowhere and in severe depression. The book, the ultimate guide to getting over depression explained how ignoring your problems and allowing them to accumulate can be the primary source for depression. Some people face problems as soon as they encounter them while others bury them deeply in their subconscious minds or throw them behind their backs. When they do so their subconscious minds usually responds back with depression.

(7) Sublimation. Sublimation is satisfying your socially unacceptable needs in a socially accepted way. For example, becoming a boxer in order to satisfy your hidden need for violence.

(8) Regression. Regression is returning to a previous state of development. Crying instead of taking actions to solve your problems means you have returned to the stage of childhood.

(9) Identification. By identifying with something or someone else you can increase your sense of self-worth. Saying that a famous singer is a friend of yours can make you feel good about yourself.

(10) Undoing. This means trying to fix your mistake, like sending a SMS to apologize to a friend you've recently had a fight with.

(11) Fantasy. It is pretty much self-explanatory. Imagining yourself beating up your boss with a chair after he shouts at you is a perfect example of fantasizing.

(12) Reaction formation. Taking actions that are the opposite of your real desires, such as greeting one of your enemies warmly just to show that you do not hate him.

(13) Humor. Looking at the funny side of a situation can help you forget about the real problem.

(14) Compensation. Hiding your weaknesses by acting as a beacon of strength; saying something like "I am never scared after watching a horror movie.

(15) Affiliation. Affiliation is to seek the help of another person in getting over your problem.

(16) Dissociation. Dissociating yourself from reality is another famous defense mechanism.

2.5   The life and death instincts

In his later theory Freud argued that humans were driven by two conflicting central desires: the life drive (Eros) (incorporating the sex drive) and the death drive (Thanatos).

Freud's description of Eros, whose energy is known as libido, included all creative, life-producing drives. The death drive (or death instinct), whose energy is known as mortido, represented an urge inherent in all living things to return to a state of calm: in other words, an inorganic or dead state.

He recognized Thanatos only in his later years, developing his theory on the death drive in Beyond the Pleasure Principle. Freud approached the paradox between the life drives and the death drives by defining pleasure and unpleased.

According to Freud, unpleased refers to stimulus that the body receives (for example, excessive friction on the skin's surface produces a burning sensation; or, the bombardment of visual stimuli amidst rush hour traffic produces anxiety.). Conversely, pleasure is a result of a decrease in stimuli (for example, a calm environment the body enters after having been subjected to a hectic environment). If pleasure increases as stimuli decreases, then the ultimate experience of pleasure for Freud would be zero stimulus, or death.

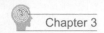

Given this proposition, Freud acknowledges the tendency for the unconscious to repeat unpleasable experiences in order to desensitize, or deaden, the body. This compulsion to repeat pleasurable experiences explains why traumatic nightmares occur in dreams, as nightmares seem to contradict Freud's earlier conception of dreams purely as a site of pleasure, fantasy, and desire.

On the one hand, the life drives promote survival by avoiding extreme unpleased and any threat to life. On the other hand, the death drive functions simultaneously toward extreme pleasure, which leads to death. Freud addresses the conceptual dualities of pleasure and unpleased, as well as sex/life and death, in his discussions on masochism and sadomasochism. The tension between Eros and Thanatos represents a revolution in his manner of thinking.

2.6　Psychoanalytic therapy

Psychoanalytic therapy is one of the most well-known treatment modalities, but it is also one of the most misunderstood by mental health consumers. This type of therapy is based upon the theories and work of Sigmund Freud.

Freud's theories and research methods were controversial during his life and still are so today, but few dispute his huge impact on the development of psychotherapy. Most importantly, Freud popularized the "talking-cure"—an idea that a person could solve problems simply by talking over them. Even though many psychotherapists today tend to reject the specifics of Freud's theories, this basic mode of treatment comes largely from his work.

Most of Freud's specific theories—like his stages of psychosexual development—and especially his methodology have fallen out of favor in modern cognitive and experimental psychology. Figure 3-2 depicts the couch used in Freud's apartment, for the psychoanalytic therapy.

Some psychotherapists, however, still follow an approximately Freudian system of treatment. Many more have modified his approach, or joined one of the schools that branched from his original theories, such as the Neo-Freudians. Still others reject his theories entirely, although their practice may still reflect his influence.

Psychoanalytic therapy looks at how the unconscious mind influences thoughts and behaviors. Psychoanalysis frequently involves looking at early childhood experiences in order to discover how these events might have shaped the individual and how they contribute to current actions. People undergoing psychoanalytic therapy often meet with their therapist at least once a week and may remain in therapy for a number of weeks, months or even years.

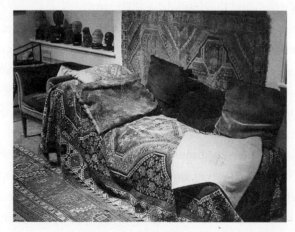

Figure 3-2　Couch in Freud's apartment used for psychoanalytic therapy

2.6.1   Free association

Freud used a new method for indirectly studying unconscious processes. In this technique, known as free association, a patient said everything that came to mind—no matter how absurd or irrelevant it seemed—without attempting to produce logical or meaningful statements. The person was instructed not to edit or censor the thoughts. Freud's role, that of psychoanalyst, was to be objective; he merely sat and listened and then interpreted the associations. Free association, Freud believed, revealed the operation of unconscious processes.

Free association is a technique used in psychoanalytic therapy to help patients learn more about what they are thinking and feeling. Freud used free association to help his patients discover unconscious thoughts and feelings that had been repressed or ignored. When his patients became aware of these unconscious thoughts or feelings, they were better able to manage them or change problematic behaviors.

The goal of free association is not primarily to uncover hidden memories but to identify genuine thoughts and feelings about life situations that might be problematic, yet not be self-evident. For example, a woman might tell herself and others that she loves the people she works with but ends up avoiding her colleagues most of the time. Free association would be a helpful technique to explore the conflict or tension between these two competing attitudes.

Free association is typically performed in a therapy setting by first having the patient get into a relaxed position (sitting or lying down). It can be done with the eyes open or closed; although, most people find closing their eyes helpful to avoid surrounding distractions. The person then begins to talk, saying the first things that come to mind. There is no effort made to tell a linear story or shape the ideas that come to mind. The person spontaneously says his or her first thoughts without any concern for how painful, silly or illogical it might sound to the therapist.

The therapist is listening to the patient free association and trying to identify what, if any, thoughts or feelings might be repressed. Bringing these repressed feelings or thoughts to the surface might help the patient better understand the conflict they are experiencing. For example, the woman who "loves" her colleagues but rarely engages with them may say things when free associating that she would never consciously admit to herself. She may say things such as, "I have anxiety about my performance," "I encounter unrealistic expectation at the workplace" or "I feel different from others." The therapist takes note of these potentially repressed feelings and discusses them with the patient once the free association exercise is completed.

The previously unconscious thoughts and feelings become conscious as they are discussed. This new awareness can be used to make deliberate changes in behavior. For example, once the woman is aware that she is feeling anxious about her performance, she could approach her boss and ask for feedback. This not only provides a reality check for her performance, which could lower her anxiety, but also increases her relational contact with colleagues, which was part of the original tension she was feeling.

2.6.2   Dream interpretation

Freud also believed that dreams are expressions of the most primitive unconscious urges. To learn more about these urges, he used dream analysis—basically an extension of free association—in which he applied the same technique to a patient's dreams. While working out his ideas, Freud took careful, extensive notes on all his patients and treatment sessions. He used these records, or case studies, to develop and illustrate a comprehensive theory of personality.

Dream analysis, in psychoanalysis, provides the possibility to decipher the mystery of neurotic disorders, specifically hysteria, and secondly, it opens the road towards the unconscious. Freud's phrase: "The interpretation of dreams is the royal road to a knowledge of the unconscious" has become famous.

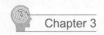

The first great dream interpreted by Freud that leads him to his great discoveries was materialized in 1895. It is the famous dream of Irma's injection, which Freud almost thoroughly analyzed and published in his grandiose work The Interpretation of Dreams. Dream was approached in a manner, which was to become specific for the practitioners of psychoanalysis: by means of the dreamer's associations.

Dream analysis reveals Freud's feelings of guilt towards Irma, one of his young patients, whose treatment had not yielded the expected results. Freud defends himself from these negative feelings in his dream, blaming his very patient who, apparently, was not a submissive and compliant patient, or Dr. Otto, one of his colleagues, guilty of a careless medical intervention.

After analyzing his dream, most coherent as it proved, Freud justly declared that dreams are not meaningless, they are not absurd; they do not imply that one portion of our store of ideas is asleep while another portion is beginning to wake. On the contrary, they are psychical phenomena of complete validity-fulfillments of wishes. Dreams therefore require integration into the range of intelligible waking mental acts; "they are constructed by a highly complicated activity of the mind".

This assertion in fact expresses a great opening towards the activity of abysmal psyche, and mostly the belief in psychic determinism, in the idea that all psychic deeds have their own meaning and connect to day activities, even in a somewhat less visible manner. Contrary to the general opinion of his time's scientific world, Freud thinks dreams are a coherent psychic activity that can be analyzed in depth.

This definition emphasizes two key aspects of the theory of dreams: Dreams are a disguised fulfillment of a wish, and this is a repressed wish. We can therefore conclude that disguise is caused by repression. That is the reason why all dream researchers before Freud were not able to discover these facts: they only analyzed the manifest content of the dream, that is its outer shape at wakening time, its facade, not caring about latent thoughts giving rise to its becoming, thoughts we reach by means of the method of associations devised by Freud.

Freud went even further to analyze the nature of distortion by the dream, partially the work of dream-censorship and partly of dream-work, a complex process by means of which latent thoughts are turned into dreams as such. Freud's analysis includes dream-work, and the end of his book also provides us with his opinions concerning the psychology of the dream process: primary and secondary processes, repression, unconsciousness, etc.

Freud listed the distorting operations that he claimed were applied to repressed wishes in forming the dream as recollected: it is because of these distortions (the so-called "dream-work") that the manifest content of the dream differs so greatly from the latent dream thought reached through analysis—and it is by reversing these distortions that the latent content is approached.

The operations included:

(1) Condensation one dream object stands for several associations and ideas; thus "dreams are brief, meagre and laconic in comparison with the range and wealth of the dream-thoughts."

(2) Displacement a dream object's emotional significance is separated from its real object or content and attached to an entirely different one that does not raise the censor's suspicions.

(3) Visualization a thought is translated to visual images.

(4) Symbolism a symbol replaces an action, person, or idea.

That is why the interpretation of dreams represents the major work on dreams and unconscious life, not equaled so far. It remains an essential stage in the study of psychoanalysis. In spite of the importance of dream-analysis for the discovery of abysmal psyche functioning as well as for therapy as such, this crucial field of psychoanalysis has no more concerned psychoanalysts after Freud's research.

In many areas of psychology today, Freud's view of unconscious motivation remains a powerful and

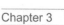

controversial influence. Modern psychologists may support, alter, or attempt to disprove it, but most have a strong opinion about it. The technique of free association is still used by psychoanalysts, and the method of intensive case study is still a major tool for investigating behavior.

2.7   Evaluation

Psychoanalytic perspective is an orientation toward understanding behavior based on unconscious motivation concerned with the basic instincts, sex and aggression. Freud's theory has had enormous influence, as well as considerable criticism, both now and during his era.

The school of psychoanalysis is the first systematic theory that describes the development of behavior from causes to results. It has made a significant impact on both psychology and cultures. Freudian terms such as, "slip of the tongue," and "repression," are popular in our everyday language. Freud's ideas changed how we think about the human mind and behavior. Many of the theories of personality developed by psychoanalytic thinkers are still influential today, including Freud's theory of psychosexual stage and Erikson's theory of psychosocial stages. His work and writings contributed to our understanding of personality, clinical psychology, human development, and abnormal psychology.

There are some weaknesses in this perspective. Both Freud and psychoanalysis have been criticized in very extreme terms. Exchanges between critics and defenders of psychoanalysis have often been so heated that they have come to be characterized as the Freud Wars.

Many of the concepts proposed by psychoanalytic theorists are difficult to measure and quantify. Many of Freud's observations and theories were based on case studies that make his findings difficult to generalize to a larger population. Freud overemphasized that behavior is shaped by unconscious impulses such as desires or instincts, and the studied sample was primarily abnormal. It is limited when extending these results to explain and understand behaviors in a certain culture and class. Although there are many criticisms of Freud's theory, there is no question that he had an enormous impact on the field of psychology. His work had a profound influence on a number of disciplines, including sociology, anthropology, literature, and art.

And in treatment, costs are often cited as the biggest downside of psychoanalytic therapy. Many patients are in therapy for years, so the financial and time costs associated with this treatment modality can be potentially very high.

3. Behaviorism and behavior therapy

The pioneering work of Russian physiologist Ivan Pavlov (1849—1936) charted another new course for psychological investigation. Behaviorism, also known as behavioral psychology, is a theory of learning based on the idea that all behaviors are acquired through conditioning. Psychologists who stressed investigating observable behavior became known as behaviorists. Their position, as formulated by psychologist John B. Watson (1878—1958), was that psychology should concern itself only with the observable facts of behavior. Watson further maintained that all behavior, even apparently instinctive behavior, is the result of conditioning and occurs because the appropriate stimulus is present in the environment.

3.1   Classical conditioning

In a famous experiment, Pavlov rang a tuning fork each time he gave a dog some meat powder. The dog would normally salivate when the powder reached its mouth. After Pavlov repeated the procedure several times, the dog would salivate when it heard the ring of the tuning fork, even if no food appeared. It had been conditioned to associate the sound with the food.

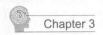

The conditioned reflex was a response (salivation) provoked by a stimulus (the tuning fork) other than the one that first produced it (food). The concept was used by psychologists as a new tool, as a means of exploring the development of behavior. Using this tool, they could begin to account for behavior as the product of prior experience. This enabled them to explain how certain acts and certain differences among individuals were the result of learning.

Classical conditioning is a technique frequently used in behavioral training in which a neutral stimulus is paired with a naturally occurring stimulus. Eventually, the neutral stimulus comes to evoke the same response as the naturally occurring stimulus, even without the naturally occurring stimulus presenting itself. The associated stimulus is now known as the conditioned stimulus and the learned behavior is known as the conditioned response.

Ivan Pavlov showed that classical conditioning applied to animals. Did it also apply to humans? In a famous (though ethically dubious) experiment, Watson and Rayner (1920) showed that it did.

Little Albert was a 9-month-old infant who was tested on his reactions to various stimuli. He was shown a white rat, a rabbit, a monkey and various masks. Albert described as "on the whole stolid and unemotional" showed no fear of any of these stimuli. However, what did startle him and cause him to be afraid was if a hammer was struck against a steel bar behind his head. The sudden loud noise would cause little Albert to burst into tears. When Little Albert was just over 11 months old the white rat was presented and seconds later the hammer was struck against the steel bar. This was done 7 times over the next 7 weeks and each time Little Albert burst into tears. By now little Albert only had to see the rat and he immediately showed every sign of fear. He would cry (whether or not the hammer was hit against the steel bar) and he would attempt to crawl away. In addition, the Watson and Rayner found that Albert developed phobias of objects that shared characteristics with the rat; including the family dog, a fur coat, some cotton wool and a Father Christmas mask. This process is known as generalization.

Watson and Rayner had shown that classical conditioning could be used to create a phobia. A phobia is an irrational fear that is out of proportion to the danger. Over the next few weeks and months Little Albert was observed and 10 days after conditioning his fear of the rat was much less marked. This dying out of a learned response is called extinction. However, even after a full month it was still evident, and the association could be renewed by repeating the original procedure a few times.

3.2   Operant conditioning

Operant conditioning (sometimes referred to as instrumental conditioning) is a method of learning that occurs through reinforcements and punishments. Through operant conditioning, an association is made between a behavior and a consequence for that behavior. When a desirable result follows an action, the behavior becomes more likely to occur again in the future. Responses followed by adverse outcomes, on the other hand, become less likely to happen again in the future.

Most behavior of humans cannot easily be described in terms of individual responses reinforced one by one, and B. F. Skinner devoted a great deal of effort to the problem of behavioral complexity, which now called Skinner box (Figure 3-3). Some complex behavior can be seen as a sequence of relatively simple responses, and here Skinner invoked the idea of "chaining." Chaining is based on the fact, experimentally demonstrated, that a discriminative stimulus not only sets the occasion for subsequent behavior, but it can also reinforce a behavior that precedes it. That is, a discriminative stimulus is also a "conditioned reinforcer." For example, the light that sets

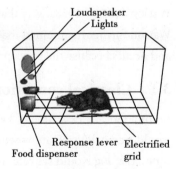

Figure 3-3   Skinner box

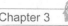

the occasion for lever pressing may also be used to reinforce "turning around" in the presence of a noise. This results in the sequence "noise-turn-around-light-press lever-food." Much longer chains can be built by adding more stimuli and responses.

Skinner created the operant chamber as a variation of the puzzle box originally created by Edward Thorndike.

The structure forming the shell of a chamber is a box large enough to easily accommodate the animal being used as a subject. (Commonly used model animals include rodents—usually lab rats—pigeons, and primates). It is often sound-proof and light-proof to avoid distracting stimuli.

Operant chambers have at least one operandum (or "manipulandum"), and often two or more, that can automatically detect the occurrence of a behavioral response or action. Typical operanda for primates and rats are response levers; if the subject presses the lever, the opposite end moves and closes a switch that is monitored by a computer or other programmed device. Typical operanda for pigeons and other birds are response keys with a switch that closes if the bird pecks at the key with sufficient force. The other minimal requirement of a conditioning chamber is that it has a means of delivering a primary reinforcer (a reward, such as food, etc.) or unconditioned stimulus like food (usually pellets) or water. It can also register the delivery of a conditioned reinforcer, such as an LED signal as a "token".

Despite such a simple configuration, one operandum and one feeder, it is possible to investigate many psychological phenomena. Modern operant conditioning chambers typically have many operanda, like many response levers, two or more feeders, and a variety of devices capable of generating many stimuli, including lights, sounds, music, figures, and drawings. Some configurations use an LCD panel for the computer generation of a variety of visual stimuli.

Some operant chambers can also have electrified nets or floors so that shocks can be given to the animals; or lights of different colors that give information about when the food is available. Although the use of shock is not unheard of, approval may be needed in countries that regulate experimentation on animals.

However, Skinner recognized that a great deal of behavior, especially human behavior, cannot be accounted for by gradual shaping or the construction of response sequences. Complex behavior often appears suddenly in its final form, as when a person first finds his way to the elevator by following instructions given at the front desk. To account for such behavior, Skinner introduced the concept of rule-governed behavior. First, relatively simple behaviors come under the control of verbal stimuli: the child learns to "jump", "open the book", and so on. After a large number of responses come under such verbal control, a sequence of verbal stimuli can evoke an almost unlimited variety of complex responses.

Skinner identified 3 types of responses or operant that can follow behavior:

(1) Neutral operants. Responses from the environment that neither increase nor decrease the probability of a behavior being repeated.

(2) Reinforcers. Responses from the environment that increase the probability of a behavior being repeated. Reinforcers can be either positive or negative.

(3) Punishers. Responses from the environment that decrease the likelihood of a behavior being repeated. Punishment weakens behavior.

3.2.1   Reinforcement

Reinforcement is a basic term in operant conditioning. The term operant conditioning was introduced by B. F. Skinner to indicate that in his experimental paradigm the organism is free to operate on the environment. Reinforcement is a consequence that will strengthen an organism's future behavior whenever that behavior is preceded by a specific antecedent stimulus. In this paradigm the experimenter cannot trigger the desirable response; the experimenter waits for the response to occur (to be emitted by the organism) and then a

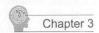

potential reinforcer is delivered. In the classical conditioning paradigm the experimenter triggers (elicits) the desirable response by presenting a reflex eliciting stimulus, the Unconditional Stimulus (UCS), which he pairs (precedes) with a neutral stimulus, the Conditional Stimulus (CS).

(1) Positive reinforcement. It occurs when a desirable event or stimulus is presented as a consequence of a behavior and the behavior increases. A positive reinforcer is a stimulus event for which the animal will work in order to acquire it. Whenever a rat presses a button, it gets a treat. For example, if the rat starts pressing the button more often, the treat serves to positively reinforce this behavior.

(2) Negative reinforcement. Negative reinforcement occurs when the rate of a behavior increases because an aversive event or stimulus is removed or prevented from happening. A negative reinforce is a stimulus event for which an organism will work in order to terminate, to escape from, to postpone its occurrence. For example: A child cleans his or her room, and this behavior is followed by the parent stopping "nagging" or asking the child repeatedly to do so. Here, the nagging serves to negatively reinforce the behavior of cleaning because the child wants to remove that aversive stimulus of nagging.

3.2.2　Punishment

Punishment is not a mirror effect of reinforcement. In experiments with laboratory animals and studies with children, punishment decreases the likelihood of a previously reinforced response only temporarily, and it can produce other "emotional" behavior and physiological changes (increased heart rate, for example) that have no clear equivalents in reinforcement.

(1) Positive punishment. Positive punishment occurs when a response produces a stimulus and that response decreases in probability in the future in similar circumstances. Example: a mother yells at a child when he or she runs into the street. If the child stops running into the street, the yelling ceases. The yelling acts as positive punishment because the mother presents an unpleasant stimulus in the form of yelling.

(2) Negative punishment. Negative punishment occurs when a response produces the removal of a stimulus and that response decreases in probability in the future in similar circumstances. Example: a teenager comes home after curfew and the parents take away a privilege, such as cell phone usage. If the frequency of the child coming home late decreases, the privilege is gradually restored. The removal of the phone is negative punishment because the parents are taking away a pleasant stimulus and motivating the child to return home earlier.

3.3　Social learning theory

In social learning theory Albert Bandura agrees with the behaviorist learning theories of classical conditioning and operant conditioning. However, he adds two important ideas: (1) Mediating processes occur between stimuli and responses. (2) Behavior is learned from the environment through the process of observational learning.

3.3.1　Observational learning

Children observe the people around them behaving in various ways. This is illustrated during the famous Bobo doll experiment (Figure 3-4).

The participants in this experiment were 36 boys and 36 girls from the Stanford University nursery school, all between the ages of 37 months and 69 months with a mean age of 52 months. The children were organized into 4 groups and a control group. The 4 groups exposed to the aggressive model and non-aggressive model belonged to the experimental group. 24 children were exposed to an aggressive model and 24 children were exposed to a non-aggressive model. The two groups were then divided into males and females, which ensured that half children were exposed to models of their own sex and the other half were exposed to models of the opposite sex. The remaining 24 children were part of a control group.

For the experiment, each child was exposed to the scenario individually, so as not to be influenced or distracted by classmates. The first part of the experiment involved bringing a child and the adult model into a playroom. In the playroom, the child was seated in one corner filled with highly appealing activities such as stickers and stamps. The adult model was seated in another corner containing a toy set, a mallet, and an inflatable Bobo doll. Before leaving the room, the experimenter explained to the child that the toys in the adult corner were only for the adult to play with.

During the aggressive model scenario, the adult would begin by playing with the toys for approximately one minute. After this time the adult would start to show aggression towards the Bobo doll. Examples of this included hitting/punching the Bobo doll and using the toy mallet to hit the Bobo doll in the face. The aggressive model would also verbally assault the Bobo doll yelling "Sock him," "Hit him down," "Kick him," "Throw him in the air," or "Pow". After a period of about 10 minutes, the experimenter came back into the room, dismissed the adult model, and took the child into another playroom. The non-aggressive adult model simply played with the other toys for the entire 10-minute period. In this situation, the Bobo doll was completely ignored by the model, and then the child was taken out of the room.

The next stage of the experiment, took place with the child and experimenter in another room filled with interesting toys such as trucks, dolls, and a spinning top. The child was invited to play with them. After about 2 minutes the experimenter decides that the child is no longer allowed to play with the toys, explaining that she is reserving those toys for the other children. This was done to build up frustration in the child. The experimenter said that the child could instead play with the toys in the experimental room (this included both aggressive and non-aggressive toys). In the experimental room the child was allowed to play for the duration of 20 minutes while the experimenter evaluated child's play.

The first measure recorded was based on physical aggression such as punching, kicking, and sitting on the Bobo doll, hitting it with a mallet, and tossing it around the room. Verbal aggression was the second measure recorded. The judges counted each time the children imitated the aggressive adult model and recorded their

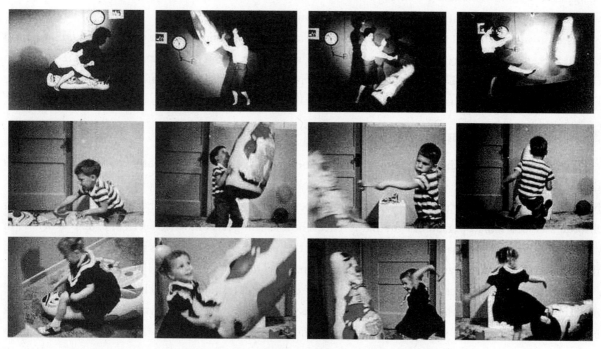

Figure 3-4   Bandura's observational learning experiment

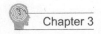

results. The third measure was the number of times the mallet was used to display other forms of aggression than hitting the doll. The final measure included modes of aggression shown by the child that were not direct imitation of the role-model's behavior.

Bandura found that the children exposed to the aggressive model were more likely to act in physically aggressive ways than those who were not exposed to the aggressive model. The results concerning gender differences strongly supported Bandura's prediction that children are more influenced by same-sex models. Results also showed that boys exhibited more aggression when exposed to aggressive male models than boys exposed to aggressive female models.

3.3.2 Mediational processes

Bandura believes that humans are active information processors and think about the relationship between their behavior and its consequences. Observational learning could not occur unless cognitive processes were at work. These mental factors mediate in the learning process to determine whether a new response is acquired.

There are four mediational processes proposed by Bandura:

(1) Attention. The extent to which we are exposed/notice the behavior. For a behavior to be imitated it has to grab our attention. We observe many behaviors on a daily basis and many of these are not noteworthy. Attention is therefore extremely important in whether a behavior has an influence in others imitating it.

(2) Retention. How well the behavior is remembered. The behavior may be noticed, but it is not always remembered which obviously prevents imitation. It is important therefore that a memory of the behavior is formed so that the observer can perform it later. Much of social learning is not immediate so this process is especially vital in those cases. Even if the behavior is reproduced shortly after seeing it, memory should be there to perform it.

(3) Reproduction. This is the ability to perform the behavior that the model has just demonstrated. We see much behavior on a daily basis that we would like to be able to imitate but that this not always possible. We are limited by our physical ability and for that reason, even if we wish to reproduce the behavior, we cannot. This influences our decisions whether to try and imitate it or not. Imagine the scenario of a 90-year-old-lady who struggles to walk after watching Dancing on Ice. She may appreciate that the skill is a desirable one, but she will not attempt to imitate it because she physically cannot do it.

(4) Motivation. The will to perform the behavior. The rewards and punishment that follow a behavior will be considered by the observer. If the perceived rewards outweigh the perceived costs (if there are any) then the behavior will be more likely to be imitated by the observer. If the vicarious reinforcement is not seen to be important enough to the observer, then they will not imitate the behavior.

3.4 Behavior therapy

The behavioral approach to therapy assumes that behavior that is associated with psychological problems develops through the same processes of learning that affects the development of other behaviors. Therefore, behaviorists see personality problems in the way that personality was developed. They do not look at behavior disorders as something a person has but that it reflects how learning has influenced certain people to behave in a certain way in certain situations. Understanding how the process of learning takes place comes from research that has been done on operant and classical conditioning.

Behavior therapy is based upon the principles of classical conditioning developed by Ivan Pavlov and operant conditioning developed by B.F. Skinner. Classical conditioning happens when a neutral stimulus comes right before another stimulus that triggers a reflexive response. The idea is that if the neutral stimulus or any other stimulus that triggers a response is paired together often enough, the neutral stimulus will produce the reflexive response. Operant conditioning has to do with rewards and punishments and how they can either strengthen or weaken certain behaviors. There has been a good deal of confusion on how these two conditionings differ and whether the various techniques of behavior therapy have any common scientific base.

Contingency management programs are a direct product of research from operant conditioning. These programs have been highly successful with those suffering from panic disorders, anxiety disorders, and phobias.

Systematic desensitization and exposure and response prevention both evolved from respondent conditioning and have also received considerable research.

Behavior avoidance test (BAT) is a behavioral procedure in which the therapist measures how long the patient can tolerate an anxiety-inducing stimulus. The BAT falls under the exposure-based methods of behavior therapy.

Exposure-based methods of behavioral therapy are well suited to the treatment of phobias, which include intense and unreasonable fears (of spiders, blood, and public speaking). The therapist needs some type of behavioral assessment to record the continuing progress of a patient undergoing an exposure-based treatment for phobia.

The simplest possible assessment approach for this is the BAT. The BAT approach is predicted on the reasonable assumption that patient's fear is the main determinant of behavior in the testing situation. BAT can be conducted virtually, or physically, depending on the patients' maladaptive behavior. Its application is not limited to phobias; it is applied to various disorders such as post-traumatic stress disorder and obsessive-compulsive disorder.

However, behavioral therapy is an umbrella term for types of therapy that treat mental health disorders. This form of therapy seeks to identify and help change potentially self-destructive or unhealthy behaviors. It functions on the idea that all behaviors are learned and that unhealthy behaviors can be changed. The focus of treatment is often on current problems and how to change them.

There are a number of different types of behavioral therapy:

(1) Cognitive-behavioral therapy. Cognitive-behavioral therapy is extremely popular. It combines behavioral therapy with cognitive therapy. Treatment is centered on how someone's thoughts and beliefs influence their actions and moods. It often focuses on a person's current problems and how to solve them. The long-term goal is to change a person's thinking and behavioral patterns to healthier ones.

(2) Cognitive-behavioral play therapy. Cognitive-behavioral play therapy is commonly used with children. By watching children play, therapists are able to gain insight into what a child is uncomfortable expressing or unable to express. Children may be able to choose their own toys and play freely. They might be asked to draw a picture or use toys to create scenes in a sandbox. Therapists may teach parents how to use play to improve communication with their children.

(3) System desensitization. System desensitization relies heavily on classical conditioning. It is often used to treat phobias. People are taught to replace a fear response to a phobia with relaxation responses. A person is first taught relaxation and breathing techniques. Once mastered, the therapist will slowly expose them to their fear in heightened doses while they practice these techniques.

(4) Aversion therapy. Aversion therapy is often used to treat problems such as substance abuse and alcoholism. It works by teaching people to associate a stimulus that's desirable but unhealthy with an extremely unpleasant stimulus. The unpleasant stimulus may be something that causes discomfort. For example, a therapist may teach you to associate alcohol with an unpleasant memory.

(5) Flooding. Flooding (also known as implosion therapy) works by exposing the patient directly to

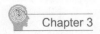

their worst fears. For example a claustrophobic will be locked in a closet for 4 hours or an individual with a fear of flying will be sent up in a light aircraft. What flooding aims to do is expose the sufferer to the phobic object or situation for an extended period of time in a safe and controlled environment. Unlike systematic desensitization that might use in vitro or virtual exposure, flooding generally involves vivo exposure.

3.5　Evaluation

Behavioral perspective is an orientation toward understanding observable behavior in terms of conditioning and reinforcement. Behavioral principles have many effective practical applications especially in mental health settings, where therapists and counselors use these techniques to explain and treat a variety of illnesses. The behavioral perspective is becoming the dominant framework for experimental research because it is very objective, and with high levels of reliability. Both classical conditioning and operant conditioning have never been shown to be wrong, but they have been shown to be incomplete.

The behavioral perspective ignores mental processes such as thoughts and feelings, and discounts the qualitative difference between humans and animals on research. Nonetheless, the behavioral perspective has grown in popularity for some fifty years, and is still influential today.

In treatment, Behavior therapy sometimes is seen not humanistic. For example flooding is rarely used and if you are not careful it can be dangerous. It is not an appropriate treatment for every phobia. It should be used with caution as some people can actually increase their fear after therapy, and it is not possible to predict when this will occur.

4. Cognitivism and cognitive therapy

Cognitivism is the psychology of learning that emphasizes human cognition or intelligence as a special endowment enabling man to form hypotheses and develop intellectually. Cognitivism is also known as cognitive development. The underlying concepts of cognitivism involve how we think and gain knowledge. Cognitivism involves examining learning, memory, problem solving skills, and intelligence. Cognitive theorists may want to understand how problem solving changes throughout childhood, how cultural differences affect the way we view our own academic achievements, language development, and much more. Cognitive Psychology specializes in extensive articles that have a major impact on cognitive theory and provide new theoretical advances. The cognitive perspective developed largely as a reaction to the behavioral perspective. Both cognitive perspective and behavioral perspective are interested in what happens in the mind between the stimulus and the response. Cognitive psychologists argue that individuals' thoughts and beliefs about how the world works determine their behaviors and emotions, while behaviorists hold that individuals passively respond to stimuli. The cognitive perspective believes that individuals actively process information in their brain before responding to the information.

4.1　Information processing theory

Information processing theory describes how information is received, processed, stored and then retrieved in the human brain. It is interesting to note that this theory compares processing of information by humans to those by computers. The information processing theory is an approach to the cognitive development of a human being, which deals with the study and the analysis of the sequence of events that occur in a person's mind while receiving some new piece of information.

George Miller compared the information processing in humans to that in a computer model. He also said that learning is simply a change in the knowledge that has been stored by the memory. In short, it is the analysis of the way a human being learns something new. There is a fixed pattern of events that take place in such a situation, and by knowing this pattern we can enable children and adults with special abilities to learn new things faster.

This theory claims that the human mind is very similar to that of computers, as far as information processing and analysis are concerned. It also states that any new piece of information that enters the brain is first analyzed and then put through the test of several benchmarks before being stored in some vestibules of the memory. Since these actions occur at a very fast speed, we are unable to notice them in action. The sensory perceptors of a human being function in the same way as the hardware of a computer does, and the mindset and the rules and strategies adopted by the person while learning, are equivalent to the software used by computers. The information processing system of a person can thus be enhanced if these perceptors and rules are altered.

4.2 Schema

In psychology and cognitive science, a schema describes a pattern of thought or behavior that organizes categories of information and the relationships among them. It can also be described as a mental structure of preconceived ideas, a framework representing some aspect of the world, or a system of organizing and perceiving new information (Figure 3-5).

Schemata influence attention and the absorption of new knowledge: People are more likely to notice things that fit into their schema, while re-interpreting contradictions to the schema as exceptions or distorting them to fit. Schemata have a tendency to remain unchanged, even in the face of contradictory information. Schemata can help in understanding the world and the rapidly changing environment. People can organize new perceptions into schemata quickly as most situations do not require complex thought when using schema, since automatic thought is all that is required.

People use schemata to organize current knowledge and provide a framework for future understanding. Examples of schemata include academic rubrics, social schemas, stereotypes, social roles, scripts, worldviews, and archetypes. In Paget's theory of development, children construct a series of schemata, based on the interactions they experience, to help them understand the world.

For example, a young child may first develop a schema for a horse. She knows that a horse is large, has hair, four legs, and a tail. When the little girl encounters a cow for the first time, she might initially call it a horse. After all, it fits in with her schema for the characteristics of a horse; it is a large animal that has hair, four legs, and a tail. Once she is told that this is a different animal called a cow, she will modify her existing schema for a horse and create a new schema for a cow.

Now, let's imagine that this girl encounters a miniature horse for the first time and mistakenly identifies it as a dog. Her parents explain to her that the animal is actually a very small type of horse, so the little girl must at this time modify her existing schema for horses. She now realizes that while some horses are very large animals, others can be very small. Through her new experiences, her existing schemas are modified and new information is learned.

The processes through which schemas are adjusted or changed are known as assimilation and accommodation. In assimilation, new information is incorporated into pre-existing schemas. In accommodation, existing schemas might be altered or new schemas might be formed as a person learns new information and has new experiences.

While the use of schemas to learn in most situations occurs automatically or with little effort, sometimes an existing schema can hinder the learning of new information. Prejudice is one example of schema that prevents people from seeing the world as it is and inhibits them from taking in new information. By holding

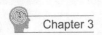

certain beliefs about a particular group of people, this existing schema may cause people to interpret situations incorrectly. When an event happens that challenges these existing beliefs, people may come up with alternative explanations that uphold and support their existing schema instead of adapting or changing their beliefs.

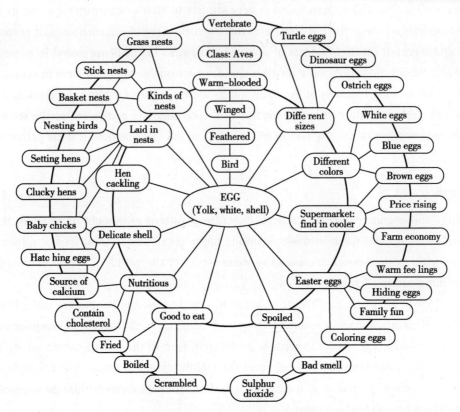

Figure 3-5 A schema of "egg"

4.3 Cognitive-behavioral theory and therapy

Cognitive-behavioral theories are best conceptualized as a general category of theories, or a set of related theories, which have evolved from the theoretical writings, clinical experiences, and empirical studies of behavioral and cognitively oriented psychologists. There is no single definition of cognitive-behavioral theory. The individual theories are tied together by common assumptions, techniques and research strategies, but maintain a diversity of views about the role cognitions play in behavior change. The hyphenated term "cognitive-behavioral" reflects the importance of both behavioral and cognitive approaches to understanding and helping human beings. Cognitive-behavioral theories and counseling interventions are currently highly influential. There are many different cognitive-behavioral intervention techniques and the number is likely to grow as the theories continue to be developed and tested for effectiveness with a variety of psychological problems.

4.3.1 Beck's cognitive therapy

Cognitive therapy (CT) is a type of psychotherapy developed by American psychiatrist Aaron T. Beck. CT is one of the therapeutic approaches within the larger group of cognitive-behavioral therapies (CBT) and was first expounded by Beck in the 1960s. Cognitive therapy seeks to help the patient overcome difficulties by identifying and changing dysfunctional thinking, behavior, and emotional responses. This involves helping patients develop skills for modifying beliefs, identifying distorted thinking, relating to others in different ways, and changing behaviors. Treatment is based on collaboration between patient and therapist and on testing beliefs. Therapy may consist of testing the assumptions which one makes and identifying how certain of one's usually unquestioned thoughts are distorted, unrealistic and unhelpful. Once those thoughts have been challenged, one's feelings about the subject matter of those thoughts are more easily subject to change. Beck initially focused on depression and developed a list of "errors" in thinking that he proposed could maintain depression, including arbitrary inference, selective abstraction, over-generalization, and magnification (of negatives) and minimization (of positives).

An example of how CT works is this: having made a mistake at work, a man may believe, "I am useless and cannot do anything right at work." Strongly believing this then tends to worsen his mood. The problem may be worsened further if the individual reacts by avoiding activities and then behaviorally confirming the negative belief to himself. As a result, any adaptive response and further constructive consequences become unlikely, which reinforces the original belief of being "useless." In therapy, this example could be identified as a self-fulfilling prophecy or "problem cycle," and the efforts of the therapist and patient would be directed at working together to change it. This is done by addressing the way the patient thinks and behaves in response to similar situations and by developing more flexible ways to think and respond, including reducing the avoidance of activities and the practicing of positive activities (Mood repair strategies). If, as a result, the patient escapes the negative thought patterns and dysfunctional behaviors, the negative feelings may be relieved over time.

4.3.2   Cognitive-behavioral therapy

Cognitive-behavioral Therapy (CBT) is a psychotherapy that integrates the approaches of behavior therapy and cognitive therapy. It is based on modifying everyday thoughts and behaviors, with the aim of positively influencing emotions. The general approach developed out of behavior modification and cognitive therapy, and has become widely used to treat mental disorders. The particular therapeutic techniques vary according to the particular kind of patient or issue, but commonly include keeping a diary of significant events and associated feelings, thoughts and behaviors; questioning and testing assumptions or habits of thoughts that might be unhelpful and unrealistic; gradually facing activities which may have been avoided; and trying out new ways of behaving and reacting. Relaxation and distraction techniques are also commonly included. CBT is widely accepted as an evidence-based, cost-effective psychotherapy for many disorders. It is sometimes used with groups of people as well as individuals, and the techniques are also commonly adapted for self-help manuals and, increasingly, for self-help software packages.

4.3.3   Rational emotive behavior therapy

Rational emotive behavior therapy (REBT), previously called rational therapy and rational emotive therapy, is a comprehensive, active-directive, philosophically and empirically based psychotherapy which focuses on resolving emotional and behavioral problems and disturbances and enabling people to lead happier and more fulfilling lives. REBT was created and developed by the American psychotherapist and psychologist Albert Ellis who was inspired by many of the teachings of Asian, Greek, Roman and modern philosophers. REBT is one of the first and foremost forms of cognitive behavior therapy and was first expounded by Ellis in the mid-1950s and continues its development to this day.

In REBT the ABC model is used for systematically analyzing a patient's problems into its cognitive components:

A. The activating event.

B. The mediating evaluative beliefs.

C. The emotional and behavioral consequences.

This is sometimes extended to ABCDE by the addition of

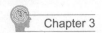

D. Disputing.

E. The effect of practicing rational thinking.

A, adversity (or activating event) that contributes to disturbed and dysfunctional emotional and behavioral Cs, consequences, but also what people B, believe about the A, adversity. A, adversity can be either an external situation or a thought or other kind of internal event, and it can refer to an event in the past, present, or future.

The Bs, beliefs that are the most important in the A-B-C model are explicit and implicit philosophical meanings and assumptions about events, personal desires, and preferences. The Bs, beliefs that are most significant are highly evaluative and consist of interrelated and integrated cognitive, emotional and behavioral aspects and dimensions.

According to REBT, if a person's evaluative B, belief about the A, activating event is rigid, absolutistic and dysfunctional, the C, the emotional and behavioral consequence, is likely to be self-defeating and destructive. Alternatively, if a person's evaluative B, belief is preferential, flexible and constructive, the C, the emotional and behavioral consequence is likely to be self-helping and constructive.

Through REBT, by understanding the role of their mediating, evaluative and philosophically based illogical, unrealistic and self-defeating meanings, interpretations and assumptions in upset, people often can learn to identify them, begin to D, dispute, refute, challenge and question them, distinguish them from unhealthy constructs, and subscribe to more constructive and self-helping constructs.

4.4   Evaluation

The cognitive perspective emphasizes that cognitive processes can actively organize information we receive, and the cognitive experiences are key points to understand individuals' behaviors. Cognitive psychologists study mental processes by using rigorous scientific methods. It makes it possible to understand mental processes and behaviors more scientifically. However, it is overly simplistic that the working model of the human mind is seen as an analog of the computer model. This ignores the complexity of the human mind. Today, psychologists often prefer to combine cognitive perspective with other perspectives, such as neuroscience and the behavioral approach, to strengthen its explanations. Cognitive psychology is used in many different ways, such as suggestions on how to improve memories, improving performance in situations that require concentration, such as air traffic controllers and so on.

In general, there are many different ways to think about human thoughts and behaviors. Each perspective has strengths and weaknesses in both its theoretical assumptions and clinical applications. There is not any perspective that can adequately explain all of psychological phenomena in various cultural contexts or classes. For example, behaviorists claim that human behavior is largely shaped by environmental stimuli while psychoanalysts argue that behavior is shaped by unconscious impulses beyond individual's control. Both of these perspectives have a powerful explanation to behavior in certain conditions, but they are sometimes not adequate to explain certain mental processes.

5. Humanism and humanistic therapy

Humanistic psychology is a psychological perspective that rose to prominence in the mid-20th century in answer to the limitations of Sigmund Freud's psychoanalytic theory and B. F. Skinner's behaviorism. With its roots running from Socrates through the Renaissance, this approach emphasizes individual's inherent drive towards self-actualization, the process of realizing and expressing one's own capabilities and creativity.

It helps the patient gain the belief that all people are inherently good. It adopts a holistic approach to human existence and pays special attention to such phenomena as creativity, free will, and positive human potential. It encourages viewing ourselves as a "whole person" greater than the sum of our parts and encourages self-exploration rather than the study of behavior in other people. Humanistic psychology acknowledges spiritual aspiration as an integral part of the human psyche. It is linked to the emerging field of trans-personal psychology.

In the 20th century, humanistic psychology was referred to as the "third force" in psychology, distinct from earlier, even less humanistic approaches of psychoanalysis and behaviorism. In our postindustrial society, humanistic psychology has become more significant; for example, neither psychoanalysis nor behaviorism could have birthed emotional intelligence.

5.1　Maslow's hierarchy of deeds

When your need for water go unsatisfied and your thirst will preoccupy you. But if you were deprived of air, your thirst would disappear. This example illustrate that some needs take priority over others. The particular needs that motivate our behavior depend on which needs are not met.

Abraham Maslow (1970) proposed on such hierarchy of needs (Figure 3-6). Maslow was a humanist psychologist who believed humans are driven to achieve their maximum potential. He did not discount the biological aspects of motivation but proposed that there were basic needs, psychological needs and self-fulfillment needs. Maslow suggested that before more sophisticated, higher-order needs can be met, certain primary needs must be satisfied. The original version of hierarchy of needs model comprised five needs, which remains for most people the definitive hierarchy of needs. In fact, 1970's adapted version included cognitive and aesthetic needs, and 1990's version added transcendence needs. Altogether, the hierarchy of needs consist of physiological, safety, belongingness and love, esteem, cognitive, aesthetic, self-actualization, and transcendence needs. A pyramid can represent the hierarchy of needs model, with the more basic needs at the bottom and the higher-order needs at the top (Figure 3-6).

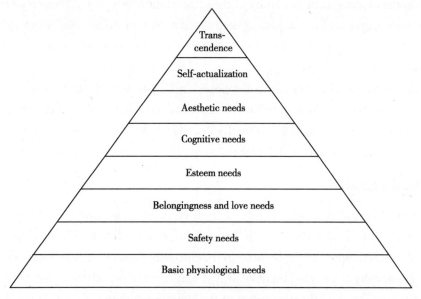

Figure 3-6　Maslow's hierarchy of needs

Physiological needs consist of needs for oxygen, food, water, warmth, rest, sex, and so on. To move up the hierarchy, a person must first meet these basic physiological needs. Physiological needs are the strongest needs because if a person were deprived of all needs, the physiological ones would come first in person's search for satisfaction.

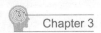

Safety needs are the needs for order, predictability, shelter, physical security, freedom from fear, etc. Adults have little awareness of their safety needs except in times of emergency or periods of disorganization in the social structure (such as widespread rioting). Children often display the signs of insecurity and the need to be safe. According to Maslow, physiological and safety needs compose the low-order needs.

Belongingness and love needs include the need to obtain and give affection such as, affiliation with friends, a supportive family, an intimate relationship, and the need for group or social identification.

Esteem needs involve needs for esteem, such as prestige, feelings of accomplishment, and social acceptance. Esteem needs involve needs for both self-esteem and for the esteem a person gets from others. Maslow stated that esteem relates to the need to develop a sense of self-worth by knowing that others know and value one's competence.

Cognitive needs are the expression of the natural human needs to learn, explore, discover and create to get a better understanding of the world around them. Once the first four classes of needs are fulfilled, cognitive needs can become dominant. Maslow believed that humans have the need to increase their intelligence and thereby chase knowledge.

Aesthetic needs means humans need to refresh themselves in the presence and beauty of nature while carefully absorbing and observing their surroundings to extract the beauty that the world has to offer.

Self-actualization is a state of self-fulfillment in which people realize their highest potentials, each in his or her own unique way. Although Maslow first suggested that only a few famous individuals, such as Thomas Jefferson and Abraham Lincoln, achieved self-actualization, he later expanded the concept to encompass everyday people. For example, a teacher who creates an environment that maximizes students' opportunities for success may be self-actualized.

Transcendence is at the top of the pyramid, also sometimes referred to as spiritual need. It may lead some individuals to higher states of consciousness and a cosmic vision of one's part in the universe.

Maslow's hierarchy of needs integrates virtually the other theoretical approaches to motivation. Though some researches on the theory—such as a study of the satisfaction of needs in 88 countries from 1960—1994 (Hagerty, 1999)—have supported his sequence of need achievement, we do not always replace a higher priority on lower-level needs. For example, many prisoners in Nazi concentration camps gave their food, clothing, and even their lives for others.

Note that Maslow's hierarchy of needs was developed in U.S. an individualist culture, and was reflective of a mainly male-oriented view of human behavior. In general, cross-cultural studies indicate similar human needs, but the sequence of needs might be culturally dependent. Maslow's theory can be modified to better reflect people's attitudes and values from different cultures.

5.2 Self-actualization

"Self-actualization" represents a concept derived from Humanistic psychological theory and, specifically, from the theory created by Abraham Maslow. Self-actualization, according to Maslow, represents the growth of an individual toward fulfillment of the highest needs, especially those for meanings in life. Carl Rogers also created a theory implicating a "growth potential" whose aim was to integrate congruently the "real self" and the "ideal self" thereby cultivating the emergence of the "fully functioning person". It was Maslow, however, who created a psychological hierarchy of needs, the fulfillment of which theoretically leads to a culmination of fulfillment of "being values", or the needs that are on the highest level of this hierarchy, representing meaning.

Instead of focusing on psychopathology and what goes wrong with people, Maslow (1943) formulated a more positive account of human behavior, which focused on what goes right. He was interested in human potential, and how we fulfill that potential. Maslow (1943, 1954) stated that human motivation is based on people seeking fulfillment and change through personal growth. Self-actualized people are those who were fulfilled and doing all they were capable of. The growth of self-actualization refers to the need for personal growth and discovery that is present throughout a person's life. For Maslow, a person is always "becoming" and never remains static in these terms. In self-actualization a person comes to find a meaning to life that is important to them.

As each individual is unique the motivation for self-actualization leads people in different directions. For some people self-actualization can be achieved through creating works of art or literature, for others through sport, in the classroom, or within a corporate setting.

Maslow (1962) believed self-actualization could be measured through the concept of peak experiences. This occurs when a person experiences the world totally for what it is, and there are feelings of euphoria, joy and wonder.

By studying 18 people he considered to be self-actualized (including Abraham Lincoln and Albert Einstein) Maslow (1970) identified 15 characteristics of a self-actualized person. Characteristics of self-actualizers include:

(1) They perceive reality efficiently and can tolerate uncertainty;

(2) Accept themselves and others for what they are;

(3) Spontaneous in thought and action;

(4) Problem-centered (not self-centered);

(5) Unusual sense of humor;

(6) Able to look at life objectively;

(7) Highly creative;

(8) Resistant to enculturation, but not purposely unconventional;

(9) Concerned for the welfare of humanity;

(10) Capable of deep appreciation of basic life-experience;

(11) Establish deep satisfying interpersonal relationships with a few people;

(12) Peak experiences;

(13) Need for privacy;

(14) Democratic attitudes;

(15) Strong moral/ethical standards.

Behaviors leading to self-actualization include:

(1) Experiencing life like a child, with full absorption and concentration;

(2) Trying new things instead of sticking to safe paths;

(3) Listening to your own feelings in evaluating experiences instead of the voice of tradition, authority or the majority;

(4) Avoiding pretense ("game playing") and being honest;

(5) Being prepared to be unpopular if your views do not coincide with those of the majority;

(6) Taking responsibility and working hard;

(7) Trying to identify your defenses and having the courage to give them up.

Erikson created a theory of psychosocial dichotomies represented as "trust versus mistrust" and "autonomy versus shame and doubt", as examples. In terms of Erikson's final stage of development, that of "ego integrity versus despair", the successful resolution of this stage corresponds with a sense of life's meaning. It is clear that the self-actualized person might be in danger of dying, but nevertheless may find meaning in life. This means that lower level needs might be unfulfilled even in situations represented by "being values", such as a sense of meaning in life. Note, however, that Maslow asserted that one's needs may be only partially fulfilled at any given moment.

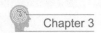

5.3　Positive psychology

Several humanistic psychologists—such as Abraham Maslow, Carl Rogers, and Erich Fromm—developed theories and practices pertaining to human happiness and flourishing. More recently, positive psychologists have found empirical support for the humanistic theories of flourishing. In addition, positive psychology has moved ahead in a variety of new directions.

In 1998 Martin Seligman, president of American Psychological Association, suggested that psychology turn toward understanding and building human strengths to complement the traditional emphasis on healing damage. Psychology had neglected the positive side of life, having spent much of the last half century primarily concerned with psychopathology. As a result, psychologists and psychiatrists can now measure with considerable precision, and effectively treat, a number of major mental illnesses. However, this progress came at a cost. Relieving life's miseries made building the states that make life worth living less of a priority.

Positive psychology is the branch of psychology that uses scientific understanding and effective intervention to aid in the achievement of a positive outlook when it comes to subjective experiences, individual traits, and events that occur throughout one's lifetime. The goal of positive psychology is to step away from the pathological thoughts that may arise in a hopeless mindset, and to instead, maintain a sense of optimism that allows for people to understand what makes life worth living.

Positive psychology is concerned with three issues: positive emotions, positive individual traits, and positive institutions.

Positive emotions are concerned with being content with one's past, being happy in the present and having hope for the future. Positive individual traits focus on one's strengths and virtues. Finally, positive institutions are based on strengths to better a community of people.

Positive psychology can have a range of real-world applications in areas including education, therapy, self-help, stress management, and workplace issues. Using strategies from positive psychology, teachers, coaches, therapists, and employers can motivate others and help individuals understand and develop their personal strengths.

5.4　Carl Rogers and person-centered therapy

Person-centered therapy (PCT) is also known as person-centered psychotherapy, person-centered counseling, patient-centered therapy and rogerian psychotherapy. PCT is a form of psychotherapy developed by psychologist Carl Rogers in the 1940s and 1950s. The goal of PCT is to provide patients with an opportunity to realize how their attitudes and behavior are being affected.

Although this technique has been criticized by behaviorists for lacking structure and by psychoanalysts for actually providing a conditional relationship, it has proven to be an effective and popular treatment.

Primarily, this type of therapy encourages a self-awareness and mindfulness that helps the patient change their state of mind and behavior from one set of reactions to a healthier one with more productive self-awareness and thoughtful actions. Essentially, this approach allows the merging of mindfulness and behavioral therapy, with positive social support.

Rather than identifying persons as "sick" or fundamentally flawed from childhood as the Freudians did, Rogers was interested in how he and other mental health professionals could recognize the health in people. Mentally robust people, in Rogers's view, exist in the here and now, free of defense mechanisms that would make it difficult for them to accept reality as it is. Called "the quiet revolutionary," Rogers went where no mental health professional had been before. His 1942 innovation of the tape-recording of psychotherapeutic interviews was far ahead of his time, but this method has now become standard practice for those providing mental health services. Many of these remarkable taped interviews done by Rogers over the years have been donated to the American Academy of Psychotherapists' tape library. These invaluable teaching tools are available to therapists all over the world.

In an article from the Association for Humanistic Psychology, the benefits of humanistic therapy are described as having a "crucial opportunity to lead our troubled culture back to its own healthy path. More than any other therapy, Humanistic-Existential therapy models democracy. It imposes ideologies of others upon the patient less than other therapeutic practices. Freedom to choose is maximized. We validate our patients' human potential."

The person-centered therapist learns to recognize and trust human potential, providing patients with empathy and unconditional positive regard to help facilitate change. The therapist avoids directing the course of therapy by following patient's lead whenever possible. Instead, the therapist offers support, guidance, and structure so that the patient can discover personalized solutions within themselves.

Two primary goals of person-centered therapy are increased self-esteem and greater openness to experience. Some of the related changes that this form of therapy seeks to foster in patients include closer agreement between patient's idealized and actual selves; better self-understanding; lower levels of defensiveness, guilt, and insecurity; more positive and comfortable relationships with others; and an increased capacity to experience and express feelings at the moment they occur.

Rogers stated that there are six necessary and sufficient conditions required for therapeutic change:

(1) Therapist-patient psychological contact, a relationship between patient and therapist must exist, and it must be a relationship in which each person's perception of the other is important.

(2) Patient incongruence that exists between patient's experience and awareness.

(3) Therapist congruence or genuineness, the therapist is congruent within the therapeutic relationship. The therapist is deeply involved him- or herself and they can draw on their own experiences (self-disclosure) to facilitate the relationship.

(4) Therapist unconditional positive regard (UPR), the therapist accepts the patient unconditionally, without judgment, disapproval or approval. This facilitates increased self-regard in the patient, as they can begin to become aware of experiences in which their view of self-worth was distorted by others.

(5) Therapist empathic understanding, the therapist experiences an empathic understanding of patient's internal frame of reference. Accurate empathy on the part of the therapist helps the patient believe therapist's unconditional love for them.

(6) Patient perception that the patient perceives, to at least a minimal degree, therapist's UPR and empathic understanding.

Rogers believed that the most important factor in successful therapy was not therapist's skill or training, but rather his or her attitude. Three interrelated attitudes on the part of the therapist are central to the success of person-centered therapy: congruence; unconditional positive regard; empathy; as listed below:

(1) Congruence refers to therapist's openness and genuineness—the willingness to relate to patients without hiding behind a professional facade. Therapists who function in this way have all their feelings available to them in therapy sessions and may share significant emotional reactions with their patients. Congruence does not mean, however, that therapists disclose their own personal problems to patients in therapy sessions or shift the focus of therapy to themselves in any other way.

(2) Unconditional positive regard means that the therapist accepts the patient totally for who he or she is without evaluating or censoring, and without disapproving of particular feelings, actions, or characteristics. The therapist communicates this attitude to the patient by a willingness to listen without interrupting, judging, or giving advice. This attitude of positive regard creates a nonthreatening context in which the

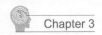

patient feels free to explore and share painful, hostile, defensive, or abnormal feelings without worrying about personal rejection by the therapist.

(3) Empathy. The third necessary component of a therapist's attitude is empathy ("accurate empathetic understanding"). The therapist tries to appreciate patient's situation from patient's point of view, showing an emotional understanding of and sensitivity to patient's feelings throughout the therapy session. In other systems of therapy, empathy with the patient would be considered a preliminary step to enabling the therapeutic work to proceed; but in person-centered therapy, it actually constitutes a major portion of the therapeutic work itself. A primary way of conveying this empathy is by active listening that shows careful and perceptive attention to what the patient is saying. In addition to standard techniques, such as eye contact, that are common to any good listener, person-centered therapists employ a special method called reflection, which consists of paraphrasing and summarizing or both what a patient has just said. This technique shows that the therapist is listening carefully and accurately, and gives patients an added opportunity to examine their own thoughts and feelings as they hear them repeated by another person. Generally, patients respond by elaborating further on the thoughts they have just expressed.

According to Rogers, when these three attitudes (congruence, unconditional positive regard, and empathy) are conveyed by a therapist, patients can freely express themselves without having to worry about what the therapist thinks of them. The therapist does not attempt to change patient's thinking in any way. Even negative expressions are validated as legitimate experiences. Because of this non-directive approach, patients can explore the issues that are most important to them—not those considered important by the therapist. Based on the principle of self-actualization, this undirected, uncensored self-exploration allows patients to eventually recognize alternative ways of thinking that will promote personal growth. The therapist merely facilitates self-actualization by providing a climate in which patients can freely engage in focused, in-depth self-exploration.

5.5 Evaluation

The humanistic perspective provides power to individual's growth by emphasizing the positive nature of humans, free will, and the innate ability associated with changes. The Humanistic perspective has had a profound influence on methods of therapy and counseling. Many other therapists have adopted a humanistic undertone in their work with patients. It can facilitate patients toward a positive developmental orientation.

The main weakness of humanistic perspective is its lack of concrete treatment approaches aimed at specific issues. It is difficult to both develop a concrete treatment technique, as well as exam the effectiveness of the techniques, because it emphasizes individual's subjective experiences. Some psychologists believe that the humanistic perspective has been shown to be effective but only with less severe problems, and it is not adequate to help those with more sever personality or mental health pathology. In addition, it does not pay sufficient attention to influences of both unconscious thoughts and biological factors.

6. Biological psychology

Biological perspective is an orientation toward understanding the biological bases of behavior and mental process. It focuses on how the brain and nervous systems operate on behavior and mental processes. Biological psychologists believe that all behavior is biologically determined, because the mind appears to reside in the brain. Therefore, all thoughts, feelings, and behaviors ultimately have a physiological basis. Psychologists of biological perspective argue that psychology should investigate the brain, nervous system, endocrine system, neurochemistry, and genes.

There are two primary concerns in biological perspective: one is the workings of the nervous system, and the other is the role of heredity on behavior. Biological psychologists have attempted to find out how the nervous system controls behavior and mental processes. They focus on the study of the relationship between the structure and function of the brain and specific mental processes.

One of the earliest methods used to explore the workings of the brain, especially the relations between the cerebral structure and behavior, was the detailed analysis of clinical patients who had suffered certain types of brain trauma. In the 1860s, French physician Pierra Broca discovered that speech capacity is located in a certain area of the brain. He extended the implications of his study, asserting that all behavior may be associated with some specific mechanism or structure in the brain. More recently, with the development of various tools, the biological perspective has made lots of advancements. For example, psychologists study the link between brain and behavior using neuroimaging tools, such as the functional magnetic resonance imaging, which is invaluable to observe which areas of the brain are active during a particular task. Using functional magnetic resonance imaging, which is invaluable to observe which areas of the brain are active during a particular task, the study findings suggest that people with high psychological well-being effectively recruit the ventral anterior cingulate cortex when confronted with potentially aversive stimuli, manifesting reduced activity in subcortical regions such as the amygdala. Using the positron emission tomography, studies suggested that imagination of personally saddening experiences increased regional cerebral blood flow in the inferior orbitofrontal cortex. Scientists also acquired many valuable findings when they study brain injury, in an attempt to work out normal psychological function. The biological revolution has had tremendous impact on the field of psychology. Researchers now have the ability to examine the function of neurotransmitters in the brain.

Another important aspect of contemporary biological perspective is to explore the role of heredity in psychological processes. Heredity means the biological transmission of characteristics from one generation to the other. Human genes have evolved over millions of years to adapt behavior to the environment. Therefore, much behavior has a genetic basis. Researchers investigating the interaction between genes and the environment have shown that the environment affects our genetic makeup. Biological psychologists are interested in mechanisms of inheritance of psychological phenomena, such as whether high intelligence is inherited from one generation to the next. Some studies suggested that the degree to which intelligence is attributed to heredity ranges from 40 percent to about 80 percent. Some researchers argued that the individuals with alcoholism and drug addiction should not receive too many moral criticisms, because alcoholism and drug addiction are seen as the expression of a more general psychopathological hereditary condition. Modern biology is rapidly developing today, and scientists have the ability to decipher the human genome. In future, we will understand precisely how the behavior and the personality are affected by the genetic factors.

The biological revolution has had tremendous impact on the field of psychology. This perspective has grown significantly over the last few decades. The approach is very scientific and reliable, especially with advances in the tools of study, such as functional magnetic resonance imaging and positron emission tomography scans, which allow researchers to look at the brain under a variety of conditions. The practical applications of these techniques are extremely effective.

The main weakness of biological perspective of psychology is that it often over-simplifies the huge complexity of physical systems and their interactions with the environment. It has not explained how mind and body interact because the mind and emotions are difficult to study objectively.

（朱荔芳）

Chapter 4

Clinical Interview and Evaluation

Psychological assessment is a process of testing that uses a combination of techniques to help arrive at some hypotheses about a person and his behavior, personality and capabilities. Psychological assessment also refers to as a psychological testing, or a psychological interview on a person. Psychological testing is always performed by a licensed psychologist, or a psychology trainee (such as an intern). Psychologists are the only profession that being expertly trained to perform and interpret psychological tests.

Psychological assessment should never be performed in a vacuum. A part of a thorough assessment of an individual is that he also undergoes a full medical examination, to rule out the possibilities of a medical, disease or organic cause for his symptoms. It is often helpful to have this done first, before the psychological testing.

1. Psychological assessment

1.1 Components of psychological assessment

There are several methods to help you assess your patients or patients.

1.1.1 Observations

Observations of the person being referred in their natural setting—especially if it is a child—can provide valuable assessment information. In the case of a child, how do they behave in school settings, at home, and in the neighborhood? Does the teacher treat them differently than other children? How do their friends react to them?

The answers to these and similar questions can give a better picture of a child and the settings in which they function. It can also help the professional conducting the assessment better formulate treatment recommendations.

1.1.2 Interviews

Valuable information is gained through interviewing. When it is for a child, interviews are conducted not only the child, but the parents, teachers and other individuals familiar with the child. Interviews are more open and less structured than formal testing and give those being interviewed an opportunity to convey information in their own words. A formal clinical interview is often conducted with the individual before the start of any psychological assessment or testing. This interview can last anywhere from 30 to 60 minutes, and includes questions about individual's personal and childhood history, recent life experiences, work and school history, and family background.

1.1.3 Norm-referenced tests

A standardized psychological test is a task or set of tasks given under standard, set conditions. It is designed to assess some aspect of a person's knowledge, skill or personality. A psychological test provides a scale of measurement for consistent individual differences regarding some psychological concept and serves to line up people according to that concept.

Tests can be thought of as yardsticks, but they are less efficient and reliable than actual yardsticks. A test yields one or more objectively obtained quantitative scores so that, as much as possible, each person is assessed in the same way. The intent is to provide a fair and equitable comparison among test takers.

Norm-referenced psychological tests are standardized on a clearly defined group, termed the norm group, and scaled so that each individual score reflects a rank within the norm group. Norm-referenced tests have been developed to assess many areas, including intelligence; reading, arithmetic, and spelling abilities; visual-motor skills; gross and fine motor skills; and adaptive behavior. Psychologists have a choice of many well-standardized and psychometrically sound tests with which to evaluate an individual.

Norm-referenced tests have several benefits over non-norm-referenced tests. They provide valuable information about a person's level of functioning in the areas covered by the tests. They relatively little time to administer, permitting a sampling of behavior within a few hours. Each appraisal can provide a wealth of information that would be unavailable to even the most skilled observer who did not use testing. Norm-referenced tests also provide an index for evaluating change in many different aspects of child's physical and social world.

1.1.4 Informal assessment

Standardized norm-referenced tests may at times need to be supplemented with more informal assessment procedures, such as projective tests or even career-testing or teacher-made tests. For example, in the case of a child, it may be valuable to obtain language samples from the child, test child's ability to profit from systematic cues, and evaluate child's reading skills under various conditions. The realm of informal assessment is vast, but informal testing must be used more cautiously since the scientific validity of the assessment is less known.

Psychologists seek to take the information gathered from psychological assessment and weave it into a comprehensive and complete picture of the person being tested. Recommendations are based on all the assessment results and from discussion with peers, family, and others who may shed light on person's behavior in different settings. For instance, in children, information must be obtained from parents and teachers in order for psychological assessment to be considered complete and relevant to the child. Major discrepancies among the findings must be resolved before any diagnostic decisions or recommendations for treatment are made. Psychological assessment is never focused on a single test score or number. Every person has a range of competencies that can be evaluated through a number of methods. A psychologist is there to evaluate the competencies as well as the limitations of the person, and report on them in an objective but helpful manner. A psychological assessment report will not only note weaknesses found in testing, but also individual's strengths.

1.2 Phases of psychological assessment

1.2.1 Evaluating the referral question

Clinicians rarely are asked to give a general or global assessment, but instead are asked to answer specific questions. To address these questions, it is sometimes helpful to contact the referral source at different stages in the assessment process. For example, it is often important in an educational evaluation to observe the student in the classroom environment. The information derived from such an observation might be relayed back to the referral source for further clarification or modification of the referral question. Likewise, an attorney may

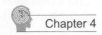

wish to somewhat alter his or her referral question based on preliminary information derived from clinician's initial interview with the patient.

1.2.2　Acquiring knowledge relating to the content of the problem

Before beginning the actual testing procedure, examiners should carefully consider the problem, the adequacy of the tests they will use, and the specific applicability of that test to an individual's unique situation. This preparation may require referring both to the test manual and to additional outside sources. Clinicians should be familiar with operational definitions for problems such as anxiety disorders, psychoses, personality disorders, or organic impairment so that they can be alert to their possible expression during the assessment procedure.

1.2.3　Data collection

After clarifying the referral question and obtaining knowledge relating to the problem, clinicians can then proceed with the actual collection of information. This may come from a wide variety of sources, the most frequent of which are test scores, personal history, behavioral observations, and interview data. Clinicians may also find it useful to obtain school records, previous psychological observations, medical records, police reports, or discuss the patient with parents or teachers. It is important to realize that the tests themselves are merely a single tool, or source, for obtaining data. The case history is of equal importance because it provides a context for understanding patient's current problems and, through this understanding, renders the test scores meaningful. In many cases, a patient's history is of even more significance in making predictions and in assessing the seriousness of his or her condition than his or her test scores.

1.2.4　Interpreting the data

The end product of assessment should be a description of patient's present level of functioning, considerations relating to etiology, prognosis, and treatment recommendations. Etiologic descriptions should avoid simplistic formulas and should instead focus on the influence exerted by several interacting factors. These factors can be divided into primary, predisposing, precipitating, and reinforcing causes, and a complete description of etiology should take all of these into account. Further elaborations may also attempt to assess the person from a systems perspective in which the clinician evaluates patterns of interaction, mutual two-way influences, and the specifics of circular information feedback.

2. Clinical interview

Imagine that you are a psychologist and a patient comes to see you. Just looking at him/her, you cannot tell what's wrong with him/her or why s/he has come to your office. What do you do? You probably answered, "I talk to him/her, of course!" Talking to your patients is a good first step in figuring out what's wrong and how to treat her.

The clinical interview, also called the intake interview, allows the psychologist to speak with the patient in person and form a professional opinion of patient's personality and any disorders he might be suffering from. The psychologist can learn not only from patient's answers but from his body language and other subtle factors the patient might not be directly aware of. Clinical interviews can follow either a structured or unstructured format. They can be conducted for the purpose of making a diagnosis or simply to gain a better.

Probably the most important means of data collection during psychological evaluation is the assessment interview. Without interview data, most psychological tests are meaningless. The interview also provides potentially valuable information that may be otherwise unobtainable, such as behavioral observations, idiosyncratic features of the patient, and person's reaction to his or her current life situation. In addition, interviews are the primary means for developing rapport and can serve as a check against the meaning and validity of test results.

2.1   Structure of interview

A clinical interview is a dialogue between psychologist and patient that is designed to help the psychologist diagnose and plan treatment for the patient. It is often called "a conversation with a purpose." What's the difference between you, as a psychologist, talking to the patients and their best friends talking to them? There are several key differences in a normal conversation and a clinical interview.

Sometimes an interview is mistakenly thought to be simply a conversation. In fact, the interview and conversation differ in many ways. An interview typically has a clear sequence and is organized around specific, relevant themes because it is meant to achieve defined goals. Unlike a normal conversation, the assessment interview may even require the interviewer and interviewee to discuss unpleasant facts and feelings. Its general objectives are to gather information that cannot easily be obtained through other means, establish a relationship that is conducive to obtaining the information, develop greater understanding in both the interviewer and interviewee regarding problem behavior, and provide direction and support in helping the interviewee deal with problem behaviors. The interviewer must not only direct and control the interaction to achieve specific goals, but also have knowledge about the areas to be covered in the interview.

A basic dimension of an interview is its degree of structure. Some interviews allow the participants to freely drift from one area to the next, whereas others are highly directive and goal oriented, often using structured ratings and checklists. The more unstructured formats offer flexibility, possibly high rapport, the ability to assess how patients organize their responses, and the potential to explore unique details of a patient's history. Unstructured interviews, however, have received frequent criticism, resulting in widespread distrust of their reliability and validity. As a result, highly structured and semi-structured interviews have been developed that provide sound psychometric qualities, the potential for use in research, and the capacity to be administered by less trained personnel.

Regardless of the degree of structure, any interview needs to accomplish specific goals, such as assessing patient's strengths, level of adjustment, the nature and history of the problem, diagnosis, and relevant personal and family history. Techniques for accomplishing these goals vary from one interviewer to the next. Most practitioners use at least some structured aids, such as intake forms that provide identifying data and basic elements of history. Obtaining information through direct questions on intake forms frees the clinician to investigate other aspects of the patient in a more flexible, open-ended manner. Clinicians might also use a checklist to help ensure that they have covered all relevant areas. Other clinicians continue the structured format throughout most of the interview by using one of the formally developed structured interviews, such as the Schedule for Affective Disorders and Schizophrenia (SADS) or Structured Clinical Interview for the DSM-IV (SCID).

2.2   Structured and unstructured interviews

Structured clinical interviews use simple questions to get detailed and specific information from the patient. Some questions are phrased so that the patient can only answer yes or no. Others are phrased so that the patient must agree, disagree or partially agree with a statement made by the psychologist. Use structured clinical interviews when you want to make an official diagnosis.

Structured interviews are a means of collecting data for a statistical survey. In this case, the data is collected by an interviewer rather than through a self-administered questionnaire. Interviewers read the questions exactly as they appear on the survey questionnaire. The choice of answers to the questions is often fixed (close-ended) in advance, though open-ended questions can also be included within a structured interview.

A structured interview also standardizes the order in which questions are asked of survey respondents, so the questions are always answered within the same context. This is important for minimizing the impact of context effects, where the answers given to a survey question can depend on the nature of preceding questions. Though context effects can never be avoided, it is often desirable to hold them constant across all respondents.

Unstructured clinical interviews ask more open-ended questions where the patient is encouraged to expand on her answers. Use unstructured interviews when you want to get a broader picture of patient's personality and issues.

An unstructured interview or non-directive interview is an interview in which questions are not prearranged. These non-directive interviews are considered to be the opposite of a structured interview. The form of the unstructured interview varies widely, with some questions being prepared in advance in relation to a topic that the researcher or interviewer wishes to cover. They tend to be more informal and free flowing than a structured interview, much like an everyday conversation. This nature of conversation allows for spontaneity and for questions to develop during the course of the interview, which are based on the interviewee's responses.

Unstructured interviews are a lot more time consuming in comparison to other methods. This is due because there are typically no prearranged questions asked during an unstructured interview and if there are questions prepared, they are open ended questions which prioritize elaborated answers. As a result, the unstructured interview is sometimes expensive and only feasible with small samples.

When conducting a clinical interview, whether it is structured or unstructured, you should try to pick up on as many nonverbal clues as possible. For example, notice whether the patient looks you in the eyes or avoids eye contact, and whether he appears calm, anxious or hostile. A patient who avoids eye contact might be experiencing anxiety or suspicion, while excessive eye contact might be an expression of hostility. You should also try to pick up on what psychologists refer to as "para-verbal" cues. These are factors such as how fast or slow the patient talks, how well he enunciates words, and his tone of voice. All of these factors can affect the accuracy of your diagnosis. For example, a patient who has difficulty enunciating might be suffering from a neurological condition.

2.3　Types of clinical interviews

Again, imagine that you are a psychologist. How might your clinical interview be different for a first-time patient, and a long-term patient that you've had for years? How might it be different for someone, who does not appear to have anything wrong with him/her, and a patient who is forced to come see you because s/he keeps talking to trees and other inanimate objects? There are many types of clinical interviews that can be used at different times and with different people.

2.3.1　The intake interview

The intake interview happens the first time someone comes to see you. This is the interview where you, as the psychologist, ask what brings them to you, what their mental and physical health history is and what they would like to get out of their time with you.

When you talk to a female, for example, you might start by asking why she has come to see you. She says that, even though everyone else sees her and thinks she's fine, she feels like a mess. She's stressed out all the time and has been experiencing panic attacks. You might then go on to ask questions about when the panic attacks started and ask her to elaborate on her life and problems.

To another woman who talks to trees? Unlike the former, she appears to have something wrong with her from the get-go. Not only that, but when you begin to talk to her, you realize that she's not answering your questions in a logical way; she's making no sense whatsoever.

2.3.2 Mental status exam

A mental status exam is a clinical interview that looks at more than just the answers to your questions. You can look at a patient's behaviors, appearance, attitude and movements, as well as their answers to your questions. All of these things will give you a good view of what their mental health is like. Of course, a mental status exam can be used on any patient, but it is often used on patients who are not able to talk clearly about their problems.

2.4 How to conduct a clinical interview

Whether you are doing an intake interview, a mental status exam or one of many other types of clinical interviews, there are several elements that are important.

First of all, psychologists conducting clinical interviews need to offer a safe space for discussion. The patient needs to be in a nonjudgmental space in order to open up. In addition, reminding a patient that you will not share their information with others unless there is an immediate danger to the patient or someone else will help to build trust and allow the patient to be honest.

Asking open-ended questions is much more valuable than asking yes or no questions. Allowing the patient time to think about and answer open-ended questions will give much better insight. For example, the closed-ended question "Do you feel depressed?" can be answered with a simple yes or no. It does not really give your insight into patient's thoughts and feelings.

Compare that to the open-ended question, "How do you feel?" They might say depressed, stressed out, like the weight of the world is on their shoulders, completely uninterested in all the things they used to love or any number of other things. But, the answers to the open-ended question can tell you much more about a patient than a simple yes or no.

Finally, psychologists conducting a clinical interview should listen to more than just the words of the patient. Non-verbal clues, like patient's posture and tone of voice, can tell you a lot. For example, what if you asked a patient how they're feeling and they respond, "I am fine." The words by themselves might lead you to believe the patient. But wait! What if the patient said those words in an angry tone of voice? What if she was twisting her hands around in her lap when she said them? These are signs that there is something else going on behind the words.

2.5 Checklist for an interview

Clinical psychological interview questions should cover the following aspects (Table 4-1):

Table 4-1 Clinical psychological interview aspects

	Description of the problem
	Initial onset
	Changes in frequency
History of the Problem	Antecedents/consequences
	Intensity and duration
	Previous treatment
	Attempts to solve
	Formal treatment

(Continued)

Family Background		Socioeconomic level Parent's occupation(s) Emotional/medical history Married/separated/divorced Family constellation Cultural background Parent's current health Family relationships Urban/rural upbringing
Personal History	Infancy	Developmental milestones Family atmosphere Amount of contact with parents Early medical history Toilet training
	Early and Middle Childhood	Adjustment to school Academic achievement Hobbies/activities/interests Peer relationships Relationship with parents Important life changes
	Adolescence	All areas listed for early and middle Childhood Presence of acting out (legal, drugs, sexual) Early dating Reaction to puberty
	Early and Middle Adulthood	Career/occupational Interpersonal relationships Satisfaction with life goals Hobbies/interests/activities Marriage Medical/emotional history Relationship with parents Economic stability
	Late Adulthood	Medical history Ego integrity Reaction to declining abilities Economic stability
Miscellaneous		Self-concept (like/dislike) Happiest/saddest memory Earliest memory Fears Somatic concerns Events that create happiness/sadness Recurring/noteworthy dreams

3. Psychological test

Psychological test is an essentially objective and standardized measure of a sample of behavior. Another conception of scale usually used in a title of psychological test, such as Wechsler Adult Intelligence Scale. Scales relate raw scores on a test to some defined theoretical or empirical distribution.

Psychological testing is not the same as psychological assessment which is a process that involves the integration of information from multiple sources, including psychological tests, personal and medical history, description of current symptoms and problems by either self or others, and interviews with other persons about the person being assessed. A psychological test is one of the sources of data used within the process of assessment; usually more than one test is used.

3.1   Types of tests

There are more than 4500 published psychological tests in Psychology Resource Centre of York University Library. Psychological tests can be classified into different categories, such as group or individual test based on performance type, verbal or non-verbal test based on the content, commercial or non-commercial Tests. Generally, Psychological tests fall into several categories:

(1) Achievement and aptitude tests. Its attempts to evaluate knowledge or special capacity in a particular area are used in educational or employment settings, such as Scholastic Aptitude Tests (SAT) for college admission, and the Graduate Record Examination (GRE).

(2) Intelligence tests. It is focus on measuring your intelligence. The famous tests include the Stanford-Binet Scale, the Wechsler Scale, and Raven's Test.

(3) Personality tests. It is focus on measuring individual basic personality traits. The most well-known personality tests are: the Minnesota Multiphasic Personality Inventory (MMPI), NEO Personality Inventory (NEO) and the Rorschach inkblot test.

(4) Neuropsychological Tests. It is tries to measure deficits in cognitive functioning and help clinical doctors identify whether there is related brain damage. For example the Halsted-Reitan Neuropsychological Battery, Luria-Nebraska Neuropsychological battery, and Wechsler Memory Scale.

(5) Occupational tests. It is attempts to match individual interests with the demands of persons in known careers.

(6) Specific clinical assessment. It is focus on measuring specific clinical matters, such as current level of anxiety or depression, including Zung Self-Rated Depression or Anxiety Scale.

3.2   Uses of tests

The main domains of psychological tests are diagnosis of "Exceptionality", screening devices, career counseling and research. In clinics or hospitals, psychological tests may be used for purposes of diagnosis, treatment planning and to evaluate the degree of rehabilitation. Clinical tests can provide information about overall personality functioning and the need for psychotherapy. Decisions about treatment do not depend exclusively on psychological test results but are based on the judgment of relevant staff members with whom the psychologist collaborates. In educational settings, intelligence and achievement tests are usually used to assess individual accomplishment and to improve instruction and curriculum planning. Elementary schools use kindergarten and first-grade screening procedures to determine readiness for reading and writing programs. Screening tests also identify developmental, visual, and auditory problems for which the child may need special assistance. If child's progress in school is unusually slow, or if he or she shows signs of a learning disability or behavior disorder, testing may clarify whether the difficulty is neurologically or emotionally based. Many high schools administer interest inventories and aptitude tests to assist in the students educational or vocational planning.

Tests are also used in military, industrial and organizational settings, primarily for selection and classification. Selection procedures provide guidelines for accepting or rejecting candidates for jobs. Classification

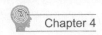

procedures, which are more complex, aim to specify the types of positions for which an individual seems best suited. Intelligence testing is usually supplemented by methods devised expressly to meet the needs of the organization.

3.3 Requirements for a good test

Nowadays, more and more psychological tests are applied in many fields. It is essential that they measure what they are intended to measure and that the scores accurately reflect the test taker's knowledge and skills. The features that make a test useful, however, are the same regardless of the test's purpose; the requirements for a good test apply equally to all psychological tests. The features of good tests must involve in standardization, reliability and validity. Reliability, validity, and uniform testing procedures are essential requirements for any test whether the test is designed to measure personality characteristics, mastery of a specific subject matter, job skills, or the probability of succeeding in college or professional school.

3.3.1 Item-selection

There are two chief ways to select test items. One way is to choose novel items, which provide an uneducated child with just as much chance to succeed as a child who has been taught at home or in school. In this particular test, the child is asked to choose figures that are alike, on the assumption that the designs are unfamiliar to all children. The other way is to choose familiar items, on the assumption that all those for whom the test is designed have had the requisite prior experience to deal with the items.

Many of the items on intelligence tests assume general knowledge and familiarity with the language of the test. However, such assumptions can never be strictly met. The language spoken in one home is never exactly the same as that spoken in another; the available reading material and the stress on cognitive abilities also vary. Even the novel items test perceptual discriminations that may be acquired in one culture and not in another. Despite these difficulties, items can be chosen that work reasonably well. The items included in contemporary intelligence tests have survived in practice after many others have been tried and found ineffective. It should be remembered, however, that intelligence tests have been validated according to their success in predicting school performance within a particular culture.

3.3.2 Standardization

How are test scores of different individuals comparable? Testing conditions must be the same for each one, which is one step of standardization. Standardization implies uniformity of procedure in administering and scoring the test. The standardized test administration procedures are important because testing situation is influenced by many factors and administrator's characteristics as well. The standardized test is a test administered and scored in a consistent manner. Test Administration must be uniform by means of using a Test manual which contains important source information, only individuals with training and experience can be examiners. In giving instructions orally, the rate of speaking, tone of voice, inflections, pauses, and facial expression should be considered.

Raw score of an individual in a special test is meaningless. For example, Wang's mathematic mark is 60 and his literature mark is 80, and 100 is full mark. Does Wang learn literature better than mathematics? If the literature average mark in Wang's class is 90, his literature is not good. If mathematic average mark is 40, Wang's mathematic is better than his classmates. To interpret the raw scores of a psychological test, a very important step of standardization is to establish norms that are the normal or average performance obtained from a group of subjects. This group called the standardization sample should be great and representative. "The norms are thus empirically established by determining what the persons in a representative group actually do on the test. Any individual's raw score is the referred to [as] the distribution of scores obtained by the standardization sample, to discover where he or she falls in that distribution." (Anastasi, A., 1988). Percentile, standard score, and intelligence quotient (IQ) are important norms and relate to the normal curve, which is always divided in the same respective manner.

A percentile is the value of a variable below which a certain percent of observations fall. Therefore, the 50th percentile is the value (or score) below which 50 percent of the observations may be found. The term percentile and percentile rank are often used in descriptive statistics as well as in the reporting of scores from norm-referenced tests.

Standard scores that is called z-scores, is a dimensionless quantity derived by subtracting the population mean from an individual raw score, and then dividing the difference by the population standard deviation. The standard score indicates how many standard deviations an observation is above or below the mean. It allows comparison of observations from different normal distributions, which is done frequently in research.

Some concepts attempt to measure intelligence, such as mental age, IQ. The term was introduced in Binet-Simon scale in 1905. A child's performance on a test of mental ability expressed as the average age of children who achieved the same level in a standardization age group. "IQ" was mentioned first by German psychologist William Stern (1871—1938) in 1912. IQ refers to a ratio of mental age (MA) to chronological age (CA). However, the conception of Stern's original IQ was this MA/CA. The US psychologist Lewis Madison Terman (1877—1956) modified Stern's formula to (MA/CA) × 100 to express mental age as a percentage of chronological age and to eliminate decimals of scores. Anne age 4, had passed the scores of 11 year olds on a psychological test, therefore, her IQ was 275. In 1944, the standard definition of IQ was used by David Wechsler in Wechsler Adult Intelligence Scale. Deviation IQ refers to a standard deviation of 15 and a mean of 100. Terman's IQ was called the ratio IQ. By the definition, an IQ of 100 is average; approximately 68 per cent of IQ scores fall between 85 and 115, approximately 95 per cent fall between 70 and 130, approximately 99.74 falls between 55 and 145.

3.3.3   Reliability

The scores of test are reliable when they are reproducible and consistent. The reliability refers to the internal consistency and stability with which a measuring instrument performs its function.

Some factors influence the reliability of tests. The quality of a test relies on the length of the test, the clarity of items to examinee and the consistency in the administration of a test. The different scores of a test may result from differences between testing occasions or due to the difference in scoring by different administrators. If we did not know how much rubber yardstick stretched each time, the scaling results would be unreliable no matter how carefully we marked the measurement. If items that are too difficult, too easy, and have near-zero or negative discrimination are replaced with better items, the reliability of the measure will increase. Reliability may be estimated through a variety of methods because tests must be shown to be reliable if the results are to be used with confidence.

Test-retest reliability is estimated as the Pearson correlation coefficient between two administrations of the same measure. In the alternate forms method, reliability is estimated by the Pearson's correlation coefficient of two different forms of a measure. Single-administration methods include split-half and internal consistency. This can be done by repeating the test, and by giving the test in two different but equivalent forms, or by treating each half of the test separately, therefore named the split-half reliability. The split-half method treats the two halves of a measure as alternate forms. This "halves reliability" estimate is then stepped up to the full test length using the Spearman-Brown prediction formula. If each individual tested achieves roughly the same score on both measures, then the test is reliable. The coefficient of correlation between paired scores for the

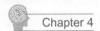

same group of examinees on a given test is called a reliability coefficient. Well-constructed tests usually have a reliability coefficient of r = 0.90 or greater.

Cronbach's alpha, first named as alpha by Cronbach in 1951, and indicates the degree of internal consistency of items within a test. It is usually interpreted as the mean of all possible split-half coefficients. Cronbach's alpha will generally increase when the correlations between the items increase. For this reason the coefficient is also called the internal consistency or the internal consistency reliability of the test. A test could be regarded as good structure if Cronbach's alpha is more than 0.70.

3.3.4　Validity

In psychometrics validity is the extent to which a test measures which it purports to measure, or the extent to which specified inferences from the test's scores are justified or meaningful. The valuation of a test's validity must take into account the intended uses of the test and the inferences to be made from its scores. Test validity is important and differs from reliability. A college examination in philosophy that is full of questions containing complex or tricky wording might be a test of a student's verbal ability rather than of the philosophy learned in the course. Such an examination might be reliable, but it would not be a valid test of achievement for the course. Criterion validity, construct validity, content validity, face validity are usually used to describe test validity.

Criterion validity reflects the success of measures used for prediction or estimation. To measure validity, we must also obtain two scores for each person: the test score and some other measure of the ability in question which is called a criterion. There are two types of criterion-related validity: Concurrent and predictive validity. For concurrent validity, suppose that a test is designed to predict success in learning. To determine whether the test is valid, it is given to a group of individuals before they study typing. After completing the course, the students are tested on the number of words per minute that they can type accurately. This is a measure of their success and serves as a criterion. A coefficient of correlation between the early test scores and the scores on the criterion can now be obtained. This correlation coefficient, known as a validity coefficient, tells something about the value of a given test for a given purpose. The higher the validity coefficient, the more accurate will be the prediction made from the test results. For predictive validity, tests are intended to predict abilities that are more wide-ranging and difficult to measure than typing skills. Scores on the Medical College Admissions Test (MCAT), a standard test in USA, are used to select medical students. If the purpose of MCAT is to predict success in medical school, a person's grade point average could be used as a criterion; correlating his or her MCAT score with the grade point average would be one way of validating the test. The important point to remember here is that the evaluation of a test's validity must take into account the intended uses of the test and the inferences to be made from its scores.

Construct validity refers to whether a test measures or correlates with a theorized psychological construct, such as intelligence. It is related to the theoretical ideas behind the personality trait under consideration; a non-existent concept in the physical sense may be suggested as a method of organizing how personality can be viewed.

A construct is not restricted to one set of observable indicators or attributes. It is common to a number of sets of indicators. Thus, "construct validity" can be evaluated by statistical methods that show whether or not a common factor can be shown to exist underlying several measurements using different observable indicators. This view of a construct rejects the past idea that a construct is neither more nor less than the operations used to measure it.

Content validity is a non-statistical type of validity that involves "the systematic examination of the test content to determine whether it covers a representative sample of the behavior domain to be measured". A test has content validity built into it by careful selection of which items to include. Items are chosen so that they comply with the test specification which is drawn up through a thorough examination of the subject domain. By using a panel of experts to review the test specifications and the selection of items the content validity of a test can be improved. The experts will be able to review the items and comment on whether the items cover a representative sample of the behavior domain. Content validity is related to face validity, though content validity should not be confused with face validity. Face validity is very closely related to content validity. While content validity depends on a theoretical basis for assuming if a test is assessing all domains of a certain criterion (e.g., does assessing addition skills yield a good measure for mathematical skills? To answer this you have to know, what different kinds of arithmetic skills mathematical skills include) face validity relates to whether a test appears to be a good measure or not. This judgment is made on the face of the test, thus it can also be judged by the amateur.

3.4   Tests of intellectual ability

Intelligence tests are often tests that measure general intellectual ability, but as we noted earlier, many psychologists consider that term inappropriate. There is no general agreement as to what constitutes intelligence, and intelligence cannot be considered apart from an individual's culture and experiences. During this discussion of intelligence tests, these qualifications should be kept in mind.

3.4.1   Binet's method

Binet proposed that a slow or "dull" child was like a normal child retarded in mental growth. He devised a scale of mental age to measure intelligence in terms of the kinds of changes that are ordinarily associated with growing older. If one rises above the others and to how many degrees, if one rises above the average level of other individuals considered as normal, or if he remains below. Average mental age (MA) scores correspond to chronological age (CA), which is the age determined from child's date of birth; a bright child's MA is above his or her CA; a slow child's MA is below his or her CA. For example, a 6 year-old child who passed all the tasks usually passed by 7 year-olds, but nothing beyond, would have a mental age that exactly matched his chronological age, 7.0. The mental age scale is easily interpreted by teachers and others who deal with children of differing mental abilities.

Some items of the Binet-Simon Scale (1905) are as follows:

(1) Follows a moving object with the eyes.

(2) Grasps a small object which is seen.

(3) Recognizes the difference between a square of chocolate and a square of wood.

(4) Points to familiar named objects, e.g., "Show me the cup."

(5) Compares two lines of markedly unequal length.

(6) Repeats three spoken digits.

(7) Tells how two common objects are different, e.g., "paper and cardboard."

(8) Compares two lines of slightly unequal length.

(9) Puts three nouns, e.g., "Paris, river, fortune" (or three verbs) in a sentence.

(10) Reverses the hands of a clock.

(11) After paper folding and cutting, draws the form of the resulting holes.

Binet and Simon began to revise a modern version, developing a test primarily for kids ages 3 to 15 that would compare their intellectual capabilities to other children of the same age, and they published this second version in 1908. The version of 1911 was extended to an adult range, and applied mental age scoring, even quotient later, however, it was not unpublished before Binet died in 1911.

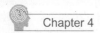

3.4.2 Stanford-Binet Intelligence Scale

In 1908, after studying abroad, Goddard HH brought the Binet-Simon scale to the United States and translated it into English. Following Goddard in the U.S. the test items developed by Binet were adapted for American school children by Lewis Terman, a professor of cognitive psychology at Stanford University. He standardized the administration of the test and developed age-level norms by giving the test to thousands of children. In 1916, he published the Stanford revision of the Binet tests, now referred to as the Stanford-Binet Intelligence Scale. This test has become one of the best-known and widely used intelligence tests.

Terman kept the concept of Binet's mental age. Each test item was age-graded at the level at which a substantial majority of the children passed it. A child's mental age could be obtained by summing the number of items passed at each age level. Terman adopted William Stern's suggestion that mental age/chronological age multiplied by 100 (to get rid of the decimal) be made the intelligence quotient or IQ. It expresses intelligence as a ratio of mental age (MA) to chronological age (CA): $IQ = MA/CA \times 100$. The 100 is used as a multiplier so that the IQ will have a value of 100 when MA is equal to CA. If MA is lower than CA, then the IQ will be less than l00; if MA is higher than CA, then the IQ will be more than 100.

In 1937, Terman created two parallel forms of the Stanford-Binet, these parallel forms were published as Form L (for Lewis) and Form M (for Maud) of the Stanford-Binet. In 1950s, Merrill, the first student of Terman and later a fellow professor and research collaborator at Stanford University, took the lead in revising the Stanford-Binet, selecting the best items from Forms L and M to include in a new version of the test. The new form was published in 1960 and was later used to re-collected normative data in 1973. The test form in 1973 added alternate items at all levels, however, it remained similar to the 1937 forms.

In 1986, the Fourth Edition of the Stanford-Binet Intelligence Scale moved from the age-scale format introduced by Binet to a point-scale format. Many of the items and item-types from the prior editions were included, and extended scales were created using the same types of items and activities. Besides the new and expanded tests, the Fourth Edition provided several factors, including Verbal Reasoning, Abstract/Visual Reasoning, Quantitative Reasoning, and Short-Term Memory, in addition to IQ.

In 2003, the Fifth Edition (SB5) was published. According to the publisher's website, "The SB5 was normed on a stratified random sample of 4,800 individuals aged 2 to 85 or more matched the 2000 U.S. Census." SB5 attempts to carry on the tradition of the prior editions while taking advantage of current research in measurement and cognitive abilities. Multiple factors of SB5 are modified from those on the Fourth Edition, but represent abilities assessed by all former versions of the test. The use of routing subtests continues, with a nonverbal routing test added to complement vocabulary. The SB5 re-accepts the age-scale format for the body of the test, presenting a variety of items at each level of the test. The five factors assessed in the test are: Fluid Reasoning, Knowledge, Quantitative Reasoning, Visual-Spatial Processing, and Working Memory. Each is assessed in two separate domains, verbal and nonverbal, in order to accurately assess individuals with deafness, limited English, or communication disorders. The reliability coefficients were high ranging from 0.91 to 0.98. Correlation was relatively high, (approximately 0.90) when compared to earlier versions of the Stanford Binet. Correlation were in the high 0.70 to mid-0.80 range when compared to other tests, such as the Bender-Gestalt, the WAIS-III, the WIAT-II, the WISC-III, and the WPPSI-R. Testing time takes 45 to 60 minutes depending on child's age and how many subtests are administered. Some controversy remains to the accuracy of bias in this test.

3.4.3 Wechsler Intelligence Scales

Stanford-Binet Scale (1905) was not adapted to identify particular intellectual abilities appropriate for adults, and depended too heavily on language ability. David Wechsler (1896—1981), born in a Jewish family in Romania and immigrated with his parents to the United States as a child, had experience of the Army Alpha test during World War I and the Stanford-Binet Scale later. He contacted with several pioneers in the field of intelligence theory, and thought Intelligence as, "the aggregate or global capacity of the individual to act purposefully, to think rationally and to deal effectively with his environment". He developed one of the first intelligence tests named the Wechsler-Bellevue Intelligence Test to measure separate abilities, in 1939, when Wechsler became chief psychologist at Bellevue Psychiatric Hospital. From these he derived, the Wechsler Intelligence Scale for Children (WISC) in 1949, Wechsler Adult Intelligence Scale (WAIS) in 1955, and the Wechsler Preschool and Primary Scale of Intelligence (WPPSI) in 1967.

In 1949, Wechsler published WISC as a downward extension of the Wechsler Adult Intelligence Scale which was the Wechsler-Bellevue Intelligence Test before 1955. The WISC was revised in 1974 as the WISC-R, and the third edition of the WISC-III was published in 1991. The current version, the WISC-IV, was produced in 2003. There are ten core subtests and five supplemental ones in the WISC-IV. The supplemental subtests are used to accommodate children in certain rare cases, or to make up for spoiled results which may occur from interruptions or other circumstances. The subtests generate a Full Scale score (FSIQ,) and four composite scores known as indices: Verbal Comprehension (VCI,) Perceptual Reasoning (PRI,) Processing Speed (PSI) and Working Memory (WMI.) Each of the ten core subtests is given equal weighting towards full-scale IQ. There are three subtests for both VCI and PRI, thus they are given 30% weighting each; in addition, PSI and WMI are given weighting for their two subtests each.

WAIS was published in 1955 as a revision of the Wechsler-Bellevue test (1939). WAIS is a battery of tests that is composed from subtests Wechsler "adopted" from the Army Tests. WAIS-R was standardized in 1981 on a sample of 1,880 US subjects, applied for individual aged 16 to 89 years. WAIS-III was revised in 1997. The WAIS-IV was standardized on a sample of 2,200 people in the United States ranging in age from 16 to 90. An extension of the standardization has been conducted with 688 Canadians in the same age range. The fourth edition of the test was released in 2008 by Pearson. The structure of WAIS-IV has removed the verbal/performance subscales pattern replaced by the index scores. The General Ability Index (GAI) is now included, which consists of the Similarities, Vocabulary and Information subtests from the Verbal Comprehension Index and the Block Design, Matrix Reasoning and Visual Puzzles subtests from the Perceptual Reasoning Index. The GAI is clinically useful because it can be used as a measure of cognitive abilities that are less vulnerable to impairment. There are total of 15 subtests in WAIS-IV.

The WPPSI was developed by David Wechsler in 1967. It is a descendent of the earlier Wechsler Adult Intelligence Scale and the Wechsler Intelligence Scale for Children tests, which has been revised twice, in 1989 and 2002. WPPSI-III is published by Harcourt Assessment. WPPSI-III can provides subtest and composite scores which represent intellectual functioning in verbal and performance cognitive domains, as well as providing a composite score which represents a child's general intellectual ability. The WPPSI-III is composed of 14 subtests. Performance subtests are nonverbal (both spatial and fluid reasoning) problems, several of which are timed. Subtest scores, IQ scores, Processing Speed Quotients, and the General Language Composite scores are based on the scores of the 1700 children originally tested in a very carefully designed, nationwide sample, but still must be interpreted very cautiously for any individual, especially one who may have somewhat unusual patterns of strengths and weaknesses. As with any test, influences such as anxiety, motivation, fatigue, rapport, and experience may invalidate test scores.

3.4.4   Group tests

The Stanford-Binet and the Wechsler scales are individual ability tests that are administered to a single individual by a specially trained tester. Group ability tests, in contrast, can be administered to a large number

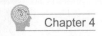

of people by a single examiner and are usually in pencil-and-paper form. The advantages of an individual test over a group test are many. The tester can be certain the subject understands the questions, can evaluate person's motivation, and can gain additional clues to intellectual strengths and weaknesses by carefully observing subject's approaches to different tasks. Group ability tests are useful when large numbers of people have to be evaluated. The armed services, for example, use a number of group tests which measure general intellectual ability and special skills and help in selecting men and women for special jobs, including pilots, navigators, electronic technicians, and computer programmers.

Raven's Progressive Matrices are multiple-choice tests of abstract reasoning, originally developed by Dr. Raven JC in 1936, and can be used to test groups as well. Three types of RPM are Standard, Colored and Advanced Progressive Matrices. In each test item, a candidate is asked to identify the missing segment required to complete a larger pattern. Many items are presented in the form of a 3×3 or 2×2 matrix.

3.4.5   Kaufman Assessment Battery for Children

The Kaufman Assessment Battery for Children (KABC) is a psychological diagnostic and standardized test that assesses intelligence and achievement in children aged two years, six months to 12 years, six months. KABC was published by Kaufman and his wife in 1983. Kaufman worked together with Wechsler on the revision of the WISC, and supervised the standardization of the WISC-R. Its construction incorporates several recent developments in both psychological theory and statistical methodology. KABC based the theories of the Luria neuropsychological model and the Cattell/Horn/Carroll (CHC) approach. The new version of KABC-II was published in 2002, which extended its age range from three to eighteen years and enhanced its usefulness. In addition, new subtests were being added and existing subtests updated. The Cattell-Horn-Carroll model of KABC-II can be chosen for children from a mainstream cultural and language background. Or if Crystallized Ability would not be a fair indicator of child's cognitive ability, the Luria model which excludes verbal ability can be chosen.

Administer the same subtests on four or five ability scales. Then, interpret the results based on your chosen model. Either approach gives you a global score that is highly valid and that shows small differences between ethnic groups in comparison with other comprehensive ability batteries. In addition, a nonverbal option allows you to assess a child whose verbal skills are significantly limited.

3.5   Tests of personality

Personality is the sum total of the behavioral and mental characteristics that are distinctive of an individual. It strongly relates to the prediction of person's behavior and performance at work, school or in marriage.

Personality is the most complicated phenomena, however, consistency that is the theoretic foundation of it assessed. We perceive consistency in the personalities of individuals we know well, and we believe that we can predict how they will behave in a variety of situations. Moreover, most personality theories also regard personality as a stable. Traits, and trait theory, refer to habitual patterns of behavior, thought, and emotion. They are relatively stable over time and influence behavior. Certain basic personality traits characterize an individual over a variety of day-to-day situations and even over the course of a lifetime. Thus, if an individual appears to behave honestly or conscientiously in situations occurred in tests, the action of he or she can be predicted in other similar situations. Psychoanalytic theory also assumes consistency of individual personality; unresolved conflicts during childhood may lead to a cluster of personality characteristics that characterize a person throughout life. Self-theories assume that the self-concept plays a central role in integrating our behavior that provides consistency. Even though we may change in important ways, we still think of ourselves as the same, stable person. Indeed, the feeling of consistency within our thoughts and behavior is essential to our well-being. The loss of a sense of consistency is characteristic of personality disorganization and labeled as abnormal.

In a large scale longitudinal studies, a total of more than 100 subjects were followed over a 35 year period. They were first evaluated in junior high school by psychologists on a number of standardized personality traits, and rated three times in senior high school, in their mid-30s, and in their mid-40s. The results found that 58 percent of personality variables showed a significant positive correlation over the three-year period from junior to senior high school. 31 percent of the items showed a significant correlation over the 30-year period from Junior high school to mid-40s.

Personality changes can be found at any time in life, especially during adolescence and early adulthood due to conflict and tension. The longitudinal study of junior high students found marked individual differences in the degree of personality consistency over the age periods studied. In fact, personality development involves both constancy and change.

The main methods that have been used to assess personality can generally be classified as observational methods, personality inventories, and projective techniques.

3.5.1   Personality inventories

A personality inventory is essentially a questionnaire in which the person reports his or her reactions or feelings in certain situations. The personality inventory resembles a structured interview in that it asks the same questions of each person and the answers are usually given in a form that can be easily scored. A personality inventory may be designed to measure a single dimension of personality or several personality traits simultaneously. The Sixteen Personality Factor Questionnaire and Eysenck Personality Questionnaire produce a personality profile showing individual's scores on 16 different traits. A different method of test construction was used in the development of the Minnesota Multiphasic Personality Inventory and California Personality inventory.

(1) The Minnesota Multiphasic Personality Inventory

Minnesota Multiphasic Personality Inventory, shorten for MMPI, is one of the most widely used paper-and-pencil tests of personality. The original MMPI was developed by Starke R. Hathaway, and J. C. McKinley, at the University of Minnesota Hospitals and first published in 1942. In 1989, the MMPI-2 was published and standardized on a new national sample of adults in the United States. The MMPI-A was a special version of the MMPI designed for adolescents, and published in 1992, which has 478 items with a short form of 350 items. In 2003, a new version of the MMPI-2 has been published.

The original MMPI has ten clinical scales and three validity scales and adapts to individuals aged 15 to adult, which is composed of approximately 550 statements about attitudes, emotional reactions, physical and psychological symptoms, and past experiences. The subject respond to each statement by answering true or false or "cannot say." Some sample test items follow: "I have never done anything dangerous for the thrill of It.", "I daydream very little." "My mother or father often made me obey, even when I thought it was unreasonable." "At times my thoughts have raced ahead faster than I could speak them."

MMPI used the technique of empirical construction, because the test items bear an actual relationship to the personality characteristic being measured. To develop a scale of items that distinguish between paranoid and normal individuals, for example, the same questions were given to two groups, the criterion group and the control group. Individuals in the criterion group were hospitalized with the diagnosis of paranoia, and had never been diagnosed as having psychiatric problems. In the control group, in which the variables were similar to the criterion group in age, sex socioeconomic status, and other important variables. Questions that at face value might seem to distinguish normal from paranoid individuals (e.g., "I think that most people would lie to get ahead") may or may not do so when put to an empirical test. In fact, patients diagnosed as paranoid were significantly less apt to respond "true" to this statement than were normal individuals. Figure 4-1 presents an illustration of MMPI results in a man.

The MMPI-2 is the first major revision of the MMPI and can be used with adults 18 and over. It has 567 items of true-or-false format and usually completes all items during 1 and 2 hours. There is an infrequently used abbreviated form of the test that consists of the MMPI-2's first 370 items. The shorter version has been mainly used in circumstances that have not allowed the full version to be completed (e.g., illness or time pressure), but the scores available on the shorter version are not as extensive as those available in the 567-item version. The MMPI-2 can be scored by compute. The scoring programs offer a range of scoring profile choices including the extended score report, which includes data on the newest and most psychometrically advanced scales—the Restructured Clinical Scales (RC scales). The extended score report also provides scores on the more traditionally used Clinical Scales as well as Content, Supplementary, and other subscales of potential interest to clinicians. Use of the MMPI is tightly controlled for financial as well as ethical reasons. The clinician using the MMPI has to pay for materials and for scoring and report services, as well as a charge to install the computerized program.

MMPI-2-RF composed of 338 items is developed by Yossef S. Ben-Porath and Auke Tellegen from

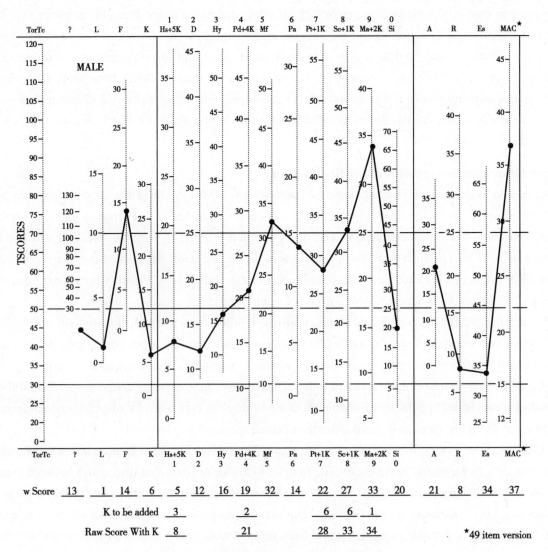

Figure 4-1 A male's testing results of MMPI

the MMPI-2 with RC Scale and published in 2003. It is linked to current models of psychopathology and personality. The MMPI-2-RF attempts to help clinicians in the assessment of mental disorders, identification of specific problem areas, and treatment planning in a variety of settings. The MMPI-2-RF normative sample is come from the MMPI-2's, which consists of 1,138 men and 1,138 women aged from 18 to 80 years from several regions and diverse communities in the U.S. The scales of MMPI-2-RF has 8 Validity Scales; 12 Higher-Order (H-O) and Restructured Clinical (RC) Scales; 14 Somatic/Cognitive and Internalizing Scales; 11 Externalizing, Interpersonal, and Interest Scales; and 5 Personality Psychopathology Five (PSY-5) Scales. MMPI-2-RF can be administrated and completed during 35-50 minutes by paper-and-pencil or 25-35 minutes by computer.

(2) California Psychological Inventory

The California Psychological Inventory (CPI), based on the method of empirical construction, is a self-report inventory created by Harrison Gough in 1956 or 1957. The CPI uses some items from the same questions of the MMPI, and concerned to measure personality traits of more "normal" individuals. The CPI scales measure such traits as dominance, sociability, self-acceptance, responsibility, and socialization.

The comparison groups for some of the scales were obtained by asking students of high school and college to nominate the classmates they would rate high or low on the trait in question. The principles of the CPI are based on that of the MMPI. Foe example of the dominance scale, the students among criterion group were described by their peers as high in dominance (aggressive, confident, self-reliant), and those among control group were described by their peers as low in dominance (retiring, lacking in self-confidence, inhibited). Items that revealed a statistically significant difference between the criterion group and the control group formed the dominance scale.

The third edition of the CPI contains 434 true-false questions, half of which were taken from the original version of the MMPI. The CPI is used to the individuals aged from 13 years to older. The test is scored on 18 scales, three of which are validity scales. Eleven of the non-validity scales were selected by comparing responses from various groups of people. The other four were content validated. The 18 scales are further grouped into four classes: 1) measures of poise, ascendancy, self-assurance, and interpersonal adequacy; 2) measures of socialization, responsibility, intrapersonal values, and character; 3) measures of achievement potential and intellectual efficiency; 4) measures of intellectual modes and interest modes. The CPI takes about 45-60 minutes to complete.

(3) The Sixteen Personality Factor Questionnaire

Raymond Bernard Cattell (1905—1998) was a British and American psychologist known for his exploration of a wide variety of substantive areas in psychology. He followed the work of Allport and Odbert, and used the computer skill to analyze the list of Allport-Odbert. He organized the list into 181 clusters and asked subjects to rate people whom they knew by the adjectives on the list. Using factor analysis Cattell generated 12 factors, and then included four factors. Thus, the Sixteen Personality Factor Questionnaire (16PF) was empirically developed to comprehensively measure all of the basic traits of normal personality, and originally published in 1949. The second to fourth editions were published in 1956, 1962, and 1967 respectively; and the fifth edition was published in 1993, and focused on the language used in the test, simplifying the answer format, creating new validity indices, improving reliability and validity of test, and developing a new standardization sample based on the U.S. Census population.

The 16PF Fifth Edition consists of 185 multiple-choice items which are non-threatening and asks simple questions about daily behavior, interests, and opinions, each item is written at a fifth-grade reading level. The administration of the 16-PF can be completed during 35 to 50 minutes for the paper-and-pencil version

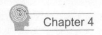

and about 30 minutes by computer. The 16PF Questionnaire was designed to be administered to adults approximately age 16 and older, and for younger, the 16PF Adolescent Personality Questionnaire can be used. The 16-PF provides scores on 16 primary scales, 5 global scales, and 3 validity scales. All personality scales are bipolar, meaning that both ends of each scale have a clear, meaningful definition (Table 4-2).

Table 4-2   The meanings of 16 PF.

Descriptors of low range	Primary factor	Descriptors of high range
Impersonal, distant, cool, reserved, detached, formal, aloof (schizothymia)	Warmth (A)	Warm, outgoing, attentive to others, easy-going, kindly, participating, likes people (affectothymia)
Concrete thinking, lower general mental capacity, less intelligent, unable to handle abstract problems (lower scholastic mental capacity)	Reasoning (B)	Abstract-thinking, more intelligent, bright, higher general mental capacity, fast learner (higher scholastic mental capacity)
Reactive emotionally, changeable, affected by feelings, emotionally less stable, easily upset (lower ego strength)	Emotional stability (C)	Emotionally stable, adaptive, mature, faces reality calmly (Higher Ego Strength)
Deferential, cooperative, avoids conflict, submissive, humble, obedient, easily led, docile, accommodating (submissiveness)	Dominance (E)	Dominant, forceful, assertive, aggressive, competitive, stubborn, bossy (dominance)
Serious, restrained, prudent, taciturn, introspective, silent (desurgency)	Liveliness (F)	Lively, animated, spontaneous, enthusiastic, happy go lucky, cheerful, expressive, impulsive (surgency)
Expedient, nonconforming, disregards rules, self indulgent (low super ego strength)	Rule-consciousness (G)	Rule-conscious, dutiful, conscientious, conforming, moralistic, staid, rule bound (High Super Ego Strength)
Shy, threat-sensitive, timid, hesitant, intimidated (threctia)	Social boldness (H)	Socially bold, venturesome, thick skinned, uninhibited (parmia)
Utilitarian, objective, unsentimental, tough minded, self-reliant, no-nonsense, rough (harria)	Sensitivity (I)	Sensitive, aesthetic, sentimental, tender minded, intuitive, refined (premsia)
Trusting, unsuspecting, accepting, unconditional, easy (alaxia)	Vigilance (L)	Vigilant, suspicious, skeptical, distrustful, oppositional (protension)
Grounded, practical, prosaic, solution oriented, steady, conventional (praxernia)	Abstractedness (M)	Abstract, imaginative, absent minded, impractical, absorbed in ideas (autia)
Forthright, genuine, artless, open, guileless, naive, unpretentious, involved (artlessness)	Privateness (N)	Private, discreet, nondisclosing, shrewd, polished, worldly, astute, diplomatic (Shrewdness)
Self-Assured, unworried, complacent, secure, free of guilt, confident, self satisfied (untroubled)	Apprehension (O)	Apprehensive, self doubting, worried, guilt prone, insecure, worrying, self blaming (guilt proneness)
Traditional, attached to familiar, conservative, respecting traditional ideas (conservatism)	Openness to Change (Q1)	Open to change, experimental, liberal, analytical, critical, free thinking, flexibility (Radicalism)
Group-oriented, affiliative, a joiner and follower dependent (group Adherence)	Self-Reliance (Q2)	Self-reliant, solitary, resourceful, individualistic, self sufficient (Self-Sufficiency)
Tolerates disorder, unexacting, undisciplined, flexible, lax, self-conflict, impulsive, careless of social rules, uncontrolled (low integration)	Perfectionism (Q3)	Perfectionistic, organized, self-disciplined, compulsive, socially precise, exacting will power, control, self-sentimental (High Self-Concept Control)
Relaxed, placid, tranquil, torpid, patient, composed low drive (low ergic tension)	Tension (Q4)	Tense, high energy, impatient, driven, frustrated, over wrought, time driven. (high ergic tension)

A shorter version of the test, the 16PF Select was developed specifically for use in employee selection settings, and involves a subset of the items and scales in the regular test in 1999. The 16PF Express in 2007 provides a very short, 15-minute, version of the test for research purposes, which has about four items per factor and a different answer-format.

The 16-PF can be applied in schools and colleges, clinical and counseling settings, career counseling and employee selection and development, as well as in basic personality research. It has been found to predict a wide range of important behaviors, such as creativity, academic achievement, cognitive style, empathy and interpersonal skills, leadership potential, conscientiousness, self-esteem, frustration tolerance, coping patterns, marital compatibility, and job performance. The test is widely used internationally. It has been translated and adapted into over 35 languages and dialects.

(4) The Eysenck Personality Questionnaire

The Eysenck Personality Questionnaire (EPQ) is a questionnaire to assess the personality traits of a person, and is created by Hans J. Eysenck (1916—1997). For a diagram of Eysenck Personality Questionnaire test please see Figure 4-2.

The EPQ reflects the PEN personality model of Eysenck's which is based primarily on physiology and genetics. With the help of the factor analysis Eysenck suggested two main personality factors, i.e. Neuroticism and Extraversion. Neuroticism was the tendency to experience negative emotions and Extraversion was the tendency to enjoy positive events. Based on these two dimensions, the Eysenck Personality Inventory was published in 1964. Eysenck noted how these two dimensions were similar to the four temperament types, Choleric, Melancholic, Sanguine and Phlegmatic which first proposed by the Greek physician Galen..In the late of 1970s, the third dimension was added to the model, psychoticism. Then, based on PEN model, Eysenck created EPQ for adults and children, with his wife S. B. G. Eysenck in 1975.

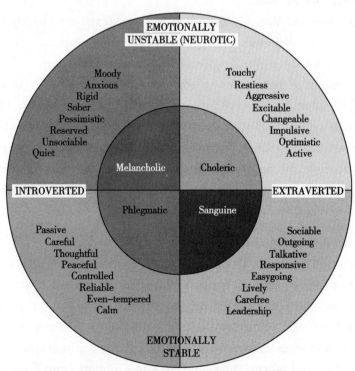

Eysenck, HJ and Eysenck, *M.W. Personatity and Individual Differences*.
Pfenum Publishing. 1958.

Figure 4-2   Diagram of Eysenck Personality Questionnaire test

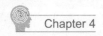

Extraversion/Introversion: Extraversion is characterized by being outgoing, talkative, high on positive affect (feeling good), and in need of external stimulation. According to Eysenck's arousal theory of extraversion, there is an optimal level of cortical arousal, and performance deteriorates as one becomes more or less aroused than this optimal level. Arousal can be measured by skin conductance, brain waves or sweating. At very low and very high levels of arousal, performance is low, but at a more optimal mid-level of arousal, performance is maximized. Extraverts, according to Eysenck's theory, are chronically under-aroused and bored and are therefore in need of external stimulation to bring them up to an optimal level of performance. Introverts, on the other hand, are chronically over-aroused and jittery and are therefore in need of peace and quiet to bring them up to an optimal level of performance.

Neuroticism/Stability: Neuroticism or emotionality is characterized by high levels of negative affect such as depression and anxiety. Neuroticism, according to Eysenck's theory, is based on activation thresholds in the sympathetic nervous system or visceral brain. This is the part of the brain that is responsible for the fight-or-flight response in the face of danger. Activation can be measured by heart rate, blood pressure, cold hands, sweating and muscular tension (especially in the forehead). Neurotic people, who have low activation thresholds, and are unable to inhibit or control their emotional reactions, experience negative affect (fight-or-flight) in the face of very minor stressors-they are easily nervous or upset. Emotionally stable people, who have high activation thresholds and good emotional control, experience negative affect only in the face of very major stressors-they are calm and collected under pressure.

Psychoticism/Socialisation: Psychoticism is associated not only with the possibility of having a psychotic episode (or break with reality), but also with aggression. Psychotic behavior is rooted in the characteristics of tough-mindedness, non-conformity, inconsideration, recklessness, hostility, anger and impulsiveness. The physiological basis suggested by Eysenck for psychoticism is testosterone, with higher levels of psychoticism associated with higher levels of testosterone.

(5) NEO Personality Inventory-Revised

The NEO Personality Inventory-Revised (NEO-PI-R) is arguably the most widely used measure designed to assess the Five-Factor Model Adjective Rating Scales of normal personality. The five robust factors of neuroticism, extraversion, conscientiousness, agreeableness, and openness represent higher-order traits that reflect the broadest dimensions of dispositions or temperaments. The NEO-PI-R provides scores on each of these five domains, as well as on six facets within each domain. Costa and McCrae (1992) report extensive reliability and validity data on the NEO-PI-R scales within normal samples. Researches have advocated the use of the FFM in research and diagnosis of personality pathology. The NEO-PI-R (precursor to the NEO-PI-R) has been shown to account for the major dimensions underlying various self-report personality disorder instruments. It is noteworthy, however, that the dimension of openness has consistently demonstrated few significant correlations with variables from these other instruments.

(6) Zuckerman-Kuhlman Personality Questionnaire

The Zuckerman-Kuhlman Personality Questionnaire (ZKPQ) was developed as the result of an attempt to define the basic factors of personality or temperament which describes five domains namely impulsive sensation seeking, neuroticism-anxiety, aggression-hostility, activity and sociability. The development of the ZKPQ began in the 1980's (Zuckerman and colleagues, 1988) before Costa and McCrae (1992), which had expanded their NEO from three to five factors to fit the popular big-five theory evolved from the lexical analyses of Goldberg (1990) and others (Norman, 1963). In a clinical sample, investigators analyzed the personality disorder symptoms assessed using the Structured Clinical Interview for DSM-III-R, and found four factors which they labeled "the four A's: Antisocial (impulsive, unstable, dramatic and easily bored),

Asocial (socially indifferent and stereotyped interests), Asthenic (anxious, fearful and dependent) and Anankastic (obsessive-compulsive, rigid and excessive perfectionism). Their findings were supported by a factor analysis using the descriptors of DSM-IV in patients with personality disorders. Reliability findings for the scales are fairly robust. Translated scales in German, Spanish, Catalan, Japanese, and Chinese have shown good factor reliabilities and internal scale reliabilities suggesting cross-cultural generality of the personality constructs. NEO-PI-R Agreeableness (-) and ZKPQ Aggression-Hostility were loaded on DAPP-BQ Dissocial; NEO-PI-R Extraversion (-) and ZKPQ Sociability (-) were loaded on DAPP-BQ Inhibition; NEO-PI-R Neuroticism and ZKPQ Neuroticism-Anxiety were loaded on DAPP-BQ Emotional Dysregualtion; NEO-PI-R Conscientiousness and ZKPQ Activity were loaded on DAPP-BQ Compulsivity (Wang et al., 2003).

(7) Five-Factor Model Adjective Rating Scales

A number of adjective rating scales are available as measures of the Five-Factor Model Adjective Rating Scales (FFM), including Goldberg's (1992) 50- and 100-item scales and John's (1990; John and colleagues, 1991) "Big Five" Inventory. Despite sound psychometric properties and excellent convergent and discriminant validities with other measures of the FFM (Briggs, 1992), however, adjective-based measures of the FFM have not been used extensively in personality disorder research. A minor exception to this statement is the Extended Interpersonal Adjective Scales-Revised-Big 5 (IASR-B5; Trapnell and Wiggins, 1990). This scale is an augmented version of the IAS-R (Wiggins and colleagues, 1988), which was developed to assess the two domains of the interpersonal circumplex model (ICM), dominance and nurturance. The IASR-B5 retains scales to assess the eight primary dimensions of the ICM, and includes scales created to measure the additional three domains of the FFM: neuroticism, conscientiousness, and openness. The measure has demonstrated excellent inter consistency (alphas ranging from 0.87 to 0.94), as well as good convergent and discriminant validity when analyzed with measures of both normal and disorder personality (e.g., NEO-PI-R or MMPI-PD) (Trapnell and Wiggins, 1990; Wiggins and Pincus, 1989, 1994).

(8) Personality Adjective Check List

The Personality Adjective Check List (PACL) is an adjective checklist developed by Strack to assess Millon's (1981) theoretical personality types in a normal population. A rational/empirical approach was employed in constructing scales to measure each of Millon's eight basic personalities plus an Experimental scale to assess features of his three severe personality types—broderline, schizotypal, and paranoid. The basic PACL scales have demonstrated acceptable internal consistency (alphas range from 0.76 to 0.89) and temporal stability, within 3-month test-retest correlations ranging from 0.69 to 0.85 (Strack, 1987). However, the Experimental scale, which combines features of three different severe personality types, have consistently demonstrated lower reliabilities (alphas and retest r's both in the lower. 60s). Consistent with Millon's theory, the PACL scales were created with item overlap. Scale intercorrelations range from 0.04 to 0.06. The PACL has demonstrated convergence and discriminant validity with other measures of normal and abnormal personality.

3.5.2 Projective tests

Projective tests are a variety of personality tests in which the examinee gives free responses to a series of stimuli such as inkblots, pictures, or incomplete sentences. When an examinee is asked to respond to an ambiguous stimulus, his or her responses may not reflect as he or she wishes and presumably revealing hidden emotions and internal conflicts. Based on projection, one type of Freud's defense mechanism, intolerable feelings, impulses or thoughts are falsely attributed to other people. Advocates of projective tests stress that the ambiguity of the stimuli presented within the tests allow examinees to express thoughts that originate on a deeper level than tapped by explicit questions. Projective tests attempt to explore the private personality and to

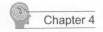

allow the individual to become much more involved in the responses. Two of the most widely used projective techniques are the Rorschach test and the Thematic Apperception Test.

(1) Rorschach Test

The Rorschach test, developed by the Swiss psychiatrist Hermann Rorschach in the 1920s, consists of ten cards, including five black inkblots, two black and red inkblots, and three multicolored, each on white paper. One image used in Rorschach test was illustrated in Figure 4-3. The use of Rorschach test spread rapidly in and after World War Ⅱ.

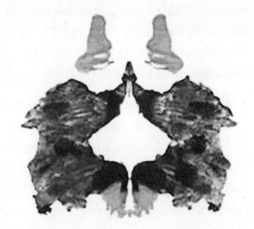

The person taking the test states what the inkblot seems to resemble as he is handed the cards one by one. Inkblot pictures of animals, people, flowers, in fact every conceivable kind of object and some which seem to be creations of imagination, as well as of the world about us, are seen. Subject's responses may be scored in various ways. Three main categories are location (whether the response involves the entire inkblot or a part of it), determinants (whether the subject responds to the shape of the blot, its color, or differences in texture and

Figure 4-3　An image used in Rorschach test

shading), and content (what the response represents). Most testers also score responses according to frequency of occurrence; for example, a response is "popular" if many people assign it to the same inkblot. The research done by Rorschach shows that the images selected and the manner of visualizing them are unique to the personality of the individual person who takes the test. By means of Rorschach's technique these images can be scored in a structure manner and interpreted to furnish a picture of individual's psychological tendencies in his relationships to himself and to others in his social environment. The Rorschach tests reveal many aspects of personality, such as the inner assets and weaknesses, emotional reactions and methods of controlling them, ways in which thinking is organized, ways in which the individual sees himself and imagines others see him, and whether he is tense in his social relations, to name but a few of the personality aspects.

Methods of interpretation differ. Rorschach scoring systems have been described as a system of pegs on which to hang one's knowledge of personality. Several elaborate scoring systems have been devised based on these categories. The most widely used method in the United States is based on the work of John E. Exner. But because these systems have proved to have a limited predictive value, many psychologists base their interpretations on an impressionistic evaluation of the response record, as well as on subject's general reaction to the test situation. Interpretation of the Rorschach requires more training and experience than interpretation of any of the other personality tests.

One problem of Rorschach test is poor reliability. It is also thought that reliability of a test should depend substantially on details of the testing procedure, such as where the tester and subject are seated; any introductory words; verbal and nonverbal responses to subject's questions or comments; and how responses are recorded. Reliability of the Rorschach Test has been generally poor because the interpretation of responses is too dependent on clinician's judgment; the same test protocol may be evaluated quite differently by two trained examiners. Exner has published detailed instructions, but Wood and colleagues cites many court cases where it was found they have not been followed. Attempts to demonstrate the Rorschachs ability to predict behavior or discriminate between groups have met with limited success.

(2) Thematic Apperception Test

The Thematic Apperception Test (TAT) was developed by the American psychologists Henry A. Murray and Christiana D. Morgan at Harvard during the 1930s and published in 1935. The original 31 cards were divided into three categories, for use with men only, with women only, or for use with subjects of either sex. One image used in Thematic Apperception Test is illustrated in Figure 4-4. The TAT intended to explore dynamics of personality and evaluate a person's patterns of thought, attitudes, observational capacity, and emotional responses to ambiguous test materials.

The TAT is usually administered to individuals in a quiet room free from interruptions or distractions. The examiner shows the subject a series of story cards. The usual number of cards shown to the subject is between 10 and 14, although Murray recommended the use of 20 cards, administered in two separate one-hour sessions with the examinee. The story is asked to include: what has led up to the event shown; what is happening at the moment; what the characters are feeling and thinking, and what the outcome of the story was. The subject is encouraged to give free rein to his or her imagination and to tell whatever story comes to mind. The test is intended to reveal basic themes that recur in a person's imaginative productions. Apperception is a readiness to perceive in certain ways based on prior experiences.

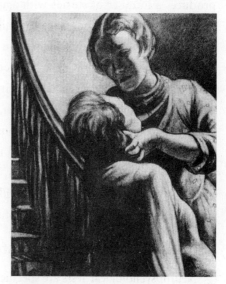

Figure 4-4   An image used in Thematic Apperception Test

People interpret ambiguous pictures according to their apperceptions and elaborate stories in terms of preferred plots or themes that reflect personal fantasies. If particular problems are bothering the subject, they may become evident in a number of the stories or in striking deviations from the usual theme in one or two stories. In addition to assessing the content of the stories that the subject is telling, the examiner evaluates subject's manner, vocal tone, posture, hesitations, and other signs of an emotional response to a particular story picture.

There are two basic approaches to interpreting responses to the TAT, called nomothetic and idiographic respectively. Nomothetic interpretation refers to the practice of establishing norms for answers from subjects in specific age, gender, racial, or educational level groups and then measuring a given subject's responses against those norms. Idiographic interpretation refers to evaluating the unique features of subject's view of the world and relationships. Most psychologists would classify the TAT as better suited to idiographic than nomothetic interpretation.

In interpreting responses to the TAT, examiners typically focus their attention on one of three areas: the content of the stories that the subject tells; the feeling theme or tone of the stories; or subject's behaviors apart from responses. These behaviors may include verbal remarks as well as nonverbal actions or signs. The story content usually reveals subject's attitudes, fantasies, wishes, inner conflicts, and view of the outside world. The story structure typically reflects subject's feelings, assumptions about the world, and an underlying attitude or themes, such as optimism or pessimism.

In analyzing responses to the TAT cards, the psychologist looks for recurrent themes that may reveal individual's needs, motives, or characteristic way of handling interpersonal relationships. Two common methods are currently used in research: Defense Mechanisms Manual (DMM) and Social Cognition and Object Relations (SCOR) scale. The DMM assesses three defense mechanisms: denial, projection, and identification. The SCOR scale assesses four different dimensions of object relations: Complexity of Representations of People, Affect-Tone of Relationship Paradigms, and Capacity for Emotional Investment in Relationships and Moral Standards, and Understanding of Social Causality.

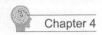

The TAT has fared somewhat better reliability contrasted to Rorschach test. When specific scoring systems are used, such as measuring achievement motives or aggressive themes, the inter-rater's scores show that reliability is fairly good. Yet the relationship of TAT scores to overt behavior is complex. A person who produces a number of stories with aggressive themes may not actually behave aggressively. The individual may be compensating for a need to inhibit aggressive tendencies by expressing such impulses in fantasy. When inhibitions about expressing aggression and the strength of aggressive tendencies are estimated from the TAT stories, the relationship to behavior becomes more predictable. The TAT is criticized as false or outdated by many professional psychologists. Their criticisms include that the TAT is unscientific because it cannot be proved to be valid or reliable. However, defenders of the TAT, including the Rorschach test, point out that it is not fair to expect accurate predictions based on test responses alone; story themes or responses to inkblots are meaningful only when considered in light of additional information, such as person's life history, other test data, and observations of behavior. The skilled clinician uses the data collected by projective tests to make tentative interpretations about individual's personality and then verifies or discards them, depending on further information. The tests are helpful in suggesting possible areas of conflict to be explored.

3.6   Neuropsychological tests

Neuropsychological Tests are specifically designed tasks used to measure a psychological function known to be linked to a particular brain structure or pathway. Its functioning refers to the ability of the nervous system and brain to process and interpret information received through the senses. The Neuropsychological Tests combine theories based on anatomical observations of neurology with the techniques of psychology, including objective observation of behavior and the use of statistical analysis to differentiate functional abilities and define impairment. Here, the Halstead-Reitan Neuropsychological Test Battery, the Luria-Nebraska Neuropsychological Battery, and the Wisconsin Cards Sorting Test will be introduced.

3.6.1   Halstead-Reitan Neuropsychological Test Battery

The Halstead-Reitan Neuropsychological Test Battery (HRNB) is typically used to evaluate individuals with suspected brain damage. The battery also provides useful information regarding the cause of damage, such as, closed head injury, alcohol abuse, Alzheimer's disorder, occurred during childhood development, and whether the damage is getting worse, staying the same, or getting better. Information regarding the severity of impairment and areas of personal strengths can be used to develop plans for rehabilitation or care.

Ward Halstead and Ralph Reitan are the developers of the Halstead-Reitan battery. Based on studies of patients with neurological impairments, Halstead recognized the need for an evaluation of brain functioning that was more extensive than intelligence testing. He began experimenting with psychological tests that might help identify types and severity of brain damage through observation of a person's behavior in various tasks involving neuropsychological abilities. Initially he chose a set of ten tests; all but three are in the current HRNB. The HRNB is a fixed set of eight tests used to evaluate brain and nervous system functioning in individuals aged 15 years and older. Children's versions are the Halstead Neuropsychological Test Battery for Older Children (ages 9 to 14).

The HRNB evaluates a wide range of nervous system and brain functions, including: visual, auditory, and tactual input; verbal communication; spatial and sequential perception; the ability to analyze information, form mental concepts, and make judgments; motor output; and attention, concentration, and memory. Interpretation of the HRNB involves: The Halstead Impairment Index and the General Neuropsychological Deficit Scale are commonly used to obtain an overall score. Each test must be interpreted in relation to other tests in the battery. Indications of lateralization and localization refer to the particular region of the brain that is damaged. Performance on sensory and motor tasks provides the necessary clues. The HRNB has been shown to discriminate normal controls from patients with brain damage with considerable accuracy (84%-98%).

Due to its complexity, the HRNB requires administration by a professional examiner and interpretation by a trained psychologist. Test results are affected by the examinee's age, education level, intellectual ability, and gender or ethnicity, which should always be taken into account. Because the HRNB is a fixed battery of tests, some unnecessary information may be gathered, or some important information may be missed. Overall, the battery requires five to six hours to complete, involving considerable patience, stamina, and cost. The battery has also been criticized because it does not include specific tests of memory; rather, memory is evaluated within the context of other tests.

3.6.2　Luria-Nebraska Neuropsychological Battery

Luria-Nebraska Neuropsychological Battery (LNNB) is a standardized test battery used in the screening and evaluation of neuropsychological impaired individuals, based on the theory of higher cortical functioning by Aleksandra R. Luria who performed pioneering theoretical and clinical work with regard to brain function.

The purposes of LNNB attempt to determine whether a significant brain injury is present or to learn more about known brain injuries and what the patient is or is not able to do with regard to neuropsychological functioning. Moreover, the LNNB can help clinician to distinguish between brain damage and functional mental disorders such as schizophrenia. Sometimes, the battery can be used for legal purposes, i.e. the presence or severity of a brain injury may be measured as part of an evaluation used in the court system.

The LNNB is appropriate for people aged 13 years and older, and takes between 90 and 150 minutes to complete. The battery consists of 269 items in 11 clinical scales, including: reading, writing, arithmetic, visual, memory, expressive language, receptive language, motor function, rhythm, tactile, and intellectual scale. The LNNB can calculate scores into three summary scales, including pathognomonic, right hemisphere, and left hemisphere. A special type of LNNB is for children aged from 8 to 12 years.

Several studies have reflected positively on the LNNB. Compared to the HRNB, they were found to be roughly equivalent in the hands of experienced clinical neuropsychologists in discriminating between a mixed group of psychiatric and brain-damaged populations. Each battery achieved an overall correspondence rate of approximately 80%. The LNNB was also found to separate brain-injured patients from pseudoneurological patients with an approximately 80% correspondence rate. Also, the intellectual processes scale has not been found to correspond well to WAIS or others.

Due to the length of the test and complexity in interpretation, the examiner must be competent and properly trained. Also, the fact that many patients are, indeed, brain damaged can make test administration difficult or frustrating.

3.7　Infants and preschool tests

3.7.1　Gesell Development Schedules

The Development Schedules were devised by Arnold Gesell (1880—1961), a physician and psychologist at the Yale Clinic of Child Development to evaluate the physical, emotional, and behavioral development of children from infancy to 6 years old. The origins of infant assessments are often traced to the work of Gesell.

Gesell was among the first to implement a quantitative study of human development from birth through adolescence. Gesell concluded that mental and physical development in infants, children, and adolescents are comparable and parallel orderly processes. In his clinic, he trained researchers to collect data and produced reports that had a widespread influence on both parents and educators. In the early 1920s, Gesell compiled a schedule of tasks for infants ages 4, 6, 9, 12, and 18 months of age and 2, 3, 4, and 5 years of age. By identifying predictable stages of development for the brain and visual and motor systems, Gesell hoped to document maturation and to include assessments of behavior and development into children's Well-child exams so that physicians could provide families with prescriptive and predictive recommendations. The results of his research were utilized in creating the Development Schedules that measures responses to standardized materials and situations both qualitatively and quantitatively. They describe typical behavior at specified ages in the following areas: ability to adapt; motor functioning; use of language; and social interaction.

The results of the test are expressed first as developmental age (DA), which is then converted into developmental quotient (DQ), representing "the portion of normal development that is present at any age." A separate developmental quotient may be obtained for each of the functions on which the scale is built.

3.7.2 Denver Developmental Screening Test

The Denver Developmental Screening Test (DDST) is a test for screening cognitive and behavioral problems in preschool children, developed by William K. Frankenburg with J.B. Dobbs in 1967. The name "Denver" reflects the fact that this screening test was created at the University of Colorado Medical Center, in Denver.

The performances of DDST are grouped into four categories, i.e. social contact, fine motor skill, language, and gross motor skill. DDST reflects what percentage of a certain age group is able to perform a certain performance. The DDST is the most widely used test for screening developmental problems in children in Canada, because it can detect severe developmental problems.

The Denver II consists of up to 125 items; divided into Social/personal, fine motor function, language and Gross motor functions. Examples of the items are: "When prone lifts head up, using forearm support (with or without hands)?"; "Child grasps raising between thumb and index finger "Copy this" (circle)."; "Give the block to Mum"; "Put it on the table": "What is a spoon/shoe/door made of?"; "While he plays with a toy, pull it away.". The tools of DDST II are simple, including Bell, Glass bottle, Set of 10 blocks, Rattle, Pencil, Tennis ball, Wool, Raisins, Bag with zip top, Cup, Doll, Baby bottle, and Interpretation card.

Sensitivity rates are reported between 56%-83% for the Denver II, but specificity may be as low as 43%, rising to 80%. However, the test has been criticized to be unreliable in predicting less severe or specific problems. Frankenburg has replied to such criticism by pointing out that the Denver Scale is not a tool of final diagnosis, but a quick method to process large numbers of children in order to identify those that should be further evaluated.

3.7.3 Bayley Scales of Infant Development

The Bayley Scales of Infant Development (BSID) was published by N. Bayley in 1969 and have been widely used in clinical assessments and research on infants. It provides overall standard scores for mental and motor development. The first revision of the BSID, the BSID-II was designed to update the normative data and published in 1993.

BSID-III is published in 2006 for children aged 1 month to 42 months. It is possible to obtain detailed information even from children who are not yet verbally functioning. Normative data collected in USA from January 2004-October 2004. Children are assessed in the five key developmental domains: Cognition, language, social-emotional behavior, motor skills, and adaptive behavior. The battery identifies infant and toddler strengths and competencies, as well as weaknesses.

Raw scores of successfully completed items are converted to five scales. Three scales are administered with child interaction, including the scale of cognitive, motor and language. Two new scales, i.e., social-emotional and adaptive behavior are conducted using parent questionnaires. Internal consistency of subtest is above 0.86. Type of Scores includes Scaled scores, Composite scores, Percentile ranks, and Growth scores.

3.8   Clinical assessments

Clinical assessments are a variety of tests that focus on measuring specific clinical matters, including the level of anxiety or depression and quality of life. Clinical assessments provide quantity tools for clinician to determine if further diagnosis and treatment of mental health conditions are needed.

3.8.1   Symptom Checklist-90-Revised

The Symptom Checklist 90 (SCL-90) is a psychiatric self-report inventory and created by Derogatis and colleagues (1973). The 90 items in the questionnaire are scored on a five-point Likert scale, indicating the rate of occurrence of the symptom during the time reference. It is intended to measure symptom intensity on nine different subscales. It has been shown to have a good reliability, as its internal consistency is high. Results concerning its validity are controversial; it discriminates patients from normal controls, thus having some rough discriminate validity, but there have been problems in replicating the original dimensions in factor analytical studies. The SCL-90 has been used widely as an outcome measure, as a measure of mental status, and as a screening instrument.

The current version of SCL-90 is Symptom Checklist-90-Revised (SCL-90-R) published in 1994. The nine scales are Obsessive-Compulsive, Interpersonal Sensitivity, Depression, Anxiety, Hostility, Phobic Anxiety, Paranoid Ideation and Psychoticism. The three global Indices are Global Severity Index (GSI) for measuring overall psychological distress, Positive Symptom Distress Index (PSDI) for measuring the intensity of symptoms, Positive Symptom Total (PST) for exploring number of self-reported symptoms. The SCL-90-R instrument is used by clinical psychologists, psychiatrists, and professionals in mental health, medical, and educational settings as well as for research purposes.

3.8.2   Test of depression and anxiety

The Zung Self-Rating Depression Scale was designed by William W.K. Zung, a psychiatrist at Duke University, to assess the level of depression for patients diagnosed with depressive disorder. The scale with 20 items is a short self-administered survey to quantify the depressed status of a patient. The four common characteristics of depression can be rated, i.e. the pervasive effect, the physiological equivalents, other disturbances, and psychomotor activities. In 1971, William WK Zung created a scale named the Zung Self-Rating Anxiety Scale (SAS) with 20 items for quantifying the level of anxiety for patients experiencing anxiety related symptoms.

The Beck Depression Inventory-II containing 21 questions was published in 1996. The test is widely used as an assessment tool by healthcare professionals and researchers in a variety of settings. The Beck Anxiety Inventory (BAI) created by Aaron T. Beck is a self-report inventory with 21-question multiple-choice and used for measuring the severity of an individual's anxiety.

3.8.3   Tests for quality of life

The term quality of life refers to experiences of illness such as pain, fatigue, and disability and also broader aspects of individual's physical, emotional, and social wellbeing. Clinical trials usually considered include the assessment of quality of life.

The EuroQol (EQ-5D) is a simple and standardized instrument for use as a measure of health outcome. The EQ-5D designed by the EuroQol Group was originally designed to complement other instruments but is now increasingly used as a "stand alone" measure. Applicable to a wild range of health conditions and treatments, the EQ-5D generates a health profile but is also capable of expressing health-related quality of life as a single index value that can be used in the clinical and economic evaluation of health care. The five dimensions of the EQ-5D are mobility, self-care, usual activities, pain/discomfort and anxiety/depression.

The SF-36 Health Survey is a multi-purpose, short-form health survey which contains 36 questions. It yields an eight-scale profile of scores as well as physical and mental summary measures. The SF-36 is a generic measure of health status as opposed to one that targets a specific age, disease, or treatment group. Accordingly, the SF-36 has proven useful in comparing general and specific populations, estimating the relative burden of different diseases, differentiating the health benefits produced by a wide range of different treatments, and screening individual patients. The SF-36 yields 8 scale profiles of functional health and well-being scores as well as psychometrically-based physical and mental health summary measures and a preference-based health utility index. The scale profiles of Physical Functioning, Role-Physical, Bodily Pain and General Health belong to Physical Component Summary. The scale profiles of Vitality, Social Functioning, Role-Emotional and Mental Health belong to Mental Component Summary. Among the most frequently studied diseases and conditions, with 50 or more SF-36 publications each, are: arthritis, back pain, cancer, cardiovascular disease, chronic obstructive pulmonary disease, depression, diabetes, gastro-intestinal disease, migraine headache, HIV/aids, hypertension, irritable bowel syndrome, kidney disease, low back pain, multiple sclerosis, musculoskeletal conditions, neuromuscular conditions, osteoarthritis, psychiatric diagnoses, rheumatoid arthritis, sleep disorders, spinal injuries, stroke, substance abuse, surgical procedures, transplantation, and trauma. In 1996, Version 2.0 of the SF-36 (SF-36v2) was introduced, to correct deficiencies identified in the original version.

4. Psychological counseling

4.1　What is counseling

Psychological counseling is a familiar concept to most of us, but difficult to define clearly. We can describe counseling as:

(1) The process that occurs when a patient and counselor set aside time in order to explore difficulties which may include the stressful or emotional feelings of the patient.

(2) The act of helping the patient to see things more clearly, possibly from a different viewpoint. This can enable the patient to focus on feelings, experiences or behavior, with a goal to facilitating positive change.

(3) A relationship of trust. Confidentiality is paramount to successful counselling. Professional counsellors will usually explain their policy on confidentiality, they may, however, be required by law to disclose information if they believe that there is a risk to life. However the counseling is not:

1) Giving advice.

2) Judgmental.

3) Attempting to sort out the problems of the patient.

4) Expecting or encouraging a patient to behave in a way in which the counsellor may have behaved when confronted with a similar problem in their own life.

5) Getting emotionally involved with the patient.

6) Looking at a patient's problems from your own perspective, based on your own value system.

Counseling psychology focuses on the normal adaptation of individuals to their environment and with helping others cope with crises, problems of daily living and mental challenges. Traditionally, counseling

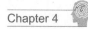

psychology has been concerned with the preventative aspects of mental health and an emphasis on patient strengths.

Counseling psychologist's help people with physical, emotional and mental health issues improve their sense of wellbeing, alleviate feelings of distress and resolve crises. They also provide assessment, diagnosis, and treatment of more severe psychological symptoms.

The problems addressed by counseling psychology are addressed from developmental (lifespan), environmental and cultural perspectives. They include, but are not limited to:

1) School and career/work adjustment concerns.

2) Making decisions about career and work, and dealing with schoolwork retirement transitions.

3) Relationship difficulties-including marital and family difficulties.

4) Learning and skill deficits. Stress management and coping with negative life events.

5) Organizational problems.

6) Dealing with and adjusting to physical disabilities, disease or injury.

7) Personal/social adjustment.

8) The development of one's identity.

9) Persistent difficulties with relating to other people in general. Mental disorders.

The procedures and techniques used within counseling psychology include, but are not limited to:

1) Individual, family and group counseling and psychotherapy.

2) Crisis intervention, disaster and trauma management.

3) Assessment techniques for the diagnosis of psychological disorders.

4) Programs/workshops that educate and inform the public about mental health, school, family, relationship and workplace issues so that problems can be prevented before they start or reduced before they get worse.

5) Consulting with organizations.

6) Program evaluation and treatment outcome.

7) Training.

8) Clinical supervision.

9) Test construction and validation.

10) Research methodologies for scientific investigations.

4.2   Difference between counseling and psychotherapy

Both "psychotherapy" and "counseling" are terms that are used to describe the same process. Both terms relate to overcoming personal difficulties and working towards positive changes. The terms Counseling and Psychotherapy are often used interchangeably.

Though they have similar meanings with considerable overlap, there are some distinctions between the two terms. Counseling is a helping approach that highlights the emotional and intellectual experience of a patient, how a patient is feeling and what they think about the problem they have sought help for. Psychotherapy, however, is based on the psychodynamic approach to counseling-it encourages the patient to go back to their earlier experiences and explore how these experiences effect their current "problem".

Counseling, sometimes called "talk therapy," is a conversation or series of conversations between a counselor and a patient. Counseling usually focuses on a specific problem and taking the steps to address or solve it, such as addiction or stress management. The focus may be on problem solving or on learning specific techniques for coping with or avoiding problem areas. Problems are discussed in the present tense, without too much attention on the role of past experiences. Counseling is also usually more short-term than therapy.

Though the titles "counselor" and "advisor" are often used like synonyms, counselors rarely offer advice. Instead, counselors guide patients to discover their own answers and support them through the actions they choose to take.

Psychotherapy, like counseling, is based on a healing relationship between a health care provider and patient. Psychotherapy, or therapy for short, also takes place over a series of meetings, though often it has a longer duration than counseling. Some people participate in therapy off and on over several years.

Instead of narrowing in on individual problems, psychotherapy considers overall patterns, chronic issues, and recurrent feelings. Psychotherapy is more long-term than counseling and focuses on a broader range of issues. The underlying principle is that a person's patterns of thinking and behavior affect the way that person interacts with the world. Depending on the specific type of psychotherapy that is being used, the goal is to help people feel better equipped to manage stresses, understand patterns in their behavior that may interfere with reaching personal goals, have more satisfying relationships, and better regulate their thinking and emotional responses to stressful situations. If someone has a form of mental illness such as depression, bipolar disorder, schizophrenia, or an anxiety disorder, psychotherapy also addresses ways in which the illnesses affects their daily life, focuses on how to best understand the illness and manage its symptoms and follow medical recommendations. This requires openness to exploring the past and its impact on the present. The aim of psychotherapy is to resolve the underlying issues which fuel ongoing complaints. Psychotherapists help to resolve past experiences as part of laying the foundation for a satisfying future. Many psychotherapists are open to and interested in wisdom from a variety of sources: the body, the unconscious, and the inner child, to name a few possibilities. Therapists should be comfortable working with strong feelings, traumatic memories, and the therapeutic relationship.

4.3   The role of the counselor

First and foremost the counselor is aware that no two people are alike. No two people understand the same language in the same way; their understanding will always be linked to their personal experience of the world.

Therefore, during the counseling process, it is important that the counselor does not try to fit patients into his/her idea of what they should be and how they should act.

The role of the counselor is to enable the patient to explore many aspects of their life and feelings, by talking openly and freely. Talking in such a way it is rarely possible with family or friends, who are likely to be emotionally involved and have opinions and biases that may be detrimental to the success of the counseling. It is important that the counselor is not emotionally involved with the patient and does not become so during counseling sessions. The counselor neither judges, nor offers advice. The counselor gives the patient an opportunity to express difficult feelings such as anger, resentment, guilt and fear in a confidential environment.

The counselor may encourage the patient to examine parts of their lives that they may have found difficult or impossible to face before. There may be some exploration of early childhood experiences in order to throw some light on why an individual reacts or responds in certain ways in given situations. This is often followed by considering ways in which the patient may change such behaviors.

Effective counseling reduces confusion, allowing the patient to make effective decisions leading to positive changes in their attitude and behavior or both. Effective counseling is not advice-giving and is not acting on someone else's behalf (these are more the roles of a life coach). The ultimate aim of counseling is to enable the patient to make their own choices, reach their own decisions and to act upon them accordingly.

（段熙明）

Chapter 5

Stress

Stress is a fact of nature in which forces from the inside or outside world which affect the individual, on either one's emotional or physical well-being, or both. The individual responds to stress in ways that affect the individual, as well as his environment. In general, stress is related to both external and internal factors. External factors include the physical environment, including job, relationships with others, family, and all kinds of the situations, challenges, difficulties, and expectations confronted with an individual on a daily basis. Internal factors determine the body's ability to response to and deal with the external stress-inducing factors. Internal factors which influence the ability to handle stress including the nutritional status, overall health and fitness levels, emotional well-being, and the amount of sleep and rest accomplished.

1. General concept of stress

In humans, stress often refers to a condition in which environmental demands exceed an individual's coping abilities. In animal models of psychiatric disorders, stress can be defined broadly as a forced exposure to aversive events or conditions that are normally avoided. In daily life, we often use the term "stress" to describe negative situations. This leads many people to believe that all stress is bad for you, which is not true. Stress is not always a bad thing. Stress is simply body's response to changes that create taxing demands.

Stress roughly the opposite of relaxation is a medical term for a wide range of strong external stimuli, both physiological and psychological, which can cause a physiological response called the general adaptation syndrome, first described in 1936 by Hans Selye in the journal Nature (Selye, 1936).

Selye was able to separate the physical effects of stress from other physical symptoms suffered by patients through his research. He observed that patients suffered physical effects not caused directly by their disease or by their medical condition.

Selye described the general adaptation syndrome as having three stages:

(1) Alarm reaction, where the body detects the external stimulus.

(2) Adaptation, where the body engages defensive countermeasures against the stressor.

(3) Exhaustion, where the body begins to run out of defenses.

Stress includes distress, the result of negative events, and eustress, and the result of positive events. Despite the type, stress is addictive. If your dog dies and you win the lottery, one does not cancel the other, both are stressful events.

Stress can directly and indirectly contribute to general or specific disorders of body and mind. Stress can have a major impact on the physical functioning of the human body. Such stress raises the level of adrenaline and corticosterone in the body, which in turn increases the heart-rate, respiration, and blood-pressure and puts more physical stress on bodily organs. Long-term stress can be a contributing factor in heart disease, high blood pressure, stroke and other illnesses. The Japanese phenomenon of Karoshi, or death from overwork, is

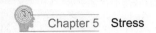

believed to be due to heart attack and stroke caused by high levels of stress.

About the time of Selye's work, the gradual realization dawned that age-old if sometimes ill-defined concepts such as worry, conflict, tiredness, frustration, distress, overwork, pre-menstrual tension, over-focusing, confusion, mourning and fear could all come together in a general broadening of the meaning of the term stress. The popular use of the term in modern folklore expanded rapidly, spawning an industry of self-help, personal counseling, and sometimes quackery.

The use of the term stress in serious recognized cases such as those of post-traumatic stress disorder and psychosomatic illness has scarcely helped clear analysis of the generalized "stress" phenomenon. Nonetheless, some varieties of stress from negative life events, or distress, and from positive life events, or eustress, can clearly have a serious physical impact distinct from the troubles of what psychotherapists call "the worried well".

1.1   Theoretical perspectives on stress

1.1.1   Fight or flight

This was one of the earliest theories on stress. It was described by Walter Cannon (1871—1945), and states that when the organism perceives a threat, the body is rapidly aroused and motivated, via the sympathetic nervous system, and the endocrine system. This concerted physiological response mobilizes the organism to attack the threat, or to flee. This response to the threat is called, Fight or Flight response. For Cannon, the Fight or Flight response is adaptive. However, the stress can be harmful to the organism due to the emotional and physiological disruption it can cause.

1.1.2   General adaptation syndrome

Hans Selye (1956, 1976) worked on rats and was surprised that all stressors, regardless of type, produced essentially the same pattern of physiological response. Selye found that all stressors led to an enlarged adrenal cortex, shrinking of the thymus and lymph glands, and ulceration of the stomach and duodenum. From that observation, Selye developed the general adaptation syndrome (GAS) concept of stress. Selye's model explains the short term effects of exposure to stressors, and accounts for the long term implications of prolonged exposure to stress. GAS consists of three phases, or stages, that illustrate the general response of the body to stress. They are: Alarm Reaction, Resistance and Exhaustion. When the body perceives the stressors as the alarm, it prepares to action, bring a brief period of arousal to physical damage. The body prepares then to cope with the stressor by using up available energy and protective stress hormones to defense, and then it returns to normal state. However, if the stressor persists, the resistance level increases beyond normal. Stress hormones are secreted at high doses and allow the body to cope with stress (phase of resistance). Certain physiological changes such as rapid heartbeat, increased blood pressure, and secretion of adrenaline are noted in this phase. Then the stressors no longer exist, the body ceases to resist. After prolonged stress, the system resources become depleted; the body fails to overcome the threat and has no more physiological resources for trying, it will face the adrenaline exhaustion and immune system weakened. This is called the Stage of Exhaustion.

1.1.3   Lazarus's model

No significant difference exists between the models of Lazarus and Seyle. By working more with humans Lazarus came to the conclusion that neither the stressor, nor the response could define stress. Rather, it was individual's perception and appraisal of the stressor that would determine if it would create stress. He realized that different people under the same situation experience different kinds of stress, whether positive or negative.

1.1.4 Tend-and-befriend

Taylor and colleagues (2000) developed a theory stress response called "tend-and-be friend." This theory is especially characteristic of females. It states that normal sympathetic arousal, thought to underlie the fight-or-flight response to stress, may be down regulated in females in ways that lead to social and nurturing behavior.

1.2 Concept of stress in psychology

Stress problems are very common. The American Psychological Association's 2007 "Stress in America" poll found that one-third of people in the United States report experiencing extreme levels of negative stress. In addition, nearly one out of five people report that they are experiencing high levels of negative stress 15 or more days per month. Impressive as these figures are, they represent only a cross-section of people's stress levels at one particular moment of their lives. When stress is considered as something that occurs repeatedly across the full lifespan, the true incidence of stress problems is much higher. Being "stressed out" is thus a universal human phenomenon that affects almost everyone.

What are we talking about when we discuss stress? Generally, most people use the word stress to refer to negative experiences that leave us feeling overwhelmed. Thinking about stress exclusively as something negative gives us a false impression of its true nature, however. Stress is a reaction to a changing, demanding environment. Properly considered, stress is really more about our capacity to handle change than it is about whether that change makes us feel good or bad. Change happens all the time, and stress is in large part what we feel when we are reacting to it.

We can define stress by saying that it involves the "set of emotional, physical, and cognitive (i.e., thought) reactions to a change." Thinking about stress as a reaction to change suggests that it is not necessarily bad, and sometimes, could even be a good thing. Some life changes such as getting a new job, moving in with a new romantic partner, or studying to master a new skill are generally considered positive and life-enhancing events, even though they can also be quite stressful. Other life changes such as losing a job or an important relationship are more negative, and also stressful.

Our experience of stress varies in intensity between high and low. How intensely stressed we feel in response to a particular event has to do with how much we need to accomplish in order to meet the demands of that situation. When we do not have to do much in order to keep up with demands, we do not experience much stress. Conversely, when we have to do a lot, we tend to feel much more stressed out.

Generally speaking, people do not like experiencing the extremes of stress. This is true for each end of the spectrum of stress intensity, both high and low. Few people enjoy the feeling of being overwhelmingly stressed in the face of great change. However, most people do not like a total absence of stress either, at least after a while. There is a word for such a condition (i.e., a lack of stress and challenge) that conveys this negative meaning: boredom. What most people tend to seek is the middle ground; a balance between a lack of stress and too much stress. They want a little challenge and excitement in life, but not so much that they feel overwhelmed by it.

A variety of events and environmental demands cause us to experience stress, including: routine hassles (such as getting the family out the door in the morning, or dealing with a difficult co-worker), one-time events that alter our lives (such as moving, marriage, childbirth, or changing jobs), and ongoing long-term demands (such as dealing with a chronic disease, or caring for a child or sick family member). Though different people may experience the same type of events, each of them will experience that event in a unique way. That is, some people are more vulnerable to becoming stressed out than others are in any given situation. An event like getting stuck in traffic might cause one person to become very stressed out while it might not affect another person much at all. Even "good" stressors such as getting married can impact individuals differently. Some

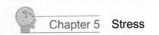

people become highly anxious while others remain calm and composed.

How vulnerable you are personally to becoming stressed out depends on a variety of factors, including your biological makeup; your perception of your ability to cope with challenges; characteristics of the stressful event (e.g., the "stressor") such as its intensity, timing, and duration; and your command of stress management skills. While some of these factors (such as your genetics and often, the characteristics of the stressor itself) are not under your direct control, some of the other factors are.

The term stress includes three related elements: stressors, stress responses, and genetic and environmental factors that modulate the effect of stressors on the organism. Stressors are events, physical or psychological, that profoundly interferes with the organism's normal steady state. These disruptions generate a stress response manifested at the physiological (e.g., activation of the sympathetic nervous system), psychological (e.g., anxiety, depression), and behavioral (e.g., performance deficits) levels. Factors that modulate the stress response include, among others, genetic predisposition to stress reactivity and predictability and controllability of the stressors.

2. Stressors

A stressor is a chemical or biological agent, environmental condition, external stimulus or an event that causes stress to an organism.

Stressors have physical, chemical and mental responses inside of the body. Physical stressors produce mechanical stresses on skin, bones, ligaments, tendons, muscles and nerves that cause tissue deformation and in extreme cases tissue failure. Chemical stresses also produce biomechanical responses associated with metabolism and tissue repair. Physical stressors may produce pain and impair work performance. Chronic pain and impairment requiring medical attention may result from extreme physical stressors or if there is not sufficient recovery time between successive exposures.

An event that triggers the stress response may include:

(1) Environmental stressors (hypo or hyper-thermic temperatures, elevated sound levels, over-illumination, overcrowding).

(2) Daily stress events (e.g., traffic, lost keys, quality and quantity of physical activity).

(3) Life changes (e.g., divorce, bereavement).

(4) Workplace stressors (e.g., high job demand vs. low job control, repeated or sustained exertions, forceful exertions, extreme postures).

(5) Chemical stressors (e.g., tobacco, alcohol, drugs).

(6) Social stressor (e.g., societal and family demands).

We mentioned it earlier and it bears repeating: stress is not always a bad thing. Stress is simply body's response to changes that create taxing demands. The previously mentioned Dr. Lazarus (building on Dr. Selye's work) suggested that there is a difference between eustress, which is a term for positive stress, and distress, which refers to negative stress.

2.1 Eustress vs. distress

Eustress, or positive stress, has the following characteristics: motivates, focuses energy; is short-term; is perceived as within our coping abilities; feels exciting; improves performance.

In contrast, distress, or negative stress, has the following characteristics: causes anxiety or concern; can be short- or long-term; is perceived as outside of our coping abilities; feels unpleasant; decreases performance; can lead to mental and physical problems.

Examples of Eustress and Distress:

It is somewhat hard to categorize stressors into objective lists of those that cause eustress and those that cause distress, because different people will have different reactions to particular situations. However, by generalizing, we can compile a list of stressors that are typically experienced as negative or positive to most people, most of the time.

(1) Examples of negative personal stressors include: 1) the death of a spouse; 2) filing for divorce; 3) losing contact with loved ones; 4) the death of a family member; 5) hospitalization (oneself or a family member); 6) injury or illness (oneself or a family member); 7) being abused or neglected; 8) separation from a spouse or committed relationship partner; 9) conflict in interpersonal relationships. 10) bankruptcy/money problems; 11) unemployment; 12) sleep problems; 13) children's problems at school; 14) Legal problems.

(2) Examples of positive personal stressors include: 1) receiving a promotion or raise at work; 2) starting a new job; 3) marriage; 4) buying a home; 5) having a child; 6) moving; 7) taking a vacation; 8) holiday seasons; 9) retiring; 10) taking educational classes or learning a new hobby; 11) work and internal sources of distress.

(3) Work and employment concerns such as those listed below are also frequent causes of distress: 1) excessive job demands; 2) job insecurity; 3) conflicts with teammates and supervisors; 4) inadequate authority necessary to carry out tasks; 5) lack of training necessary to do the job; 6) making presentations in front of colleagues or patients; 7) unproductive and time-consuming meetings; 8) commuting and travel schedules.

Stressors are not always limited to situations where some external situation is creating a problem. Internal events such as feelings and thoughts and habitual behaviors can also cause negative stress.

(4) Common internally caused sources of distress include: 1) fears (e.g., fears of flying, heights, public speaking, chatting with strangers at a party); 2) repetitive thought patterns; 3) worrying about future events (e.g., waiting for medical test results or job restructuring); 4) unrealistic, perfectionist expectations.

(5) Habitual behavior patterns that can lead to distress include: 1) over scheduling; 2) failing to be assertive; 3) procrastination and failing or both to plan ahead.

2.2　Acute vs. episodic vs. chronic stresses

For a better understanding of stress and its influence to an individual, psychologists categorize stress into three different types: acute stress, episodic stress, and chronic stress. In this section, we will discover the characteristics and attributes of each type of stress.

2.2.1　Acute stress

Of all forms of stress, acute stress is the most widely experienced one, since it typically is caused by the daily demands and pressures encountered by each one of us. While the word "stress" connotes a negative impression, acute stress is what actually brings about excitement, joy and thrill in our lives. Riding a roller coaster in a theme park, for instance, is a situation that brings about acute stress, yet brings excitement. However, riding a higher and longer roller coaster can bring so much stress that you wish it would end sooner, or that you should have not gone for the ride in the first place. When the long and windy ride is over, you might feel the effects of too much acute stress, such as vomiting, tension headaches, and other psychological and physiological or both symptoms.

Because acute stress occurs only at a very short period of time, these symptoms might only come out when the stress has already accumulated:

(1) Emotional distress, such as anger, anxiety, irritability, and acute periods of depression.

(2) Physical problems, such as headache, pain, stomach upset, dizziness, heart palpitations, shortness of breath, hypertension and bowel disorders.

like yourself, not feeling like things are real, and a sense of being out of control/not being in control), and perceptual stress (beliefs, roles, stories, attitudes, world view).

2.3.3 Psychosocial stress

Psychosocial stress: relationship/marriage difficulties (partner, siblings, children, family, employer, co-workers, employer), lack of social support, lack of resources for adequate survival, loss of employment/ investments/savings, loss of loved ones, bankruptcy, home foreclosure, and isolation.

2.3.4 Psycho-spiritual stress

Psycho-spiritual stress: A crisis of values, meaning, and purpose; joyless striving (instead of productive, satisfying, meaningful and fulfilling work); and a misalignment within one's core spiritual beliefs.

Overall, improperly or ineffectively managed stress usually takes a toll on the body. When stress-related feelings, moods, emotions are pushed into the body, the soma, this is usually termed psychosomatic or psychogenic illness, including headaches, heart palpitations, physical/cognitive/emotional pain and suffering, constricted throat and shallow, constricted breathing, clammy palms, fatigue, nausea, anxiety, allergies, asthma, autoimmune syndromes related to an ineffective functioning of the immune system, hypertension (high blood pressure), and gastrointestinal disturbances such as diarrhea, upset stomach, duodenal ulcers and esophageal reflux syndrome.

Prolonged stress can result in suppressed immune function, increased susceptibility to infectious and immune-related diseases and cancer. Emotional stress can also result in hormonal imbalances (adrenal, pituitary, thyroid, and etcetera) that further interfere with healthy immune functioning.

2.4 Five categories of stress

Stress is usually thought of as psychological. But there are many different types, which can be divided into the five categories of stress: mental, physical, emotional, nutritional, and toxic. I have developed these general categories to help my patients better understand the various stressors in their lives. The body undergoes stress anytime it encounters a challenge that is not easily overcome. What types of challenges and stressors do we commonly face?

2.4.1 Mental

Mental stressors are those in which the thought process provokes the stress response. Of all five categories of stress, this is the category that people most commonly think of. When I ask patients and friends about the sources of stress in their lives, most reply that work is their biggest stressor. This makes sense, because sustained mental focus and effort is obviously challenging, particularly in a competitive environment. Similarly, school can be a source of mental stress due to the demands of problem solving and creative thought production, especially when you are being graded on your performance. But work and school are not the only mental stressors. Other worries, like relationships with others, communication, and self-presentation are common examples. Thoughts like "What should I do for my birthday this weekend?" or "What if she does not like what I am wearing?" or "I hope I say the right thing!" are all expressions of mental stress.

2.4.2 Physical

Technically, all stress fits into this category, as stress is measured by physical changes in the body. However, the physical category specifically refers to challenges like lifting heavy objects, hiking up a hill, and other forms of exercise. Another example is sustaining an injury such as a broken bone or cut. These events require an immediate increase in energy, and they have an obvious beginning, middle, and end.

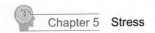

2.4.3　Emotional

It is important to separate emotional challenges from mental ones. Emotional processing occurs in a different, more primitive part of the brain. The emotional brain precedes the cognitive portion of the brain in the signal chain. If the emotional brain perceives a threat, it will trigger the fight or flight response before you even have a chance to think. Examples of emotionally challenging events are experiencing the death of a loved one, witnessing violence, or even watching a horror film. There is a blurry line between mental and emotional stress, as the most exaggerated and common mental stress occurs when there is anticipation of an outcome that could represent success or failure—and this is when it becomes a thought-induced emotional stress.

2.4.4　Nutritional

Nutritional stress is a more complex category. Out of all five categories of stress, it is one of the most important to understand because diet and nutrition have such a huge impact on health. A nutritional challenge can be in the form of a missed meal or insufficient intake of calories. It can also be a deficiency of a specific nutrient, such as protein or certain vitamins and minerals. A third possibility is that the foods you consume are difficult to break down and thus create a demand on your body which exceeds the available energy for digestion. The end result in all cases is an interruption in the material necessary to balance the demand placed on the body and to maintain function. To help reduce nutritional stress, I recommend a diet that is high in fruits and whole foods.

2.4.5　Toxic

A good example of a toxic stressor is the ingestion of or environmental exposure to a poison, such as arsenic or snake venom. The body will have a certain ability to resist the poison. But if the poison level exceeds your threshold of tolerance, it will become stressful and require significant action from body's immune and detoxification systems. Other substances that fit into this category are parasites, irritating portions of foods, microorganisms, and byproducts of bacteria and viruses. Even some of the byproducts of your own metabolism and bodily functions are toxic, such as lactic acid and nitric oxide.

3.　Mediating mechanism of stress

3.1　Physiological mediating mechanism of stress

The first person to study stress scientifically was a physiologist named Hans Selye. Dr. Selye spent many years studying the physical reactions of animals to injury and disease. Based on his research, Selye concluded that human beings and animals share a specific and consistent pattern of physiological responses to illness or injury. These changes represent our body's attempt to cope with the demands imposed by the illness or injury process.

Stage 1: Recognition of environmental demand

Every event in the environment, from the weather to the ringing telephone, has some sort of impact on us. Some of these events are predictable. For instance, the rent/mortgage payment will be due on the first of the month. You'll be expected to make small talk if you go to a party. Others are entirely unpredictable. It is hard to know when the baby will suddenly wake up sick and cannot go to daycare, when another driver will cut you off in traffic, or when you will spill coffee on your new pants. Regardless of whether we can predict an event or not, the instant we become aware of that event taking place, we have recognized a demand.

Stage 2: Appraisal of the demand

Understanding that a demand has occurred does not automatically cause us to experience stress. In over 30 years of research, psychologists Richard Lazarus and Susan Folkman found that it is our lightening fast, and largely unconscious and automatic appraisal or judgment of our ability to meet the demand that determines just how stressful we will experience it to be. The appraisal process partially explains why a particular event may be negatively stressful to one person but not to another.

We appraise a demand by asking ourselves two questions: 1) Does this event present a threat to me? 2) Do I have the resources to cope with this event? If we come to believe that the event is a threat to our well-being, or if we come to believe that we lack the means to effectively respond to the event, we then subsequently feel stressed. We will return to a more detailed discussion of the appraisal stage in a later section of this document.

Stage 3: Mobilization of the nervous system

To understand what happens at this stage, you need to know a little bit about the functioning of the human nervous system. The autonomic nervous system (ANS), controls all of the automatic functions in our body. For example, your heartbeat, our body temperature, rate of breathing and digestion are all regulated by the ANS.

If we appraise an event as threatening, one branch of the ANS called the sympathetic nervous system (SyNS) automatically signals our body to prepare for action. During this mobilization phase, the SyNS prepares us for fighting or fleeing (two primary biologically driven and useful means of reacting to a physical threat) by triggering or activating the hypothalamic-pituitary-adrenal axis (HPA) (sometimes called the brain's "stress circuit"). The HPA axis involves a complex set of interactions between multiple parts of the brain and nervous system, including the hypothalamus, the pituitary gland, and the adrenal glands. This system controls body's reactions to stress, and also handles a few other vital functions such as regulating digestion, the immune system, mood, sexual behavior, and body's overall energy usage.

In response to a stressor, the hypothalamus (which is a centrally located part of the brain that sits above the brain stem, but below the cortex) releases corticotropin-releasing hormone (CRH). In turn, CRH acts on the pituitary gland, triggering the release of another hormone called adrenocorticotropin (ACTH) into the bloodstream. Next, ACTH triggers the adrenal glands (which are situated above the kidneys), to release the hormones cortisol and cortisone as well as epinephrine (otherwise known as adrenaline) and norepinephrine (otherwise known as noradrenaline). Both epinephrine and norepinephrine are neurotransmitters or chemical messengers that serve the brain and nervous system. Hormones are also chemical messengers, but they work primarily within the blood stream, rather than inside the brain.

The presence of cortisol works to immediately increase the amount of energy the body has available by raising glucose levels in the bloodstream. Glucose is a variety of sugar, which is body's primary fuel. Cortisol also increases levels of glucose within the brain, which helps to sharpen our attention and quicken our thinking process (just like stepping on the gas in a car causes more fuel to go into the engine, causing it to produce more power). At the same time cortisol dumps fuel into the body, it also functions to shut down body systems which are not immediately important for handling a physical threat, such as digestion, reproduction, and growth. This mobilizing effect of cortisol is generally temporary in nature, because in addition to everything else it does, cortisol tells the hypothalamus to gradually slow down production of CRH.

Similar to cortisol, elevated levels of epinephrine and norepinephrine increase your heart rate, elevate your blood pressure, speed up your reaction time, and boost your energy level. Under the combined effects of cortisol, epinephrine, and norepinephrine, the body diverts blood away from digestion and towards the muscles and the brain (to enhance physical functioning); increases oxygen levels in the blood (for an energy boost); increases the rate of perspiration (to help cool us down); releases blood clotting chemicals into the blood stream (in case of injury); and dilates the pupils (to help us see better in the dark). At the same time that cortisol and epinephrine exert their effects, both the pituitary gland (see below) and the brain are also busy releasing chemicals called endorphins and enkephalins which help relieve pain and enhance a sense of well-being.

Stage 4: Response to the threat

Once your body has been prepared for action by the various hormones and neurotransmitters described in Stage 3 (above), you are ready to respond to the stressor by taking physical action. Physiologists call what happens next the "fight-or-flight" response to highlight the two most common forms that this physical response tends to take. When we fight, we try to influence or neutralize the source of stress by striking out at it. Alternatively, we can flee and reduce our stress by escaping from the place where the stress is occurring, leaving the fighting for another day. Psychologists who conduct research on stress often add a third response possibility to the classic fight and flight options. Sometimes, rather than fighting or fleeing, we simply freeze instead. In many sports, this response is called "choking."

The fight-or-flight response is automatic and fast, which was helpful to our ancestors because it provided them with automatic responses to threats when they did not have time to think logically about how best to handle a situation. Remember that herd of charging buffalo? Spending a long time debating the dangers of and potential responses to such a situation would probably be fatal. When faced with such an intensely physical threat, either fighting or fleeing as quickly as possible made the most sense in terms of survival.

The fight or flight response is optimized for responding to physical threats. It is not very useful with the sort of intangible threats that are most common in today's world. It is never appropriate to punch your boss in the face, for instance, no matter how many times he piles work on you, or passes you over for a raise. Fleeing your workplace will not necessarily help you either, as you still need to get a paycheck!

Stage 5: Return to baseline

Once a stressor has been neutralized (or has been avoided successfully), the parasympathetic nervous system (PaNS; the other branch of the ANS besides the SyNS), starts to undo the stress response by sending out new signals telling your body to calm down. The PaNS slows your heartbeat and breathing, causes your muscles to relax, and gets your digestive juices flowing again. The PaNS system is designed to promote growth, energy storage and other processes important for long-term survival.

The speeding up and slowing down activity is a characteristic of the stress response, is controlled by a gland in your brain called the hypothalamus. The main job of the hypothalamus is to maintain the homeostasis (i.e., the set-point) of important body systems including blood pressure, body temperature, fluid balance, body weight, sexual activity, sleep/wakefulness, and emotions. The hypothalamus is like a thermostat that receives inputs from other parts of the brain and body about body's internal environment. If body functions are out of balance, the hypothalamus sends messages to the ANS and to the pituitary gland to speed up or slow down relevant glands and organs to bring the body back into balance at the set-point appropriate to each system. The pituitary gland, sometimes referred to as the "master gland", secretes hormones that are responsible for the regulation of all other endocrine glands (glands that secrete hormones directly into the blood) in the body.

Some of the hormones secreted by the hypothalamus and pituitary gland stimulate the limbic system, a complex collection of sub-cortical brain structures that control emotions, motivation, and the formation of long-term memories. The limbic system is heavily interconnected with the brain's frontal cortex, which is the part of the brain that controls judgment, attention, and decision-making. The limbic system and the frontal lobes work together to make possible the appraisals or judgments regarding whether or not a stressor is dangerous or exceeds our coping ability that were described above in the section concerning Stage 2. The combined limbic/frontal system also influences whether we fight, flee, or freeze in the presence of a stressor.

3.2　Psychological mediating mechanism of stress

3.2.1　Arousal vs. anxiety

The mobilization of our stress response involves the integration of multiple organs and glands controlling both the nervous and endocrine systems. Ideally, these systems communicate and coordinate to make sure that our bodies are aroused enough to effectively deal with challenges but not so aroused that we become hyper-aroused or otherwise experience incapacitating anxiety. However, this balancing act is a tricky business, and the body and brain do not always get it right.

Physiological arousal is necessary to prime our bodies for taking action. As we become more aroused in response to stressors, our alertness increases and our attention sharpens. We become increasingly focused on the stressor itself, while other aspects of the environment fade into the background. A narrowed focus of attention towards a threat is typically adaptive, as it allows us to quickly eliminate some of the available responses we might otherwise make. This decreases the likelihood that we will become overwhelmed by choices at a critical time, and allows us (ideally) to choose the best option. For instance, we can quickly move from six possible choices (which could take a substantial amount of time to sort through in our minds) to two (fight or flee). On the other hand, too much arousal may narrow our focus so drastically that we overlook the best options.

It is helpful to visualize the relationship between our level of arousal and our subsequent performance as the upside-down "U" shaped curve attributable to research performed by psychologists Robert Yerkes and J. D. Dodson (often called the "Yerkes-Dodson Curve"). Increasing levels of arousal initially improve performance, but there quickly comes a point of diminishing returns. At high levels of stress, performance ability declines dramatically.

Arousal levels are influenced by multiple factors, including: the amount of mental energy a demand requires, our baseline level of anxiety (e.g., how anxious we are in general; sometimes referred to as our level of "trait" anxiety), and our level of anticipatory anxiety (how worried we are in advance of an upcoming event).

Stressful activities that require more concentration will seem overwhelming much sooner than activities we are skilled at and can do without almost automatically. In sports, for example, running is considered a relatively simple activity because it normally does not require much conscious thought. Stress seems to improve running performance for a long period of time before a decline sets in. Other activities, like swinging a golf club, are more complex because they require a good deal of conscious thought. In this case, stress results in a much earlier decline in performance.

3.2.2　Primary and secondary appraisal

Dr. Lazarus and Dr. Folkman described the importance of the cognitive appraisal process in determining whether stress is positive or negative. According to Lazarus and Folkman, there are two aspects to cognitive appraisal: primary appraisal and secondary appraisal.

In primary appraisal, we evaluate whether we have anything at stake in an encounter (e.g., by asking ourselves "Does this matter for me?"). A stressor that is perceived as important is more likely to cause a stress reaction than a stressor that is viewed as relatively trivial.

In secondary appraisal, we evaluate our existing coping resources (e.g., how healthy we are, how much energy we have, whether family and friends can help, our ability to rise to the challenge, and how much money or equipment we have), our available options, and the possibilities we have for controlling our situation. If we believe that we lack the coping resources necessary to deal with the situation, we will perceive it as negative

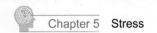

stress. Conversely, if we believe that we have the necessary coping resources, the stressor will not overwhelm us and may instead be perceived as eustress. For example, an adolescent girl with limited social and financial support might view being pregnant as a negative stress, while a middle-aged woman with adequate financial and social support might see pregnancy as an exciting and hopeful time.

3.2.3 Appraisals influence how you feel: the cognitive model

According to the highly influential and widely accepted cognitive theory of emotions, based on the seminal work of Dr. Albert Ellis and Dr. Aaron Beck, your beliefs (driven by your appraisal process) strongly influence your subsequent mood state. If you believe that you have the ability and resources to handle the stressors you are faced with, your mood will be generally positive, and vice versa, if you believe that you do not have what it takes to meet the demands you are faced with, your mood will turn negative and sour, possibly causing you to become anxious or depressed.

That your thoughts determine your mood is a good thing, because while it is difficult to alter your feelings at any given moment, it is always possible to re-evaluate and change your thoughts. If you can find a way to see your situation in a more positive light, you can alter your mood from negative to positive. This insight has been incorporated into a therapeutic technique called Cognitive Reframing, which we will elaborate upon in greater detail later in this document.

As preparation for our later discussion of cognitive reframing, we can talk now about an easy way to visualize the process of how thoughts and beliefs that result from the appraisal process end up causing feelings to change. According to Dr. Ellis, the relationship between thoughts and emotion can be represented by the simple equation A+B=C.

In this equation, the letter "A" stands for an "Activating Event." Activating Events are the triggers or stressors that create demands on us and therefore cause us potential stress. As previously mentioned, there are different types of stressors, including life events and daily hassles.

The letter "B" in the equation stands for "Beliefs." We come into the world with no preconceived beliefs or opinions. From the moment we start interacting with the environment, we start to learn the opinions of our parents, our peers, schools, etc., and also start forming opinions of our own. All of these opinions eventually become internalized into a consistent (but often biased) worldview that we use as a measuring stick against which to interpret and appraise ourselves, other people, and the world around us. The degree of bias and rigidity in our belief system is important, because, as a general rule, the more biased and rigid our beliefs are, the more often we will find ourselves becoming stressed out. Beliefs, which are accurate, flexible and optimistic in nature, help to reduce stress, while beliefs, which are rigid, negative, inflexible and pessimistic, tend to exacerbate stress.

The final letter "C" in the A+B=C equation stands for "Consequences." Consequences refer to the feelings that occur as a result of our beliefs and self-talk in response to the activating event. The consequences we experience can include stress, anxiety, depression, anger, irritability, aggression, frustration, etc.

3.2.4 Self-efficacy

Dr. Albert Bandura, an influential social psychologist, coined the term "self-efficacy" to describe people's internal beliefs about their ability to have an impact on events that affect their lives. Your self-efficacy is your belief in your own effectiveness as a person, both generally in terms of managing your life, and specifically with regard to competently dealing with individual tasks. In the context of stress, self-efficacy describes your beliefs about your ability to handle stressful situations. A large amount of research has demonstrated quite convincingly that possessing high levels of self-efficacy acts to decrease people's potential for experiencing negative stress feelings by increasing their sense of being in control of the situations they encounter. The perception of being in control (rather than the reality of being in or out of control) is an important buffer of negative stress. When people feel that they are not in control, they start feeling stressed, even if they actually are in control and simply do not know it. Another reason that people feel stressed is when they feel out of control because they do not possess the appropriate coping skills, resources, etc. to adequately cope with the situation.

When a given demand (e.g., passing an exam, winning a race) is perceived as something you can handle because you expect you will do well based on preparation or past experience (e.g., because you have studied for the exam or trained for the race), you are likely to perceive the demand as a challenge and as an exhilarating experience. After the event is over, you may even have a resulting boost in self-esteem because you worked hard to meet the demand and succeeded. If, however, the demand seems beyond your abilities, you will likely experience distress. Across time, feeling unable to respond effectively to stressful situations can further decrease your sense of self-efficacy, making you even more prone to experience distress in the future.

3.2.5 Coping skills

A coping skill is a behavior or technique that helps a person to solve a problem or meet a demand. Coping skills are problem-solving techniques or tools; they make it possible to solve problems or meet demands more easily and efficiently than might otherwise be possible.

People who have learned a variety of different coping skills are able to handle demands and solve problems more easily and efficiently than people who are not as knowledgeable about how to cope. Because they are more easily able to meet demands, people with good coping skills are less likely to experience negative stress reactions than are people with more poorly developed coping skills. In addition, people with well-developed coping skills typically develop a higher sense of self-efficacy than do their peers who have poorer coping skills, and thus are less likely to suffer the negative impact of stress reactions.

Coping skills are something that can be learned. If you do not have good coping skills, you can study techniques that will allow you to get better at coping over time. All of the stress-reduction techniques that we will shortly be presenting in this document (in the sections below covering Stress Management and Stress Prevention strategies) can be thought of as coping skills. In essence, they are tools that you can learn and then "carry around" in your personal toolbox to help you become better at managing your stress.

3.2.6 Stressor characteristics

Coping skills, self-efficacy, and appraisal are all characteristics that people bring to a stressful circumstance. They are internal to the person, meaning that they "reside in" the person who needs to respond to an activating event, rather than being a characteristic of the event itself. In contrast to these internal ways that people may react to stress, there are also characteristics that are inherent to the stressful event itself which have little or nothing to do with appraisals or coping skills. These external aspects of stressful events, which are listed below, also influence people's ability to meet stressful demands.

Intensity has to do with the magnitude or strength of the stressful event. The actual intensity of a stressful event has a lot to do with the context in which that stressful event is taking place. A dead cell-phone battery is generally a fairly low-intensity stressor when you have alternative ways of communicating, and your actual need to communicate is currently low. When your need to communicate is high, however, and your options for doing so are limited (e.g., if you have been injured in a car accident on a remote highway and need to call for an ambulance), it is an entirely different story. In this later circumstance, the same stressor quickly gains in intensity and ability to cause negative stress.

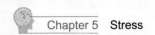

Duration has to do with how long the stressful event lasts. A short-term stressor such as a weekend houseguest will tend to cause less stress than a long-term stressor like needing to become the primary caretaker for an older relative.

Number has to do with the total quantity of stressors occurring in your life at once. A minor stressor might not be much when it occurs in isolation, but it can become a "straw that breaks the camel's back" when you are already coping with several other stressors at the same time.

Level of expertise has to do with how skilled you are in handling stressful situations. It is easier and less stressful to deal with situations and events when we are familiar with handling them. Practice with a particular kind of stress-provoking situation tends to make that situation easier to deal with. The more you practice a skill (e.g., such as playing an instrument, or rehearsing a presentation), the more automatically you can perform and the less stress you are likely to feel when an event requiring that skill occurs.

4. Stress response

People respond differently when exposed to the same stressor. Stress responses are physiological, emotional, and cognitive-behavioral, responses to an event perceived as relevant to one's well-being with some potential for harm or loss and requiring adaptation.

Within the physiological domain, two response systems are of particular importance: cardiovascular responses (indicated by blood pressure and heart rate), driven by sympathetic nervous system (SNS) activity, and output of the glucocorticoid hormone cortisol from the adrenal cortex, driven by HPA axis activity.

Emotional stress responses often include negative emotions, such as anxiety, distress, or anger, although positive emotional states related to feeling challenged and driven may also occur.

Cognitive stress responses often include rumination, distancing, paranoia, catastrophizing, flashback and intrusive memory, cognitive restructuring.

Behavioral stress responses involve actions also aimed at coping with or fleeing from the stressful event, such as actively performing a task or withdrawing effort from a situation perceived as impossible.

4.1 Physiological stress responses

Cannon proposed the "fight or flight response" as a major mechanism by which an organism responds to stress or danger. Selye subsequently expanded the definition of stress to include, "the nonspecific response of the body to any demand made upon it".

4.1.1 Stress-fight or flight response

Our body produces larger quantities of the chemicals cortisol, adrenaline and noradrenaline, which trigger a higher heart rate, heightened muscle preparedness, sweating, more rapid breathing and alertness-all these factors help us protect ourselves in a dangerous or challenging situation. Non-essential body functions slow down, such as our digestive and immune systems. All resources can then be concentrated on rapid breathing, blood flow, alertness and muscle use. The ultimate result is to quickly prime an organism for a fight-or—flight (Cannon, 1929), or freeze, response (Bracha and colleagues, 2004).

4.1.2 General adaptation syndrome theory

In the 1930s Hans Selye advanced the concept of the General Adaptation Syndrome known also as the "GAS" Theory (Selye, 1936). His theory is mainly to describe the release of hormones (glucocorticoids, GCs) from the adrenal cortex and their role in the stress response. In long term exposures to various stressors the physiological responses followed three stages: A. Alarm reaction (AR Stage); B. Stage of resistance (SR Stage); and C. Stage of exhaustion (SE Stage).

The fast AR stage involves a neural response of the autonomic sympathetic nervous system that leads to rapid secretion of adrenaline. SR stage leads to increased levels of cortisol and other corticosteroids changing the body metabolism. Long-term exposure to SE stage will eventually result in damage to body systems such as the digestive, immune, or kidney systems. Selye referred to the stress response as being nonspecific in nature. Although subsequent work would demonstrate that not all stressors result in the same physiological response (e.g., depending on factors such as type and source of stressor, duration, perception, and appraisal), Selye's invaluable contribution to the field was to pioneer the exploration of the relationship between GC physiology and stress.

4.2　Emotional response

Humans typically interpret stress with an emotional response. In response to a stressor, the sympathetic nervous system activation of visceral structures such as the heart, stomach, epidermis, and other organs generates physiological changes that may lead to a perception of an emotion (Heilman, 1994). This peripheral response is closely integrated with central nervous system components that are involved in the evaluation and regulation of emotion necessary for behavioral changes that allow an organism to adapt to the environment.

Sometimes, the stress is so strong and so powerful, that person's emotions change from that moment onward. Stress is one of the key contributing factors in increased risk of developing serious emotional conditions like anxiety and depression.

Anxiety is a feeling of nervousness, fear, apprehension, worry, or unease. It can occur in people who are unable to identify significant stressors in their life. Stress and anxiety are not always bad. In the short term, they can help you overcome a challenge or dangerous situation. However, if anxiety begins interfering with your daily life, it may indicate a more serious issue. Anxiety creates negative thinking. It is very likely that stress actually changes your brain chemistry, physical health, and your ability to cope with future issues, leading to the development of anxiety and an anxiety disorder or both. Some individuals with anxiety disorders have numerous physical complaints, such as headaches, gastrointestinal disturbances, dizziness, and chest pain.

Depression may sometimes be linked to chronic stress. Individuals with a high level of work-related stress are more than twice as likely to experience a major depressive episode, compared with people who are under less stress. Depression shares some of the symptoms of stress, including changes in appetite, sleep patterns, and concentration. Serious depression, however, is distinguished from stress by feelings of sadness, hopelessness, loss of interest in life, and, sometimes, thoughts of suicide.

There was a time when psychologists and other therapists believed that it was healthier to let angry feelings out. Various types of therapies taught patients to punch pillows while expressing pent up feelings from both the present and past. The theory was that unexpressed and pent up anger causes depression. In actuality, "letting it all out" adds to stress, promotes more anger and does nothing to relieve feelings of depression.

4.3　Cognitive responses

4.3.1　Rumination

Rumination is a cognitive response to a stressor, involving repetitive fixation on an individual's own problems, thoughts, emotions, actions, or past events (Nolen-Hoeksema, 1991). Rumination is associated with heightened self-criticism and self-blame as well as the amplification of shame, making it difficult for individuals to disengage from negative emotion (LeMoult et al., 2011). Adolescents who tend to ruminate in

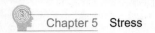

stress are more likely to be depressed and substance abusers.

4.3.2 Distancing

When attempting not to think about something distressing, the easiest alternative is likely to think about something else—that is, to be distracted. For those with a tendency to ruminate on distressing incidents distractions can be a key to recovering mentally and physically. The benefits of cognitive distancing, then or at least the prevention of cognitive fixation will come.

4.3.3 Paranoia

Stress and emotional arousal aggravate cognitive biases leading a direct increase of paranoia. Symptoms of paranoia include intense and irrational mistrust or suspicion, which can bring on sense of fear, anger, and betrayal. Some identifiable beliefs and behaviors of individuals with symptoms of paranoia include mistrust, hypervigilance, difficulty with forgiveness, defensive attitude in response to imagined criticism, preoccupation with hidden motives, fear of being deceived or taken advantage of, inability to relax, or are argumentative.

4.3.4 Catastrophizing

Catastrophizing is an irrational thought a lot of us have in believing that something is far worse than it actually is. Catastrophizing generally can take two forms.

The first of these is making a catastrophe out of a situation. In reality, it may only be a temporary situation, and there are things that you can do to change this situation.

The second kind of Catastrophizing is closely linked to the first, but it is more mental and more future oriented. This kind of Catastrophizing occurs when individuals look to the future and anticipate all the things that are going to go wrong.

Both of these types of Catastrophizing limit your opportunities in life, work, relationships and more. It can affect our entire outlook in life, and create a self-fulfilling prophecy of failure, disappointment and underachievement. It may lead you to self-pity, to an irrational, negative belief about the situation, and to a feeling of hopelessness about your future prospects.

4.3.5 Flashback and intrusive memory

Both flashbacks and intrusive memories are related to reliving a traumatic event. In a flashback, the person is actually reliving the memory and thinks they are back in the original traumatic situation. In a sense, s/he has touch with their current situation but is stuck in the past. During an intrusive memory, the person knows where and when they are, but the memory is so powerful and keeps intruding in their mind. It is the classic symptom of post-traumatic stress disorder.

4.3.6 Cognitive restructuring

There is plenty of solid evidence that how we think about what is going on in our lives can greatly contribute to whether or not we find events in our lives stressful. Cognitive distortions, or patterns of faulty thinking, can impact our thoughts, behaviors and experience of stress. Our self-talk, the internal dialogue that runs in our heads, interpreting, explaining and judging the situations we encounter, can actually make things seem better or worse, threatening or non-threatening, stressful or…well, you get the picture. Some people tend to see things in a more positive light, and others tend to view things more negatively, putting themselves at a disadvantage in life. Cognitive restructuring, a process of recognizing, challenging, and changing cognitive distortions and negative thought patterns can be accomplished with the help of other people.

4.4   Behavioral responses

4.4.1   Positive behavioral response

Positive behavioral response to a stressor is a highly adaptive, proactive, problem-focused response that is called "facing the problem head on", dealing with the negative emotions experienced by stress in a constructive manner.

Positive behavioral response includes seeking social support and using catharsis, humor and other emotional mitigation strategies. It keeps the individual away from great stress, allows distressing emotions or impulses to have a socially acceptable outlet, and redirects thoughts (cognitive energy) to good things that are either occurring or have not occurred.

New studies by scientists at the University of Southern California have found that while stress may result in a universal physiological "fight or flight response" there are gender differences in psychological and behavioral responses. Women tend to seek out, befriend and bond with other people when they are under threat or stress, whereas men generally do not. Women's enhanced abilities to gauge facial expressions and respond to them could partly underlie their tend and befriend reaction to stressful situations.

4.4.2   Negative adaptations to stress

(1) Avoidance and escape

Avoidance and escape is a maladaptive coping mechanism characterized by the effort to avoid dealing with a stressor, including drawing into oneself (avoiding relationships or social activities) and fearing commitment due to a fear of rejection. Post-traumatic stress disorder symptoms are thought to be precursors to avoidance coping.

(2) Regression

Regression is the act of returning to an earlier condition that is worse or less developed. It is a form of retreat involves taking the position of a child in some problematic situation, rather than acting in a more adult way. This is usually in response to stressful situations, with greater levels of stress potentially leading to more overt regressive acts. In a Freudian view, the stress of fixations caused by frustrations of person's past psychosexual development may be used to explain a range of regressive behaviors.

(3) Hostile and aggressive

Stress can lead to hostile and aggressive behavioral reactions. Hostility is a negative cynical attitude toward others, with a propensity for anger or aggression. Aggression is overt, often harmful, social interaction with the intention of inflicting damage or other unpleasantness upon another individual.

(4) Self pity

Self-pity is a depressing situation to be in. Feeling pity for the way you are, the kind of person you are, your life, your circumstances. Some negative fallouts of self-pity are, a general sense of negativism about yourself, lack of motivation and enthusiasm towards life, feeling of depression, feeling frustrated and helpless as you are not able to resolve the situation, suffering from poor confidence when it comes to social interaction, feeling guilty when there is absolutely no need for it.

(5) Abuse

Experiencing stressful life events is reciprocally associated with substance use and abuse. One of the ways that the individual may attempt to manage their stress is by using alcohol or drugs. Alcohol or drugs produce

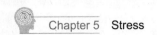

a calming effect on the body, and so the individual will feel like they have escaped their difficulties. This type of self-medication can provide temporary relief, but is ultimately self-defeating.

5. The medical consequences of stress

Stressors can also be defined as short-term (acute) or long-term (chronic). Acute stress is the reaction to an immediate threat. The threat can be any situation that is perceived, even subconsciously or falsely, as a danger. Acute stress leads to rapid changes throughout the body. Almost all body systems (the heart and blood vessels, immune system, lungs, digestive system, sensory organs, and brain) are geared up to meet the perceived danger. Under most circumstances, once the acute threat has passed, levels of stress hormones return to normal. This is called the relaxation response.

Frequently, modern life exposes people to long-term stressful situations. Stress, then, becomes chronic. Common chronic stressors include: Ongoing work pressure, long-term relationship problems, loneliness, and persistent financial worries.

5.1   The Brain

In response to acute Stress, a part of the brain called the hypothalamic-pituitary- adrenal (HPA) system is activated. The HPA systems trigger the production and release of steroid hormones (glucocorticoids), including the primary stress hormone cortisol. The HPA system also releases certain neurotransmitters (chemical messengers) called catecholamines, particularly those known as dopamine, norepinephrine, and epinephrine (also called adrenaline). Catecholamines activate an area inside the brain called the amygdala, which appears to trigger an emotional response to a stressful event. The brain releases neuropeptide S, a small protein that modulates stress by decreasing sleep and increasing alertness and a sense of anxiety. This gives the person a sense of urgency to run away.

During the stressful event, catecholamines also suppress activity in areas at the front of the brain concerned with short-term memory, concentration, inhibition, and rational thought. It also interferes with the ability to handle difficult social or intellectual tasks and behaviors during that time. At the same time, neurotransmitters signal the hippocampus to store the emotionally loaded experience in long-term memory. Long-lasting memories of dangerous stimuli would be critical for avoiding such threats in the future.

5.2   The heart, lungs, and others

The stress response also affects the heart, lungs, and circulation: the heart rate and blood pressure increase instantaneously. Breathing becomes rapid, and the lungs take in more oxygen. The spleen discharges red and white blood cells, allowing the blood to transport more oxygen throughout the body. Blood flow may actually increase 300% to 400%, priming the muscles, lungs, and brain for added demands.

The steroid hormones reduce activity in parts of the immune system, so that specific infection fighters (including important white blood cells) or other immune molecules can be repositioned. These immune-boosting troops are sent to body's front lines where injury or infection is most likely to occur, such as the skin and the lymph nodes. People who carry the herpes virus may be more susceptible to viral activation after they are exposed to stress.

Stress can cause spasms of the throat muscles, making it difficult to swallow and talk. The stress effect moves blood flow away from the skin to support the heart and muscle tissues. The physical effect is cool, clammy, sweaty skin. The scalp also tightens so that the hair seems to stand up.

5.3　Psychological disorders caused by stress

DSM-5 responded to stress events into many groups, include adjustment disorders, posttraumatic stress disorder, acute stress disorder, and other stress and related disorders.

5.3.1　Adjustment disorders

An adjustment disorder is defined as a transient maladaptive or pathological reaction to identifiable stressors or changes in life circumstances with symptoms emerging within three months of the onset of the stressor, according to DSM-5 and ICD-10. Adjustment disorders are triggered by serious, but nontraumatic, stressors, which usually are severe life events. The stressors can either be acute (e.g., loss of work, break-up of a romantic relationship, trouble with a family member), chronic (e.g., financial burden, family or occupational problems), recurring (e.g., seasonal economic slumps), or continuous (e.g., living in a criminal environment). Adjustment disorder symptom criteria include various types of behavioral symptoms, which are manifested far beyond the expected magnitude when confronted with such a burdensome event. In addition, the disorder leads to significant social, occupational, or academic performance-related impairments. The ensuing anxiety and depression can result in severe life disruption and have serious consequences such as substance abuse and suicide potential. The distinction between adjustment disorder and a normal stress response is based on the severity and the duration of symptoms or impairments.

5.3.2　Post-traumatic stress disorder symptoms

Post-traumatic stress disorder (PTSD) is a reaction to a very traumatic. The event that brings on PTSD is usually outside the norm of human experience, such as intense combat or sexual assault. Normally, symptoms occur soon after the trauma and usually get better in three months. However, some people have a longer-term form of PTSD, which can last for many years. People who experience interpersonal trauma (for example rape or child abuse) are more likely to develop PTSD, as compared to people who experience non-assault based trauma such as accidents and natural disasters. About half of people develop PTSD following rape.

The DSM-5 lists four major symptom clusters for PTSD:

Re-experiencing the event—For example, spontaneous memories of the traumatic event, recurrent dreams related to it, flashbacks or other intense or prolonged psychological distress.

Heightened arousal—for example, aggressive, reckless or self-destructive behavior, sleep disturbances, hyper-vigilance or related problems.

Avoidance—for example, distressing memories, thoughts, feelings or external reminders of the event.

Negative thoughts and mood or feelings—for example, feelings may vary from a persistent and distorted sense of blame of self or others, to estrangement from others or markedly diminished interest in activities, to an inability to remember key aspects of the event.

5.3.3　Acute stress disorder

Acute stress disorder (ASD) is a transient mental disorder caused by sudden and unusually intense stressful life events. The term ASD was first used to describe the symptoms of soldiers during World War I and II. Approximately 20% of U.S. troops displayed symptoms of CSR during WW II, and it was assumed to be a temporary response of healthy individuals to witnessing or experiencing traumatic events. Symptoms include depression, anxiety, withdrawal, confusion, paranoia and sympathetic hyperactivity. Some of the clinical symptoms of ASD are very similar to PTSD, and the main difference from PTSD is the onset time and course

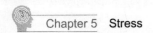

of disease. ASD onset was less than 4 weeks after 3 days to 4 weeks after the traumatic event. Symptoms for more than 4 weeks, the diagnosis should be changed to PTSD.

6. Stress management

Stress management refers to the wide spectrum of techniques and psychotherapies aimed at controlling a person's levels of stress, especially chronic stress, usually for the purpose of improving everyday functioning. The process of stress management is named as one of the keys to a happy and successful life in modern society (Paul and colleagues, 2013).

6.1　Stress vulnerability models

Stress vulnerability models describe the relation between stress and the development of (psycho-) pathology. They propose an association between (1) latent endogenous vulnerability factors that interact with stress to increase the adverse impact of stressful conditions, (2) environmental factors that influence the onset and course of (psycho-) pathology, and (3) protective factors that buffer against or mitigate the effects of stress on pathological responses. Figure 5-1 presents a stress vulnerability model.

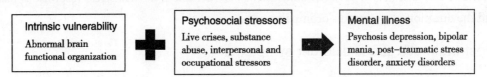

Figure 5-1　The stress vulnerability model

It is widely acknowledged that there are individual differences in how stressful people judge a particular event to be as well as in their ability to cope with adverse stressful life events. In the late 1970s, Zubin and Spring were the first to introduce this idea in the field of behavioral medicine by postulating a vulnerability model for schizophrenia. The relationship between predisposing factors (or diathesis) and development of pathology has been described in four basic stress vulnerability models.

6.1.1　Genetic vulnerability factors

Some people have genetic factors that affect stress, such as having a more or less efficient relaxation response.

In general, stress vulnerability models postulate that a genetic vulnerability interacts with adverse life events or stressors to produce pathology. This gene-environment interaction with regard to stress and the development of pathology has been most extensively investigated in mood disorders such as depression.

At the neurochemical level, the serotonin (5-HT) system has been implicated in depression. 5-HT regulates among others mood, activity, sleep, and appetite. Accumulating evidence indicates that individuals with a serotonergic vulnerability, manifested in a more sensitive brain serotonergic system, have an increased likelihood of developing mood-related disorders. Specifically, polymorphisms in the 5HT transporter system (5-HTT) have been associated with stressful life events, a heightened risk for depression, and reactivity to negative emotional stimuli. Individuals carrying two copies of the short variant of the 5-HTT allele (i.e., 5-HTTLPR), a less active gene resulting in fewer 5-HTT transporters, display an increased sensitivity to the impact of mild stressful life events, an excessive amygdala activity to fearful faces and produce elevated and prolonged levels of cortisol in response to a laboratory stressor compared to individuals with the long variant of the 5-HTT allele.

6.1.2   Individual and social vulnerability factors

(1) Personality characteristics

Certain people have personality traits that cause them to over-respond to stressful events. For example, those who are neurotic may get stressed more easily and turn to dangerous behaviors such as smoking and heavy drinking as a result.

Specific personality characteristics, such as neuroticism, openness experience and extraversion, are also stress vulnerability factors. Neuroticism is determined by some features like stress, anxiety, sensitivity, irritability, inconstancy, and intolerance. It is obvious that people having these features are prone to extreme sensitivity toward stress. Openness to experience is determined by features such as willingness to gain new experiences. Among the features of openness experience, artistic nature, creativity, and imagination can be mentioned. An artistic nature usually concurs with elegance and sensitivity. People with openness experience are sensitive toward reaction to stress and show more perception (Parvin Yadollahi and colleagues, 2014). Type A behavior (hard-driving, competitive, time-urgent, hostile-irritable) has been linked to high stress levels and the risk of eventual cardiovascular problems (i.e., coronary heart disease).

(2) Social support

The role of social support in predicting health outcomes has been widely accepted. Social support buffer effect has been suggested by the finding that the quality of spousal support moderates changes in immunological parameters in periods of interpersonal stress (Zautra and colleagues, 1998).

(3) The manner of coping with stress

Another possible source of vulnerability is the coping responses individuals use when faced with stress. Based on the general distinction between active, problem-focused coping and passive avoidance coping, research has repeatedly demonstrated that the use of more passive coping, and incidentally also the use of less active coping, prospectively predicts physical and psychological symptoms.

6.2   Measuring stress

Despite stress often being thought of as a subjective experience, levels of stress are readily measurable, using various physiological tests, similar to those used in polygraphs. In order to better manage the pressure, it is necessary to understand the stress condition through the stress test.

The Holmes and Rahe Stress Scale is used to rate stressful life events, while the Depression Anxiety Stress Scales contains a scale for stress based on self-report items. Changes in blood pressure and galvanic skin response can also be measured to test stress levels, and changes in stress levels. A digital thermometer can be used to evaluate changes in skin temperature, which can indicate activation of the fight-or-flight response drawing blood away from the extremities. Cortisol is the main hormone released during a stress response and measuring cortisol from hair will give a 60- to 90-day baseline stress level of an individual. This method of measuring stress is currently the most popular method in the clinic.

6.2.1   The Holmes and Rahe Stress Scale

In 1967, psychiatrists Thomas Holmes and Richard Rahe examined the medical records of over 5,000 medical patients as a way to determine whether stressful events might cause illnesses. Patients were asked to tally a list of 43 life events based on a relative score. A positive correlation of 0.118 was found between their life events and their illnesses.

Their results were published as the Social Readjustment Rating Scale (SRRS), known more commonly as the Holmes and Rahe Stress Scale. A modified scale has also been developed for non-adults. Similar to the adult scale, stress points for life events in the past year are added and compared to the rough estimate of how stress affects health.

The Holmes and Rahe Stress Scale (Adults)

To measure stress according to the Holmes and Rahe Stress Scale, the numbers of "Life Change Units" that apply to events in the past year of an individual's life are added and the final score will give a rough estimate of how stress affects health. The Holmes and Rahe Stress Scale is shown in table 5-1.

Table 5-1　The Holmes and Rahe Stress Scale

Life event	Life change units
Death of a spouse	100
Divorce	73
Marital separation	65
Imprisonment	63
Death of a close family member	63
Personal injury or illness	53
Marriage	50
Dismissal from work	47
Marital reconciliation	45
Retirement	45
Change in health of family member	44
Pregnancy	40
Sexual difficulties	39
Gain a new family member	39
Business readjustment	39
Change in financial state	38
Death of a close friend	37
Change to different line of work	36
Change in frequency of arguments	35
Major mortgage	32
Foreclosure of mortgage or loan	30
Change in responsibilities at work	29
Child leaving home	29
Trouble with in-laws	29
Outstanding personal achievement	28
Spouse starts or stops work	26
Beginning or end school	26
Change in living conditions	25
Revision of personal habits	24
Trouble with boss	23
Change in working hours or conditions	20
Change in residence	20
Change in schools	20
Change in recreation	19
Change in church activities	19
Change in social activities	18
Minor mortgage or loan	17

(Continued)

Life event	Life change units
Change in sleeping habits	16
Change in number of family reunions	15
Change in eating habits	15
Vacation	13
Major Holiday	12
Minor violation of law	11

Score of 300+: At risk of illness.

Score of 150-299: Risk of illness is moderate (reduced by 30% from the above risk).

Score <150: Only have a slight risk of illness.

6.2.2 Depression Anxiety Stress Scales

The Depression Anxiety Stress Scales (DASS) is available to help identify aspects of stress such as difficulty relaxing, nervous arousal and being agitated/irritable, and determine whether depression and anxiety or both are present as well. The DASS is made up of 42 self-report items to be completed over five to ten minutes, each reflecting a negative emotional symptom. The main purpose of the DASS is to isolate and identify aspects of emotional disturbance; for example, to assess the degree of severity of the core symptoms of depression, anxiety or stress.

6.3 Pressure management models

Ursin and colleagues (1978) have performed a series of studies on young paratroopers that joined the Norwegian army. Prior to jumping from airplanes, the young men were trained on ground facilities that gave them some feelings and experience of sky jumping. The men were taken to a Norwegian army base where they exercised jumping from a tower of 12 m height. Before the first jump, some biochemical parameters of stress were measured in their blood, including the levels of adrenaline, insulin, glucose, and fatty acids and were designated as resting levels. Afterwards, the soldiers were asked to climb to the top of the tower to be hooked to special ropes and jump from the tower to the ground. Most of the fall is a free fall but as they approach the surface, the ropes slow down preventing them from hitting the ground. Immediately after the jump the above stress parameters were assessed again in their blood. They were jumping for 11 consecutive days and being assessed similarly every day. It was found that in the first 3 days, especially in the second day, the levels of the above parameters increased by 200%-300% above the resting levels. However, beginning after the fourth day of jumping and all the way to the last jump on day 11, the biochemical parameters of stress were gradually reduced, but did not return back to the resting levels of the pre-jumping period.

Fear and threat usually strong negative stressors. "Practice" or repeat situations many times would turn the negative stress into a positive reaction. However, most encounters of stress are such that the individual meets those events for the first time and does not have the opportunity to "practice". How does one react positively? There are several models of stress management, each with distinctive explanations of mechanisms for controlling stress.

6.3.1 Transactional model

Richard Lazarus and Susan Folkman (1984) claim that stress can be conceived in two different ways: (1) conceived as a threat; (2) conceived as a challenge. Stress may not be a stressor if the person does not perceive the stressor as a threat but rather as positive or even challenging. Also, if the person possesses or can use adequate coping

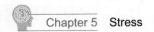

skills, then stress may not actually be a result or develop because of the stressor.

Lazarus and Folkman's interpretation of stress focuses on the transaction between people and their external environment (known as the Transactional Model). People may learn to change their perspective of the stressor and provide them with the ability and confidence to improve their lives and handle all of types of stressors.

6.3.2   Health realization/innate health model

This model of stress does not focus on individual's own coping skills of stressors (as the transactional model does), but on the nature of thought. It is ultimately a person's thought processes that determine the response to potentially stressful external circumstances. In this model, stress results from appraising oneself and one's circumstances through a mental filter of insecurity and negativity, whereas a feeling of well-being results from approaching the world with a "quiet mind" (Mills, 1995; Sedgeman, 2005).

This model proposes that helping stressed individuals understand the nature of thought—especially providing them with the ability to recognize when they are in the grip of insecure thinking, disengage from it, and access natural positive feelings—will reduce their stress.

6.4   Effective stress management

Effective stress management relies on a tested, comprehensive approach that includes the awareness of stress and the lifestyle changes. The following seven tips are designed with that in mind.

6.4.1   Identify habits and behaviors that add to stress

It is easy to identify sources of stress following a major life event such as changing jobs, moving home, or losing a loved one, but pinpointing the sources of everyday stress can be more complicated. It is all too easy to overlook your own thoughts, feelings, and behaviors that contribute to your stress levels. To identify your true sources of stress, look closely at your habits, attitude, and excuses.

A stress journal can help you identify the regular stressors in your life and the way you deal with them. Each time you feel stressed, keep track of it in your journal. As you keep a daily log, you will begin to see patterns and common themes. Write down:

(1) What caused your stress (make a guess if you are unsure)

(2) How you felt, both physically and emotionally

(3) How you acted in response

(4) What you did to make yourself feel better

6.4.2   Replace unhealthy coping strategies with healthy ones

Think about the ways you currently manage and cope with stress in your life. Are your coping strategies healthy or unhealthy, helpful or unproductive? Some coping strategies may temporarily reduce stress, but they cause more damage in the long run:

Unhealthy ways of coping with stress: Smoking, Using pills or drugs to relax, drinking too much, withdrawing from friends, family, and activities, procrastinating.

If your methods of coping with stress are not contributing to your greater emotional and physical health, it is time to find healthier ones. Focus on what makes you feel calm and in control.

6.4.3   Get moving

Physical activity plays a key role in reducing and preventing the effects of stress. Any form of physical activity can help relieve stress. While the maximum benefit comes from exercising for 30 minutes or more, you can start small and build up your fitness level gradually.

Once you are in the habit of being physically active, try to incorporate regular exercise into your daily schedule. Activities that are continuous and rhythmic are especially effective at relieving stress. Walking, running, swimming, dancing, cycling, tai chi, and aerobic classes are good choices. Instead of continuing to focus on your thoughts while you exercise, make a conscious effort to focus on your body and the physical (and sometimes emotional) sensations you experience as you are moving. Adding this mindfulness element to your exercise routine will help you break out of the cycle of negative thoughts that often accompanies overwhelming stress.

6.4.4 Connect to others

Social engagement is the quickest, most efficient way to rein in stress and avoid overreacting to internal or external events that you perceive as threatening. Expressing what you are going through can be very cathartic, even if there's nothing you can do to alter the stressful situation. There is nothing more calming to your nervous system than communicating with another human being who makes you feel safe and understood. This experience of safety—as perceived by your nervous system—results from nonverbal cues that you hear, see and feel.

The inner ear, face, heart, and stomach are wired together in the brain, so socially interacting with another person face-to-face—making eye contact, listening in an attentive way, talking—can quickly calm you down and put the brakes on defensive stress responses like "fight-or-flight." It can also release hormones that reduce stress, even if you are unable to alter the stressful situation itself. Of course, it is not always realistic to have a pal close by to lean on when you feel overwhelmed by stress, but by building and maintaining a network of close friends you can improve your resiliency to life is stressors. On the flip side, the more lonely and isolated you are, the greater your vulnerability to stress.

Reach out to family and friends and connect regularly in person. The people you talk to do not have to be able to fix your stress; they just need to be good listeners. Opening up is not a sign of weakness and it will not make you a burden to others. In fact, most friends will be flattered that you trust them enough to confide in them, and it will only strengthen your bond. And remember, it is never too late to build new friendships and improve your support network.

Reach out and build relationships as:

(1) Reach out to a colleague at work.

(2) Help someone else by volunteering.

(3) Have lunch or coffee with a friend.

(4) Ask a loved one to check in with you regularly.

(5) Accompany someone to the movies or a concert.

(6) Call or email an old friend.

(7) Go for a walk with a workout buddy.

(8) Schedule a weekly dinner date.

(9) Meet new people by taking a class or joining a club.

(10) Confide in a clergy member, teacher, or sports coach.

6.4.5 Practice the 4 A's

While stress is an automatic response from your nervous system, some stressors arise at predictable times. When handling such predictable stressors, you can either change the situation or change your reaction. When deciding which option to choose in any given scenario, it is helpful to think of the four A's: avoid, alter, adapt, or accept.

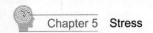

(1) Avoid unnecessary stress

A: Learn how to say "no"—Know your limits and stick to them. Whether in your personal or professional life, taking on more than you can handle is a surefire recipe for stress.

B: Avoid people who stress you out—If someone consistently causes stress in your life, limit the amount of time you spend with that person, or end the relationship.

C: Take control of your environment—If the evening news makes you anxious, turn off the TV. If traffic makes you tense, take a longer but less-traveled route.

(2) Alter the situation

If you cannot avoid a stressful situation, try to alter it. Often, this involves changing the way you communicate and operate in your daily life. If something or someone is bothering you, be more assertive and communicate your concerns in an open and respectful way. If you do not voice your feelings, the stress will increase.

Be willing to compromise. When you ask someone to change their behavior, be willing to do the same. If you both are willing to bend at least a little, you will have a good chance of finding a happy middle ground.

Manage your time better. Poor time management can cause a lot of stress. But if you plan ahead and make sure you do not overextend yourself, you will find it easier to stay calm and focused.

(3) Adapt to the stressor

Try to view stressful situations from a more positive perspective. Take perspective of the stressful situation. Ask yourself how important it will be in the long run. Will it matter in a month? A year? Is it really worth getting upset over? If the answer is no, focus your time and energy elsewhere.

Adjust your standards. Perfectionism is a major source of avoidable stress. Stop setting yourself up for failure by demanding perfection. Set reasonable standards for yourself and others, and learn to be okay with "good enough."

(4) Accept the things you cannot change

Some sources of stress are unavoidable. You cannot prevent or change stressors such as the death of a loved one, a serious illness, or a national recession. In such cases, the best way to cope with stress is to accept things as they are. Acceptance may be difficult, but in the long run, it is easier than railing against a situation you cannot change.

Do not try to control the uncontrollable. Many things in life are beyond our control—particularly the behavior of other people.

6.4.6　Maintain balance with a healthy lifestyle

In addition to regular exercise, there are other healthy lifestyle choices that can increase your resistance to stress.

Eat a healthy diet. Well-nourished bodies are better prepared to cope with stress, so be mindful of what you eat. Start your day right with breakfast, and keep your energy up and your mind clear with balanced, nutritious meals throughout the day.

Reduce caffeine and sugar. The temporary "highs" caffeine and sugar provide often end in with a crash in mood and energy.

Avoid alcohol, cigarettes, and drugs. Get enough sleep. Adequate sleep fuels your mind, as well as your body. Feeling tired will increase your stress because it may cause you to think irrationally.

（张雪琴　吴　颢）

Chapter 6

Personality Traits and Personality Disorders

Every day, we face with all kinds of people. When cont acting with them, we get to know them through their words and deeds. When we meet people, their behavioral styles and personal characteristics such as their shyness, honest, passion, talkativeness or humor, will leave us an impression, which serves as a reference for the judgment and prediction of them. These relatively stable characteristics and behaviors can be described by personality. However, evaluation of a person is just one aspect of personality psychology. The main research of the latter is to describe the origin of personality, structure, characteristics, and individual differences of it.

1. Introduction of personality

Personality comes from the Latin word persona, which refers to a mask used by actors in a play. That is, it refers to outward appearance, the public face we display to the people around. As popularly used, the word personality has a several meanings. When we say that someone has "many personalities," we usually refer to that individual's social effectiveness and appeal. Courses advertised to "improve your personality" attempt to teach social skills and to enhance your appearance or manner of speaking in order to elicit favorable reactions from others. Sometimes we use the word "personality" to describe an individual's most striking characteristic. We may refer to someone as having an "aggressive personality," or a "shy personality." When psychologists talk about personality, however, they are concerned primarily with individual differences—the characteristics that distinguish one individual from another. Personality is your characteristic pattern of thinking, feeling, and acting.

The term "character" comes from Latin. Its definition implies consistency in behavior and a tendency to act or think in a certain way, across many different situations. For example, you can probably think of an acquaintance who seldom expresses anger, no matter how others provocate him, and another who flies off the handle at the slightest irritation. Behavior is the result of the interaction between personality characteristics and the social and physical conditions of the environment. As we will see later, personality theorists differ in the extent to which they believe behavior is internally controlled (determined by the personal characteristics of the individual and therefore fairly consistent) or externally controlled (determined by the particular situation in which the behavior occurs).

2. Approaches (theories) to personality

The whole personality, like the whole elephant, is the sum of various parts. For personality, each part is explainable by an approach, representing a collection of knowledge about certain aspects of personality. At present, the field of personality seems to be separated into six parts, six distinct approaches of knowledge about human nature: psychoanalytic approach, trait approach, humanistic approach, behavioral/social

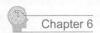

learning approach, cognitive approach and biological approach. The various views of researchers in personality do not stem from the fact that one perspective is right and the others are wrong, but rather, from the fact that they are studying different approaches of knowledge. Personality psychologists working within the various approaches often use different theoretical perspectives and focus on different facts about human nature.

Those approaches to personality are analogous to the five blind men who encounter an elephant. That is, each approach does seem to correctly identify and examine an important aspect of human personality, but they do not capture the whole person. Although not all of these perspectives are correct about every issue, each approach has something of value to offer in our quest to understand what makes each of us who we are. Nonetheless, it is still desirable at some point to integrate these diverse approaches to see how they can all fit together.

2.1　The psychoanalytic approach

Sigmund Freud created psychoanalytic theory in the early 1990s. Freud's Psychoanalytic theory proposes that personality motivated by inner forces and conflicts, which is determined by our unconscious. The unconscious region including thoughts, memories, instinctual drives, desires, demands, wishes and feelings, which cannot be observed directly. The clues to the unconscious state, such as the slips of the tongue, fantasies and dreams can help us to understand the unconscious processes that direct behavior.

2.1.1　Freudian concepts of personality structure

To describe the structure of personality, Freud proposed the theory that personality contented three interacting systems: the id, the ego, and the superego.

The id is a reservoir of unconscious psychic energy that strives to satisfy basic demands to survive, reproduce and aggress. The id is the raw, unorganized, inborn part of personality. The id operates on the pleasure principle. That is, the id is concerned only with what brings immediate personal satisfaction, regardless of any physical or social limitations. The infants, who governed by the id, cry out for satisfaction the moment they feel a need.

The ego is the largely conscious, executive part of personality, and balances the demands of the id, superego and reality world. The ego involves the conscious perceptions, memories, thoughts and judgments, which is the personality executive. The ego operates on the reality principle, which seek to satisfy id's impulses in realistic ways. That is, the primary job of the ego is to satisfy id impulses, but in a manner that takes into consideration the realities of the situation. As the ego develops, the young child learns to cope with the real world.

The superego is a voice of conscience that forces the ego to consider not only the real but also the ideal. The superego represents the rights and wrongs of society, which come from a person's parents, teachers and others. It strives perfection and judges our actions, producing positive feelings of pride or negative feelings of guilt. The superego begins around age 4 or 5. It helps the child direct the behavior more virtuous and less selfish.

The three parts of the personality are in a constant state of struggle with one another. In the healthy individual, a strong ego does not allow the id or the superego too much control over the personality. According to Freud, our unconscious mind is a continuous battlefield for these various parts of personality. The ego needs to mediate between the two more extreme delegations while also serving reality.

For more details of Freudian concepts of personality structure please see Chapter 3.

2.1.2　Freudian concepts of personality development

Freud convinced that personality forms during the first few years of life. The personality develops in childhood through the series of stages. The chief identifying characteristic of each stage concerns erogenous zones and sexual desires, and because each has an influence upon the adult personality, they have been labeled the psychosexual stages of development.

Oral stage is the first stage of development, and lasts throughout the first 18 months. The infant's mouth is the focal point of pleasure. The baby's sensual pleasures focus on sucking, biting, and chewing. Conflict experience, such as having needs ignored or being overly indulged in this period may result in the fixation of psychic energy and the development of oral personality characteristics. Fixation in oral stage might produce an adult interested in oral activities—talking, eating and smoking.

Anal stage is from 18 months to 3 years, in which a child's pleasure in centered on the anal region, and focuses on bowel and bladder elimination, retention and control. If fixation occurs in the anal stage, the adults may be orderliness, stubborn, or disorderliness and sloppiness, depending on how their toilet training progressed.

Phallic stage occurs 3 to 6 years old. The pleasure shifts to the penis or clitoris. It is during this period that the child goes through the famous Oedipus complex. Freud argued that children at this age develop a sexual attraction for their opposite-sex parent. Thus, young boys have strong incestuous desires toward their mothers, while young girls have these feelings toward their fathers. Children eventually cope with these feelings by repressing them and by identifying with the same—sex parent. On Freud's view, the identification will provide our gender identity-our sense of being male or female.

Latency stage is extending from age 6 to puberty. Sexual desires are repressed and redirected during these years, and boys and girls seem uninterested in each other. Children play mostly with peers of the same sex.

Genital stage is the last Freud's psychosexual stages, beginning in puberty. During this stage, sexuality matures and the person seeks pleasure through sexual contact with others.

For more details of Freudian concepts of personality development please see Chapter 3.

2.2   The trait approach

Psychoanalytic theory explains personality in terms of the dynamics that underlie behaviors. But trait approach describes the personality in terms of traits—people's characteristic behaviors and conscious motives.

A trait is a dimension of personality used to categorize people according to the degree to which they manifest a particular characteristic and it is a distinguishing personal characteristic or quality. It refers to any characteristic that differs from person to person in a relatively permanent and consistent way. When we informally describe others and ourselves with adjectives such as "aggressive", "cautious", "excitable", "intelligent" or "anxious", we are using trait terms.

The trait approach is concerned more with personality description, and prediction of behavior, than with personality development. Trait theories assume that people vary on a number of personality dimensions, each representing a trait. Psychologists working in the area of trait theory are concerned with determining the basic traits that provide a meaningful description of personality and finding ways to measure these traits.

2.2.1   Fundamental assumptions of the trait approach

The trait approach to personality is built upon two important assumptions. First, trait psychologists assume that personality characteristics are relatively stable over time. It would make little sense to describe people as high in self-esteem if they feel good about themselves one day but bad the next. Of course, it also defies common sense to assume that people always maintain an identical level of self-esteem regardless of circumstances. While the trait approach acknowledges that we all have our ups and downs, over a long period of time a relatively stable level of self-esteem can be identified and used to predict behavior. Second, the characteristics show stability across situations. For example, aggressive people should exhibit higher-than-average amounts of aggression during family disagreements. Again, we all act more aggressive in certain situations than in others. The trait approach assumes that over many different situations a relatively stable average degree of aggressiveness can be determined.

The trait approach generally places less emphasis on identifying the mechanisms underlying behavior. Many trait researchers focus on describing personality and predicting behavior rather than explaining why people behave the way they do. A trait description places people on a personality continuum relative to others.

2.2.2　Important trait theorists

(1) Allport's theory

Gordon Willard Allport (1897—1967) is an American psychologist. Allport defined personality in terms of identifiable behavior patterns. He was concerned more with describing and less with explaining individual traits. Allport believed that our traits have physical components in our nervous systems. He maintained that scientists would one day develop technology advanced enough to identify personality traits by examining the structure of our nervous systems.

Common traits are those aspects of personality in respect to which most people within a given culture can be profitably compared. Researchers working on common traits compare all their subjects on measures of self-esteem, anxiety, intelligence, and so on, because nearly all people can be described along these dimensions. In fact, Allport referred to nomothetic research as "indispensable" for an understanding of human personality.

Single traits are concerned with identifying the unique combination of traits that best accounts for the personality of a single individual. Allport's recommended strategy is to first determine what the important traits are for this individual and then determine where he or she falls on each of these dimensions. He referred central traits that best account for an individual's personality. Although the number of central traits varies from person to person, Allport proposed that occasionally a single trait will dominate a personality. These rare individuals can be described with a cardinal trait. Of course, there also are secondary traits that play a smaller role in the make-up of our personalities.

(2) Cattell's theory

Raymond Cattell (1905—1998) is an academic researcher who held similar viewpoints as Allport did. He also looked on traits as the basic elements of personality. Cattell found distinctions between traits common to most people in a culture and those are relatively unique to the individual.

Unlike other personality theorists, Cattell did not begin with insightful notions about the make-up of human nature and then set out to measure those features. Rather, he borrowed the approach taken by other sciences. The central goal directing much of Cattell's work is just figuring out how many different personality traits there are. Psychologists have identified, measured, and researched hundreds of personality traits. Certainly many of these traits are related. Being sociable is not entirely different from being extraverted, although we can identify some fine distinctions. By grouping together the traits related and separating those independent, Cattell reasoned that we should be able to identify the basic structure of personality. In his quest to discover this structure, Cattell employs a sophisticated statistical technique called factor analysis. He has developed a widely used personality test to measure the sixteen source traits that frequently emerge in his factor analyses.

(3) Eysenck's theory

Hans Eysenck (1916—1997) has been concerned with discovering the underlying structure of personality traits. He has also employed factor analysis to identify the basic number of what he calls types, or supertraits.

However, unlike Cattell, Eysenck's conclusion after years of research is that all traits can be subsumed within three basic personality dimensions. He calls these three dimensions extraversion-introversion, neuroticism, and psychoticism.

1) Extraversion-Introversion. The typical extravert is sociable, he likes parties, has many friends, needs to have people to talk to, and does not like reading or studying by him". An introvert is, "a quiet, retiring sort of person, introspective, fond of books rather than people; he is reserved and distant except to intimate friends". Of course, most people fall somewhere between these two extremes, but each of us is perhaps a little more of one than the other.

2) Neuroticism. High scores on this dimension are, "indicative of emotional liability and over reactivity. High-scoring individuals tend to be emotionally over responsive and to have difficulties in returning to a normal state after emotional experiences". Those falling on the other end of this dimension are less likely to fly off the handle and less prone to have large swings in emotion.

3) Psychoticism. People who score high on this dimension are described as, "egocentric, aggressive, impersonal, cold, lacking in empathy, impulsive, lacking in concern for others, and generally unconcerned about the rights and welfare of other people".

Eysenck's factor analytic research yielded evidence for two basic dimensions that could subsume all other traits: extraversion-introversion and neuroticism. Someone who scores high on extraversion and low on neuroticism possesses different traits compared with a person who scores high on both extraversion and neuroticism.

(4) The five-factor model

A central question in both Cattell's and Eysenck's theories concerns the number of dimensions needed to account for all personality traits. Using factor analysis, Cattell has produced data arguing for sixteen independent traits, whereas Eysenck has used the same statistical method to produce data arguing for three. The discrepancy comes primarily from the examination of different types of personality information. Since Cattell's and Eysenck's participants fill out different personality inventories, it is perhaps not surprising that different clusters of traits, or factors, emerge in their analyses.

Although there may never be complete agreement on this issue, recently researchers have noticed a surprisingly consistent finding in factor analytic studies of personality. Several different teams of investigators, using many different kinds of personality data, have repeatedly found evidence for five dimensions of personality. Although there is still some confusion about the fifth factor (and the possibility of small sixth and seventh factors), the researchers have consistently uncovered factors that look like the ones listed in Table 6-1.

Table 6-1   A Dimensional Model of Normal Personality: The Five-Factor Model as Measured by the Revised NEO Personality Inventory

Factors	Facet scales
Neuroticism	Anxiety, hostility, depression, self-consciousness, impulsiveness, vulnerability
Extroversion	warmth, gregariousness, assertiveness, activity, excitement seeking, positive emotions
Openness to experience	Fantasy, aesthetics, feelings, actions, ideas, values
Agreeableness	Trust, straightforwardness, altruism, compliance, modesty, tender mindedness
Conscientiousness	Competence, order, dutifulness, achievement striving, self-discipline, deliberation

If personality researchers continue to find evidence for the five-dimension model of personality, would this mean that trait theorists be better off examining only five main traits instead of the hundreds they now investigate? The answer is no. First, there is considerable debate about what the five factors mean. For example, these factors may simply represent the five dimensions that are built into our language. That is, although

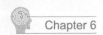

personality may in reality has a very different structure, our ability to describe personality traits is limited to the adjectives available in our language, which may fall into five primary categories. It may also be the case that our cognitive ability to organize information about others and ourselves is limited to using just these five dimensions. Thus, although people may describe personality as if all traits can be subsumed under five factors, this may not accurately capture the complexities and subtleties of human personality.

A second consideration is the usefulness of examining global personality dimensions versus more specific traits. For example, being sociable and being adventurous may be related to the larger personality concept of extraversion. However, if we want to understand how people act in social situations, it probably is more useful to examine their sociability scores than to look at the more global dimension. This is exactly what researchers found when looking at cooperative and competitive behavior. Although extraversion scores predicted who would act cooperatively and who would act competitively, researchers obtained even better predictions when they looked at scores from both of the traits that made up extraversion: sociability and impulsivity. One team of researchers found they could account for nearly twice as much of the variance in participants' behavior when they looked at sixteen specific traits than when the scores were combined into six general factors.

Third, there is still considerable disagreement about the validity of the five-factor model of personality. For example, many factor analytic studies find patterns that do not fit well within the five-factor structure. The researchers who find the five-factor structure consistently may have used similar tests to measure personality. What seems evident is that the question of how many personality traits there are remains open and that research and debate on this question will continue.

2.3 The behavioral and social learning approach

This approach, based on careful experimental research and the precise quantification of stimulus and response variables, had no place for conscious or unconscious forces because they could not be seen, manipulated, or measured. So we find no reference to anxiety, drives, motives, needs, defense mechanisms, and the other kinds of internal processes invoked by most other personality theorists. That is to say, the initial behaviorist position on personality was limited to observable behaviors. Later personality theorists expanded this position to include more cognitive and social features. In particular, Albert Bandura and Julian Rotter developed their own "social learning" theories of personality. Social-learning theory emphasizes the importance of environmental or situational determinants of behavior, including such non-observable concepts as thoughts, values, expectancies, and individual perceptions.

2.3.1 Behaviorism

John B. Watson, the founder of behaviorism. His behaviorist psychology focused on overt behavior, on the experimental research participants' responses to external stimuli. This natural science approach to psychology, based on careful experimental research and the precise quantification of stimulus and response variables, become immensely popular in the 1920s and remained a dominant force in psychology for more than 60 years.

Watson believed that whatever might be happening inside an organism—a person or an animal—between the presentation of the stimulus and the elicitation of the response had no value, meaning, or use for science. Why? Because science could not perform experiments on such internal conditions. In the behavioral approach, therefore, we find no reference to anxiety, dives, motives, needs, or defense mechanisms—the kinds of internal processes invoked by most other personality theorists. To behaviorists, personality is merely an accumulation of learned responses to stimuli, sets of overt behaviors, or habits systems. Personality refers only to what can be objectively observed and manipulated.

The behavioral approach to personality is represented here by the work of B. F. Skinner, whose ideas follow the Watsonian tradition. Skinner rejected as irrelevant any alleged internal forces or processes. His sole concern was with overt behavior and the external stimuli that shape it. Skinner attempted to understand what we call "personality" through laboratory research with rats and pigeons rather than clinical work with patients. However, his ideas have proved immensely useful in the clinical settings, through the application of behavior-modification techniques.

2.3.2 Social learning theory

The social-learning theory to personality, represented by the work of Albert Bandura, is an outgrowth of Skinner's behaviorist approach. Like Skinner, Bandura focuses on behavior rather than on needs, traits, drives, or defense mechanisms. Unlike Skinner, Bandura allows for internal cognitive variables that mediate between stimulus and response.

Bandura has investigated cognitive variables with a high degree of experimental sophistication and rigor, drawing inferences from careful observations of behavior in the laboratory. He observed the behavior of human research participants in social settings, whereas Skinner dealt with animal subjects in individual settings. Bandura agrees with Skinner that behavior is learned and that reinforcement is vital to learning, but he differ from Skinner in his interpretation of the nature reinforcement.

Bandura and Skinner both attempted to understand personality through laboratory rather than clinical work, bur their principles have been applied in the clinical setting through behavior-modification techniques. Because Bandura uses cognitive variables, his work reflected and reinforces the cognitive movement in psychology. His approach has also been called "cognitive-behavioral" in recognition of his emphasis.

For more details of the behavioral and social learning approach please see Chapter 3.

2.4 The humanistic approach

By 1960, humanistic personality psychologists focused on the "healthy" people for self-realization and self-determination that discontented with Freud's negativity and with trait psychology's objectivity. The key distinction between the humanistic approach and other theories of personality is that people are assumed to be largely responsible for their actions. Although we sometimes respond automatically to events in the environment and may at times be motivated by unconscious impulses, we have the power to determine our own destiny and to decide our actions at almost any given moment. Two pioneering psychologists illustrate these concerns on human potential: Abraham H. Maslow (1908—1970) and Carl Rogers (1902—1987).

2.4.1 Abraham H. Maslow's self-actualizing person

Maslow acknowledged the existence of unconscious motives but focused his attention on conscious aspects of personality. He conceived of people as free-willed individuals always seeking to satisfy their innate motives in a manner that fits their individual style, as well as the unique demands of their environment. It was this optimistic, psychologically healthy, and whole person that Maslow promoted during his lifetime.

Maslow proposed that we are motivated by a hierarchy of needs. If our physiological needs are met, then we get personal safety; if we achieve the security, then we seek to love, to be loved; if we become self-esteem, we ultimately seek self-actualization. Maslow believed very few adults ever reach this state of self-actualization, the point at which their potential is fully developed. But we all have the need to move toward that potential.

A peak experience is one in which time and place are transcended, in which people lose their anxieties and experience a unity of self with the universe and a momentary feeling of power and wonder. However, consistent with the humanistic notion of individuality, peak experiences are different for each person. Maslow

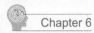

likens peak experiences to "a visit to a personally defined Heaven." Peak experiences are growth experiences, for afterward people report feeling more spontaneous, more appreciative of life, and less concerned with whatever problems they may have had.

Maslow found there were "peakers" and "nonpeakers." Each of these types of psychologically healthy people serves a different function in society. The nonpeaking self-actualizers are "the social world improvers, the politicians, the workers of society, the reformers, the crusaders." They have their feet planted firmly on the ground and have a clear direction in life. On the other hand, the "peakers" are more likely to write the poetry, the music, the philosophies, and the religions". The two types of self-actualizers play different roles in society, but both are on the way to fulfilling their potentials, each marching to a slightly different drummer.

2.4.2　Carl Roger's person-centered perspective

Rogers believed that people are basically good and are endowed with self-actualization tendencies. He was the first therapist to popularize a "person-centered" approach. His optimistic view of humanity and belief in each individual's potential for fulfillment and happiness provide a pleasant alternative to some approaches to personality covered thus far.

According to Rogers, people nurture our growth by being genuine, that is being open with their own feelings, interests, values, and needs, dropping their facades. Secondly, people also nurture our growth by being accepting with unconditional positive regard. This is an attitude that values us even knowing our failings. Under these conditions, children no longer feel a need to deny those parts of them that might otherwise have led to a withdrawal of positive regard. They are free to experience all of themselves, free to incorporate faults and weaknesses into their self-concepts, free to experience all of life. Finally, people nurture growth by being empathic, which means nonjudgmentally reflecting our feelings and meanings. Rogers said" Rarely do we listen with real understanding, true empathy".

Based on Maslow and Rogers, self-concept is the central feature of personality. Self-concept means all our thoughts and feelings about ourselves, in answer to the question, "who am I?" If our Self-concept is positive, we may perceive the world around us positively, and tend to act positively, otherwise, we will feel unhappy and dissatisfied.

For more details of the humanistic approach please see Chapter 3.

2.5　The biological approach

Researchers in this field attempt to determine the degree to which individual differences in personality are caused by genetic and environmental differences, that is, to determine the percentage of an individual difference that can be attributed to genetic differences and the percentage that is due to environment differences. However, behavioral geneticists are typically not content simply with figuring out the percentage of variance due to genetic and environmental causes. They also are interested in determining the ways in which genes and the environment interact and correlate with each other. They are interested in figuring out precisely where in the environment the effects are taking place.

The core assumption within the biological approach is that humans are, first and foremost, collections of biological systems, and these systems provide the building blocks for behavior, thought, and emotion. As personality psychologists use the term, biological approaches typically refers to three areas of research. The first area of research consists of the genetics of personality. Due to advances in behavioral genetic research, a fair amount is known about the genetics of personality. The second biological approach is best described as the psychophysiology of personality. Within this approach, researchers summarize what is known about the basis of personality in terms of nervous system functioning.

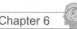

2.5.1   Genetics of personality

The word genome refers to the complete set of genes an organism possesses. Most of the genes within the human genome are the same for each individual on the planet. That is why all normally developing humans have many of the same characteristics. A small number of these genes, however, are different for different individuals. Some of genes that differ from individual to individual influence physical characteristics. The Human Genome Project has mapped human DNA sequences; in so doing, proponents of the project hope to show links between specific genes and each aspect of personality. Such fascinating new developments in molecular genetics have revived excitement and rekindled the promise of genetic approaches to personality psychology.

A heritability statistic refers to the proportion of observed variance in a group of individuals that can be accounted for by genetic variance. It describes the degree to which genetic differences between individuals cause differences in an observed property. Heritability has a formal definition: the proportion of phenotypic variance that is attributable to genotypic variance. Precisely speaking, it is just an estimate of the proportion. Phenotypic variance refers to observed individual differences; genotypic variance refers to individual differences in the total collection of genes possessed by each person. Heritability refers only to differences in a sample or population, not to an individual, and applies only to a sample or population at one point in time and in a particular array of environments. If the environments change, then heritability can change. As well, heritability can be low at one time and high at another time.

However, at the same time, genetic ideas have ignited controversy surrounding the study of genes and their influence on human behavior and personality. Part of the reason for the controversy is ideological. Many people worry about that findings from behavioral genetics will be used (or misused) to support particular political agendas. If scientists trace a behavior pattern or personality trait to a genetic component, some people worry that such findings might lead to pessimism about the possibilities for change. Another part of the controversy concerns the idea of eugenics. Eugenics is the notion that we can design the future of the human race by fostering the reproduction of persons with certain traits and by discouraging the reproduction of persons without those traits. Many people in society are concerned that findings from genetic studies might be used to support programs intended to prevent some individuals from reproducing or, even worse, to bolster the cause of those who would advocate that some people be eliminated in order to create a, "master race".

Fortunately, modern psychologists who study the genetics of personality are typically extremely careful in their attempts to educate others about the use and potential misuse of their findings. Furthermore, psychologists maintain that genetic findings need not lead to the evil consequences that some worry about. Finding that a personality characteristic has a genetic component does not mean that the environment is powerless to modify that characteristic. The percentage of observed variance in a group of individual that can be attributed to environmental differences is called environmentality. Generally speaking, the larger is the heritability, the smaller is the environmentality, and vice versa.

2.5.2   Genes and the environment

Even though some observed differences between people could be due to genetic differences, this does not mean that the environment plays no role in modifying the extent of such differences. For an individual, genes and environment are inextricably intertwined, and can't be separated. Moreover, we also cannot logically disentangle them to see which is more important. However, for the population, we can disentangle the influence of genes and environments. That is, in a sense, we can make reasonable statements about which is more important in accounting for the differences between people.

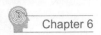

As important as it is to identify sources of environmental and genetic influence on personality, the next step requires an understanding of how genetic and environmental factors interact. More complex forms of behavioral genetic analysis involve notions such as genotype-environment interaction and genotype-environment correlation.

Genotype-environment interaction refers to the differential response of individuals with different genotypes to the same environments. Consider introverts and extraverts, who have somewhat different genotypes. Introverts tend to perform well on cognitive tasks when there is little stimulation in the room, but they do poorly when there are distractions. In contrast, extraverts do just fine with distractions. Extraversion-introversion is a perfect example of genotype-environment interaction, whereby individuals with different genotypes respond differently to the same environment to affect performance. The notion that people with different genotypes respond differently to specific environments is what is meant by genotype- environment interactions.

Genotype-environment correlation refers to the differential exposure of individuals with different genotypes to different environments. For example, parents may provide many books, intellectual discussions, crossword puzzles, and so on, to their children who are verbally inclined more than less verbally inclined children.

Plomin and colleagues describe three very different kinds of genotype-environment correlation: passive, reactive, and active. Passive genotype-environment correlation occurs when parents provide both genes and the environment to children, yet the children do nothing to obtain that environment. In sharp contrast, the reactive genotype-environment correlation occurs when parents respond to children differently, depending on child's genotypes. The last correlation is active genotype-environment correlation, which occurs when a person with a particular genotype creates, or seeks out a particular environment. The active correlation highlights the fact that we are not passive recipients of our environments; we mold, create, and select the environment we subsequently inhabit, and some of these actions are correlated with our genotypes.

These genotype-environment correlations can be positive or negative. That is, the environment can encourage the expression of the disposition, or it can discourage its expression. The key point is that environments can go against a person's genotype, resulting in a negative genotype-environment correlation, or they can facilitate the person's genotype, creating a positive genotype-environment correlation. The concepts of genotype-environment interaction and correlation are intriguing in providing a more complex picture of human personality functioning.

3. Approaches targeting personality traits

In order to study personality, regardless of the particular theoretical model methods of assessing personality variables are necessary. We make informal appraisals of personality all the time. In selecting friends, sizing up potential co-workers or candidates for political office, or deciding on a marriage partner, we make predictions about future behavior.

On many occasions, a more objective assessment of personality is desirable. In selecting individuals for high-level positions, employers need to know something about their honesty, their ability to handle stress, and so on. Decisions about the kind of treatment that will be most beneficial to a mentally ill person or that will help to rehabilitate a convicted felon require an objective assessment of individual's personality.

3.1 Observational methods

A trained observer can study an individual in a natural setting, in an experimental situation, or in the context of an interview. The interview differs from casual conversation because it has a purpose. For example, to evaluate a job applicant, to determine whether a patient is suicidal, to estimate the extent of an individual's emotional problems, or to predict whether a prisoner is apt to violate parole. The interview may be unstructured, in which case the person being interviewed largely determines what is discussed, although the interviewer usually elicits additional information through the skilled use of supplemental questions. Or, the interview may be structured, following a standard pattern, much like a questionnaire, that ensures all relevant topics are covered. The unstructured interview is used more frequently in a clinical or counseling situation; the structured interview is used more often with job applicants or research subjects when comparable data are required of all respondents.

The accuracy of the information obtained in an interview depends on factors too detailed to discuss here. However, research on the interview process has made it clear that even slight changes in the behavior of the interviewer have a marked effect on what the person being interviewed says and does. As a means of measuring personality, the interview is subject to many sources of error and bias; the success of the technique depends on the skill and awareness of the interviewer.

Impressions gained from an interview or from observing behavior can be recorded in a standardized form by means of rating scales. A rating scale is a device for recording judgments about a personality trait. For the rating to be meaningful, the rater must (1) understand the scale; (2) be sufficiently acquainted with the person being rated to make meaningful judgments, and (3) avoid the halo effect. Unless the rater knows the person fairly well or unless the behavior being rated is very specific, ratings may be influenced by social stereotypes; that is, the rater may base a judgment on how he or she believes a "suburban housewife," a "college professor," or a "high school athlete" acts and thinks rather than on the actual behavior of the subject being rated. Despite such problems, descriptions of the same person provided by different raters in different situations often yield good agreement.

3.2 Personality inventories

Another method of personality assessment relies on individual's self-observations. A personality inventory is essentially a questionnaire in which the person reports his or her reactions or feelings in certain situations. The personality inventory resembles a structured interview in that it asks the same questions of each person and the answers are usually given in a form that can be easily scored, often by a computer. A personality inventory may be designed to measure a single dimension of personality such as anxiety level, or several personality traits simultaneously.

For more information about personality inventories please see Chapter 4.

3.3 Evaluation of personality measures

Once personality measures have been identified for research, the next task is to subject them to scientific scrutiny, so that researchers determine how good the measures are. In general, three standards are used to evaluate personality measures reliability, validity and generalizability. It is important to keep in mind these standards are applicable to all measurement methods within personality research, not merely to those involving self-personality questionnaires.

3.3.1 Reliability

Reliability refers to consistency or stability of a measurement. If a test yields different results when it is administered on different occasions or scored by different people, it is unreliable. A simple analogy is a rubber yardstick. If we did not know how much it stretched each time we took a measurement, the results would be unreliable no matter how carefully we marked the measurement. Tests must be reliable if the results are to be

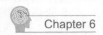

used with confidence. Personality psychologists prefer reliable measures, so that the scores accurately reflect each person's true level of the personality characteristic being measured. Since we can never measure true levels of traits we can never calculate exactly how reliable our real measures are.

It is important to demonstrate that a personality measure is reliable. To evaluate reliability, two measures must be obtained for the same individual on the same test. This can be done by repeating the test, and by giving the test in two different but equivalent forms, or by treating each half of the test separately. If individual tested achieves roughly the same score on both measures, then the test is reliable. However, this is only the first step in evaluating a personality measure. The next step is to examine whether it is valid.

3.3.2   Validity

Validity refers to the extent to which a test measures what it claims to measure. A college examination in economics that is full of questions containing complex or tricky wording might be a test of a student's verbal ability rather than of the economics learned in the course. Such an examination might be reliable (a student would achieve about the same score on a retest), but it would not be a valid test of achievement for the course. Or a test of sense of humor might be made up of jokes that are hard to understand unless the test taker is very bright and well read. This test might be a reliable measure of something (perhaps intelligence or educational achievement), but it would not be a valid test of humor.

Establishing whether a test actually measures what it is designed to measure is a complex and challenging task. There are five types of validity: face validity, predictive validity, convergent validity, discriminant validity, and construct validity.

The simplest facet of validity is called face validity. Face validity refers to whether the test, on the surface, appears to measure what it is supposed to measure. A more important component of validity is predictive validity. Predictive validity refers to whether the test predicts criteria external to the test, thus it is sometimes called criterion validity. A third aspect of validity, called convergent validity, refers to whether a test correlates with other measures that it should correlate with. A fourth kind of validity, called discriminant validity, is often evaluated simultaneously with convergent validity. Whereas convergent validity refers to what a measure should correlate with, discriminant validity refers to what a measure should not correlate with. A final type of validity is construct validity, it refers to the extent to which the instrument measures a particular construct or psychological concept such as anxiety, extroversion-introversion or neuroticism.

For more information about how to evaluate a good test, please see Chapter 4.

3.3.3   Generalizability

A third criterion for evaluating personality measures is generalizability. Generalizability is the degree to which the measure retains its validity across various contexts. One context of interest might be different groups of persons. It is critical in determining the degree to which the measure can be applied across these social and cultural contexts.

4. Personality disorder

Personality disorders are long-standing patterns of adaptive thought, behavior, and emotion. Individuals with a personality disorder show an enduring pattern of inner experience and behavior that deviates markedly from cultural expectations. These patterns are inflexible and pervasive across a wide range of social and personal situation and lead to clinically significant distress or impairment in social, occupational and other important areas of functioning.

4.1   Definition of personality disorder

The current classification system for mental disorders are including the American Psychiatric Disorders Diagnostic and Statistical Manual (DSM), and the international classification of diseases (ICD). Because of the character of mental disorders, the classification is also in constant change. This chapter focuses on the criteria and description of personality disorders in DSM-5.

The DSM-5 edition defined personality disorder as follows: A personality disorder is an enduring pattern of inner experience and behavior that deviates markedly from the expectations of individual's culture, is pervasive and inflexible, has an onset in adolescence or early adulthood, is stable over time, and leads to distress or impairment.

4.2   Classification of disorder

Each category is based around a normal personality trait, which in the disorder is manifest in an extreme and pathological manner. Most personality traits convey some kind of positive advantage provided they are tempered by recognition of the needs of others and by some kind of balance within the personality itself.

The categories of personality disorder are different in different diagnostic systems, because each classified standard focuses on its specific viewpoint. For example, group's personality disorders into nine types, the ICD-10 (international standard) classifies personality disorders into ten types, and the DSM-IV-TR (American standard) groups personality disorders into thirteen types. However, the paranoid, schizoid, antisocial, borderline, obsessive-compulsive, histrionic, and dependent personality disorder types, which will be discussed in the following section, are described similarly in different classification systems.

According to DSM-5 the personality disorders are grouped into three clusters based on descriptive similarities. Cluster A includes paranoid, schizoid, and schizotypal personality disorders. Individuals with these disorders often appear odd or eccentric. Cluster B includes antisocial, borderline, histrionic, and narcissistic personality disorders. Individuals with these disorders often appear dramatic, emotional, or erratic. Cluster C includes avoidant, dependent, and obsessive-compulsive personality disorders. Individuals with these disorders often appear anxious or fearful. It should be noted that this clustering system, although useful in some research and educational situations, has serious limitations and has not been consistently validated. Moreover, individuals frequently present with co-occurring personality disorders from different clusters. Prevalence estimates for the different clusters suggest 5.7% for disorders in Cluster A, 1.5% for disorders in Cluster B, 6.0% for disorders in Cluster C, and 9.1% for any personality disorder, indicating frequent co-occurrence of disorders from different clusters. Data from the 2001–2002 National Epidemiologic Survey on Alcohol and Related Conditions suggest that approximately 15% of the U.S. adults have at least one personality disorder. The comparisons between ICD-10 and DSM-5 are shown as follows (Table 6-2).

According to the DSM-5 guidelines, the diagnosis of personality disorders must meet the following conditions:

(1) An enduring pattern of inner experience and behavior that deviates markedly from the expectations of individual's culture. This pattern is manifested in two (or more) of the following areas:

1) Cognition (i.e., ways of perceiving and interpreting self, other people, and events).

2) Affectivity (i.e., the range, intensity, lability, and appropriateness of emotional response).

3) Interpersonal functioning.

4) Impulse control.

(2) The enduring pattern is inflexible and pervasive across a broad range of personal and social situations.

(3) The enduring pattern leads to clinically significant distress or impairment in social, occupational, or other important areas of functioning.

Table 6-2　Personality Disorder of ICD-10 vs. DSM-5

ICD-10		DSM-5	
Code	Name	Code	Name
F60.0	Paranoid	301.0	Paranoid
F60.1	Schizoid	301.20	Schizoid
F21	Schizotypal	301.22	Schizotypal
F60.2	Dissocial	301.7	Antisocial
F60.3	Emotionally unstable, borderline type	301.83	Borderline
	Emotionally unstable, impulsive type		
F60.4	Histrionic	301.50	Histrionic
		301.81	Narcissistic
F60.6	Anxious	301.82	Avoidant
F60.7	Dependent	301.6	Dependent
F60.5	Anankastic	301.4	Obsessive-compulsive
F60.89	Other specific personality disorder	301.89	Other specific personality disorder
F60.9	Other unspecific personality disorder	301.9	Other unspecific personality disorder

(4) The pattern is stable and of long duration, and its onset can be traced back at least to adolescence or early adulthood.

(5) The enduring pattern is not better explained as a manifestation or consequence of another mental disorder.

(6) The enduring pattern is not attributable to the physiological effects of a substance (e.g., a drug of abuse, a medication) or another medical condition (e.g., head trauma).

4.3　Common types of personality disorders and treatment

4.3.1　Paranoid personality disorder

(1) Clinical features of paranoid personality disorder

The defining feature of paranoid personality disorder is a pervasive and unwarranted mistrust of others. The characteristics of a paranoid personality disorder include suspiciousness, marked self-reference, feelings that other people are hostile or involved in conspiracies against the individual, a sense of injustice, preoccupation with imagined wrongs, litigious and aggressive behavior, and holding of grudges. People with paranoid personality disorder deeply believe that other people are chronically trying to deceive them or to exploit them and are preoccupied with concerns about the loyalty and trustworthiness of others. They are hypervigilant in attention to confirming evidence of their suspicions. They are often penetrating observers of situations, noting details that most other people miss. People with paranoid personality disorder tend to misinterpret or over interpret situations in line with their suspicions. For example, a wife might interpret her husband's coming home late one evening as evidence that he is having an affair with a woman at work.

(2) Theories of paranoid personality disorder

Although the etiology is unknown, both genetic and environmental aspects likely play a role. Some family history studies have shown that paranoid personality disorder is somewhat more common in the families of people with schizophrenia than in the families of healthy control subjects. This finding suggests that paranoid personality disorder may be part of the schizophrenic spectrum of disorders. Twin and adoption studies have not yet been conducted, and such studies may help tease apart the genetic influences on the development of this disorder.

Cognitive theories suggest that paranoid personality disorder results from an underlying belief that other people are malevolent and deceptive combined with a lack of self-confidence about being able to defend oneself against others. Thus, the person must always be vigilant looking for signs of others' deceit or criticism and must be quick to act against others. Research shows that patients with paranoid personality disorder endorse beliefs as predicted by this cognitive theory more than do patients diagnosed with other personality disorders.

(3) Treatments for paranoid personality disorder

Generally biological treatments and psychological treatments can be used in patients diagnosed with paranoid personality disorder.

There has been little data to suggest that pharmacologic interventions are of significant benefit. Low-dose antipsychotic medications may decrease patient's paranoia and anxiety. Under stressful situations some patients decompensate, and the paranoid ideation reaches delusional proportions, in which case antipsychotic drugs can be of more benefit.

Persons with paranoid personality disorder represent a unique challenge to the psychotherapist, because these persons often do not feel a need for treatment of their paranoia. In order to gain the trust of a person diagnosed with a paranoid personality disorder, the therapist must be calm and extremely straightforward. Although many therapists do not expect paranoid patients to achieve full insight into their problems, they hope that, by developing at least some degree of trust in the therapist, the patient can learn to trust others a bit more and thereby develop somewhat improved interpersonal relationships. Cognitive therapy for people diagnosed with this disorder focuses on increasing their sense of self-efficacy in dealing with difficult situations, thus decreasing their fear and hostility toward others.

4.3.2   Antisocial personality disorder

(1) Clinical features of antisocial personality disorder

The key features of antisocial personality disorder are impairment in the ability to form positive relationships with others and a tendency to engage in behaviors that violate basic social norms and values. People with an antisocial personality disorder have a complete disregard for the thoughts of others. They are self-centered, selfish and sometimes cruel, they are cold and affectionless. They rarely form long-term relationships and usually exploit others with whom they are involved. They are unable to appreciate the needs or feelings of others or may even gain pleasure from the humiliation or suffering of others. They often have a criminal record, which may include violent or sexual offences. Evidence of antisocial or aberrant behavior will be present from an early age. The disorder is more common in males.

A prominent characteristic of antisocial personality disorder is poor control of one's impulses. People with this disorder have a low tolerance for frustration and often act impetuously, with no apparent concern for the consequences of their behavior. They often take chances and seek thrills with no concern for danger. Drug or alcohol abuse is common, which can result in the development of short-lived psychotic states or, in the case of alcohol, long-term brain damage. These individuals may also incur brain injury because of frequent fighting or other kinds of reckless activity.

(2) Theories of antisocial personality disorder

A variety of biological and psychosocial theories of antisocial personality disorder have received some empirical support. It appears that biological, psychological and social factors are involved.

Family and twin studies support a genetic component to the etiology of antisocial personality disorder. Most theorists suggest that antisocial behavior is not the result of one gene or even a small number of genes.

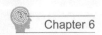

Instead, some people appear to be born with a number of genetically influenced deficits that make them ill equipped to manage ordinary life, putting them at risk for antisocial behavior.

Aggressiveness in people with antisocial personality disorders may be linked to the hormone testosterone. Although some studies have found that highly aggressive males have higher levels of testosterone than nonaggressive males, the evidence for a role for testosterone in most forms of aggression is weak. Hormones such as testosterone may play a more important role during prenatal development in organizing the fetal brain in ways that promote or inhibit aggressiveness, rather than having a direct influence on behavior in adolescence or adulthood. In addition, many animal studies have shown that impulsive and aggressive behaviors are linked to low levels of the neurotransmitter serotonin, leading to the suggestion that people with antisocial personality disorder may also have low levels of serotonin.

Research in children who show antisocial tendencies, indicates that a significant percentage, perhaps the majority, have attention-deficit/hyperactivity disorder, which involves significant problems with inhibiting impulsive behaviors and maintaining attention. The disruptive behavior of these children leads to frequent punishment and to rejection by peers, teachers, and other adults. These children then become even more disruptive, and some become overly aggressive and antisocial in their behaviors and attitudes. Thus, at least some adults with antisocial personality disorder may have lifelong problem with attentional deficits and hyperactivity, which then contribute to lifelong problems with controlling their behaviors.

People with antisocial personalities also show deficits in verbal skills and in the executive functions of the brain. These functions include, the ability to sustain concentration, abstract reasoning, concept and goal formation, the ability to anticipate and plan, the capacity to program and initiate purposive sequences of behavior, self-monitoring and self-awareness, and the ability to shift from maladaptive patterns of behavior to more adaptive ones.

(3) Treatments for antisocial personality disorder

People with this disorder tend to believe they do not need treatment. They submit to therapy when forced to because of marital discord, work conflicts, or incarceration, but they are prone to blaming others for their current situations, rather than accepting responsibility for their actions.

Evidence suggests that impulsive/aggressive behaviors in personality disorders are associated with reduced central serotonin function. SSRIs have been used to control aggressive behaviors. Lithium may also be used to reduce impulsive aggression in some patients.

Psychotherapy tends to focus on helping people with antisocial personality disorder gain control over their anger and impulsive behaviors by recognizing triggers and developing alternative coping strategies. Some therapists also try to increase individual's empathy for the effects of his or her behaviors on others.

4.3.3　Borderline personality disorder

(1) Clinical features of borderline personality disorder

The key feature of borderline personality disorder is instability, including instability of mood, instability of interpersonal relationships, and instability of self-concept. The mood of people with borderline personality disorder is unstable, with bouts of severe depression, anxiety, or anger seeming to arise frequently and often without good reason. Their self-concept is unstable, with periods of extreme self-doubt and periods of grandiose self-importance. Their interpersonal relationships are extremely unstable, and they can switch from idealizing others to despising them without provocation.

The borderline personality disorder is characterized by individuals who have explosive, short-lived emotionally charged relationships. They form intense relationships with others, which are initially idealized but then breakdown as disagreements develop. They view other as being either good or bad. Good people are those who support them and pander to their needs; bad people are those who frustrate them or do not provide enough nurturance. They are unable to tolerate frustration or disappointment; consequently, people whom they initially like and admire are soon perceived as being rejecting and unworthy as they inevitably disappoint or fail in some way. They often perceive themselves to be supportive and helpful towards others, but in reality are selfish and egocentric. They may drink heavily, take drugs or repeatedly self-harm. They are at risk of developing depressive disorders, anxiety disorders and eating disorders.

(2) Theories of borderline personality disorder

The causes of borderline personality disorder are still uncertain although there are numbers of explanations. Several family history studies of borderline personality disorder have been conducted, and the evidence that this disorder is transmitted genetically is mixed. Functional magnetic resonance imaging studies show that people with borderline personality disorder have greater activation of the amygdala in response to pictures of emotional faces, which may contribute to their difficulties in regulating their moods. Recall that the amygdala is a part of the brain that is important in the processing of emotion. Similarly, positron-emission tomography studies have found decreased metabolism in the prefrontal cortex of patients with borderline personality disorder, as is also found in patients with mood disorders.

Impulsive behaviors in people with borderline personality disorder are correlated with low levels of serotonin. Recall that impulsive behaviors in people with antisocial personality disorder have also been linked to low serotonin levels. This link suggests that low serotonin levels are associated with impulsive behaviors in general.

People with this disorder have very poorly developed views of themselves and others, stemming from poor early relationships with caregivers. These early caregivers may have encouraged children's dependence on them. They may have punished children's attempts at individuation and separation, so the children never learned to fully differentiate their views of themselves from their views of others.

(3) Treatments for borderline personality disorders

Persons with borderline personality disorder always tend to experience crises that necessitate short-term hospitalization, typically involving acute stabilization of suicidal ideation. The drug treatment has focused on reducing the symptoms of anxiety and depression. A low dose of lithium, anticonvulsants, and antidepressants can be used for acute treatments to reduce the symptoms anxiety, depression.

Psychodynamic therapy focuses on helping persons with borderline personality disorder gain a more realistic and positive sense of self, learn adaptive skills for solving problems and regulating emotions, and correct their dichotomous thinking. Group therapy can also be a useful forum in which to work with the interpersonal problems of these patients.

4.3.4   Histrionic personality disorder

(1) Clinical features of histrionic personality disorder

Histrionic personality disorder shares features with borderline personality disorder, including rapidly shifting emotions and intense, unstable relationships. People with histrionic personality disorder are overdramatic in their behavior, overly seductive, and emphasizing the positive qualities of their physical appearance, in order to pursue others' attention. People with histrionic personality disorder are overemotional and frequently moved to tears. Others see them as self-centered and shallow, unable to delay gratification, demanding, and overly independent. They are rarely happy unless surrounded by admirers. People with histrionic personality disorder are at risk of developing depression or anxiety disorders.

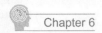

(2) Theories of histrionic personality disorder

Although discussions of histrionic personalities date back to the ancient Greek philosophers, the causes of this disorder are not well understood. Family history studies indicate that histrionic personality disorder clusters in families, along with borderline personality disorder, antisocial personality disorder, and somatization disorder. It is unclear whether this disorder is genetically related or results from processes within the family or environment. Some studies suggest that a frequent problem in parent-child relationships leads to low self-esteem. Dramatic behavior and other means to superficially impress others may be linked to individual's self-concept that he or she is not worthy of attention without special behaviors.

People with histrionic personality disorder usually want to be the center of attention. They simply want the attention of others. These individuals pursue others' attention by being highly dramatic, being overtly seductive, and emphasizing the positive qualities of their physical appearance.

(3) Treatments for histrionic personality disorder

There is little or no evidence that biological treatment is effective for histrionic personality disorder. Psychodynamic treatments focus on uncovering repressed emotions and needs, and helping people with histrionic personality disorder express these emotions and needs in more socially appropriate ways. Cognitive therapy focuses on identifying patient's assumptions that do not rely on the approval of others. Group therapy provides the members in the group comprised of similar patients, with a mirror of their own behavior and the chance to confront shallow or diverting emotional displays rather than accepting them. Moreover, these patients have considerable need for approval from others, and thus will be more likely to accept confrontations in order to avoid being rejected by other members.

4.3.5 Dependent personality disorder

(1) Clinical features of dependent personality disorder

People with a dependent personality disorder are anxious about interpersonal interactions, but their anxiety stems from a deep need to be cared for by others, rather than a concern that they will be criticized. Their desire to be loved and taken care of by others leads persons with this disorder to deny their own thoughts and feelings that might displease others, to submit to even the most unreasonable demands, and to cling frantically to others. They are overly dependent upon others, and cannot make decisions for themselves. They find it impossible to live on an independent basis and collapse emotionally whenever they have to fend for themselves. They often develop stable but imbalanced relationships with a very dominant partner, either a spouse or parent. They deeply fear rejection and abandonment and may allow themselves to be exploited and abused than lose the relationships. They are at risk of depression and anxiety disorders.

(2) Theories of dependent personality disorder

It is found that dependent personality disorder runs in families, but it is unclear whether this due to genetics or to family environment. Children with histories of anxiety about separation from their parents or of chronic physical illness appear more prone to develop dependent personality disorder. Cognitive theories suggest that people with dependent personality disorder have beliefs such as "I am needy and weak," which drive their dependent behaviors.

(3) Treatments for dependent personality disorder

People with dependent personality disorder frequently seek treatment. Person with this disorder often experience fatigue, malaise, and vague anxiety. Such symptoms may lead the person to delay efforts at establishing independence. Antidepressant or antianxiety therapy can be useful. Psychodynamic treatments focus on helping people gain insight into the early experiences with caregivers that led to their dependent behaviors through the use of free association, dream interpretation, and interpretation of the transference process. Cognitive-behavioral therapy for dependent personality disorder includes behavioral techniques designed to increase assertive behaviors and to decrease anxiety, as well as cognitive techniques designed to challenge assumptions about the need to rely on others.

4.3.6   Obsessive-compulsive personality disorder

(1) Clinical features of obsessive-compulsive personality disorder

People with an obsessive-compulsive disorder are extremely ordered, meticulous and pedantic. They often find it difficult to express emotion or show feelings towards others, although inwardly they may ruminate and worry about social encounters. They are perfectionistic and often find it difficult to complete tasks because of such high standards. They are rigid and find it difficult to adapt to change. They often have conflicts regarding sex, which they may regard as messy or dirty. They find it difficult to develop long-term relationships as most others do not live up to their high standards. They rarely have a criminal record or drink excessively. They are at risk, however, of developing depressive or obsessive illnesses and are often socially isolated.

(2) Theories of obsessive-compulsive personality disorder

There is no evidence from family history, twin, or adoption studies suggesting a genetic causes of obsessive-compulsive personality disorder. Genetic components to this disorder are still uncertain.

Early psychodynamic theorists attributed this personality disorder to fixation at the anal stage of development because the patients were subjected to an overly strict and punitive toilet training period. Other psychoanalysts argue that the obsessive-compulsive personality arises when children grow up in homes where there is much anger and niceness. The children do not develop interpersonal skills and, instead, avoid intimacy and follow rigid rules to gain a sense of self-esteem and self-control. These theories have not been empirically tested.

Cognitive theories suggest that persons with this disorder maintain beliefs that flaws, defects or mistakes are intolerable. Research found that people diagnosed with obsessive-compulsive personality disorder endorsed such beliefs significantly more often than people diagnosed with other personality disorder.

(3) Treatments for obsessive-compulsive personality disorder

Biological treatment has not been demonstrated to be effective for obsessive-compulsive personality disorder although serotonergic drugs such as selective serotonin reuptake inhibitor have been shown to be of use in the treatment of obsessive-compulsive type of anxiety. The association between obsessive-compulsive personality disorder and obsessive-compulsive disorder is not strong, and the target symptoms of improvement for the medication are not typically noted in the personality disorder.

Supportive therapies may assist people with this disorder in overcoming the crises that send them for treatment. Behavior therapies can be used to decrease the compulsive behaviors. For example, the person with this disorder may be given an assignment to alter her usual rigid schedule for the day, step by step. The person can be taught to use relaxation techniques to overcome the anxiety created by alterations in the schedule.

5. Instruments targeting personality disorder

5.1   The Dimensional Assessment of Personality Pathology

Livesley first compiled a comprehensive list of trait descriptors and behavioral acts that were characteristic of each DSM-III and DSM-III-R Axis II category. These characteristics were rated by clinicians as to the

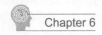

prototypically of the items for the relevant diagnoses. It is a 290-item instrument that assesses 18 dimensions of personality pathology. The Dimensional Assessment of Personality Pathology-Basic Questionnaire (DAPP-BQ) scales are internally consistent—coefficient alphas ranging from 0.08 to 0.93, and temporally stable—r's ranged from 0.82-0.93. The DAPP-BQ scales have demonstrated good convergence with other self-report measures of personality traits. According to this approach each domain is subdivided as follows (Table 6-3).

Table 6-3 A Dimensional Model of Personality Disorder: Higher basic traits of the DAPP-BQ

High traits	Sales
Emotional dysregulation	Insecure attachment, anxiousness, diffidence, affective lability, narcissism, social avoidance, passive-oppositionality
Dissocial trait	Rejection, interpersonal disesteem, conduct problems, stimulus seeking, suspiciousness
Inhibitedness	Intimacy problems, restricted expression, identity problems
Compulsivity	Compulsivity

5.2 The Schedule of Nonadaptive and Adaptive Personality

Clark (1990) compiled criteria culled from DSMs, non-DSM conceptualizations of personality disorders, and selected Axis I disorders that shared features with personality disorders (e.g., generalized anxiety disorders). Clinicians freely sorted these criteria into synonym groups that were then subjected to factor analysis, resulting in 22 consensual criterion clusters. Items were written to assess each cluster. Subsequent rounds of data collection and analysis in both normal and clinical samples yielded 12-trait dimensional scales and 3 higher-order temperament scales. The Schedule of Nonadaptive and Adaptive Personality scales (SNAP) are internally consistent (alphas ranged from 0.71 to 0.92 in both clinical and normal samples) and stable over short to moderate time periods, with 1-week to 2-month retest r's ranging from 0.68 to 0.91. In addition, to demonstrating convergence with other trait measures the SNAP scales have shown strong and systematic correlations with interview-based ratings of personality disorder.

5.3 The Parker Personality Measure

The Parker Personality Measure (PERM) was proposed for the efficient and first-level clinical description of personality disorder styles: Paranoid, Schizoid, Schizotypal, Antisocial, Borderline, Histrionic, Narcissistic, Avoidant, Dependent, Obsessive-Compulsive and Passive-Aggressive types. This refined questionnaire contains 92 items, which were factored into five higher traits. Internal reliability of PERM scales were testified in a Chinese sample (Wang et al., 2003).

（祝绮莎　王　伟）

Chapter 7

Classical Psychotherapeutic Techniques

There are hundreds of psychotherapy techniques or schools of thoughts. There were more than 250 by 1980; more than 450 by 1996; and there were over a thousand psychotherapies at the start of the 21st century—some are based on different conceptions of psychology, while others with minor different ethics (how to live) or techniques. In this chapter we will introduce three classical psychotherapeutic approaches: psychodynamic psychotherapy, behavior therapy and cognitive therapy.

1. Psychodynamic psychotherapy

The focus of psychodynamic psychotherapy is to understand how past experiences influence present behaviors. It is a form of treatment that examines defense mechanisms, such as transference, countertransference, and the internal world of fantasy and object relations and how unconscious mental functioning influences one's thoughts, feelings and behavior. A succinct definition of psychodynamic psychotherapy might be: "A therapy that involves careful attention to the therapist-patient interaction, with thoughtfully timed interpretation of transference and resistance embedded in a sophisticated appreciation of therapist's contribution to the two-person field".

Psychodynamic psychotherapy can be divided into two subtypes. One is brief or time-limited therapy of up to 6 months or 24 sessions in duration. The number of sessions is usually predetermined. Long-term or open-ended therapy can be thought of as greater than 24 sessions or 6 months and is designed to be ended more naturalistically. Therapy sessions are usually held one to three times a week, although once a week is most common.

The core concepts of psychodynamic psychotherapy include the unconscious, transference, countertransference, resistance, multiple functions, authenticity and a developmental perspective. These principles are explained in more detail later.

Basic principles of psychodynamic are:

(1) Much of mental life is unconscious.

(2) Childhood experiences in concert with genetic factors shape the adult.

(3) Patient's transference to the therapist is a primary source of understanding.

(4) Therapist's countertransference provides valuable understanding about what the patient induces in others.

(5) Patient's resistance to the therapy process is a major focus of the therapy.

(6) Symptoms and behaviors serve multiple functions and are determined by complex and often unconscious forces.

(7) A psychodynamic therapist assists the patient in achieving

(8) A sense of authenticity and uniqueness.

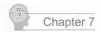

1.1 Techniques of long-term psychodynamic psychotherapy

The technique of dynamic therapy has evolved from a largely silent and nondirective role for the therapist to one in which the therapist is lively and interactive. Dynamic therapists do not hesitate to redirect patient's attention to avoided material when appropriate. They also focus as much on what is happening in the here and now as they do on childhood traumas. They collaborate with the patient in the setting of goals, knowing that the objectives may change as the therapy proceeds, and they like to offer suggestions freely without being concerned that they are departing from a rigid form of neutrality. Nevertheless, long-term psychodynamic therapy (LTTP) still operates within a frame.

1.1.1 The therapeutic frame

The therapeutic frame is best thought of as an envelope that is more flexible than a picture frame. It is composed of a set of professional boundaries that are designed to be asymmetrical so that the primary focus is on helping the patient towards enhanced understanding rather than gratifying therapist's needs. Several key components of the frame are commonly listed as professional boundaries in psychotherapy. The setting of the therapy itself, usually therapist's office or a room in a clinic or hospital, is a boundary. So is the length of the session, which is usually 45 or 50 minutes. The asymmetry of the setting is especially emphasized by the fact that the therapist is paid to deliver a service to the patient and therefore has a fiduciary responsibility to put patient's needs first. Another core boundary is the absence of dual relationships outside the therapy. In other words, the therapist should not enter into financial or business relationships (other than an agreement on the fee), social contact with the patient and certainly not romantic or sexual involvement. Indeed, the limit of physical contact in long-term dynamic therapy is generally a handshake. Confidentiality is also a cornerstone of the psychotherapy frame. Finally, although self-disclosure of therapist's feelings in a limited way is occasionally helpful, for the most part the emphasis is on patient's disclosure to the therapist.

1.1.2 Therapeutic interventions

Contemporary psychodynamic therapists tend to be spontaneous in their interactions with their patients, but a set of time-honored therapeutic interventions are particularly useful in characterizing the therapeutic strategies involved in long-term dynamic therapy. Despite of the images evoked by the names such as insight-oriented, intensive, or exploratory, when characterizing dynamic therapy, much of this treatment provides support to the patient as well as insight. In fact, the therapeutic interventions can best be conceptualized as occurring on an expressive-supportive continuum. Figure 7-1 reflects how this continuum might occurrence, with the most exploratory or insight-delivering comments on the left end of the continuum and the most supportive interventions on the right.

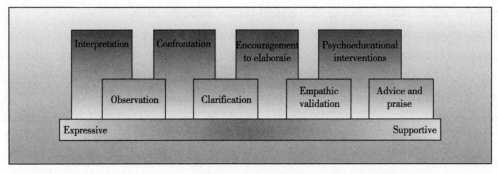

Figure 7-1 An expressive-supportive continuum of interventions

Good dynamic therapy is expressive or exploratory at some times and supportive at others. The therapist must shift flexibly along this continuum based on patient's emotional state and readiness to accept interpretations and observations about unconscious material.

Interpretation delivering insight and understanding are thus the most expressive of all interventions. It usually involves making fantasies or feelings conscious that were previously unconscious, but it is always designed to explain something to the patient. Interpretations may link relationships in patient's current life with the transference experience in the therapeutic relationship and with childhood experiences of others. At times, however, interpretations do not touch on the therapeutic relationship and are purely focused on experiences outside the therapy. At other times they address patient's defenses or resistances. One rule of thumb is not to interpret transference issues unless they are serving as a resistance to the therapy.

Observation stops short of interpretation in that it does not include an attempt to explain or link. The therapist merely watches the behavior, the sequence of a comment, a flash of affect or a pattern within the therapy. The motive or explanation is left untouched with the hope that the patient will reflect on therapist's observation.

Confrontation generally involves an attempt to draw a patient's attention to something that is being avoided. Unlike observation, which usually targets at something outside patient's awareness, confrontation usually points out the avoidance of conscious material.

Clarification is the next methods of intervention along the continuum (Figure 7-1). This type of comment is a way of bringing clarity to issues that are vague, diffusing or disconnected. It can be a way of helping a patient recognize a pattern or of checking the correctness of a therapist's understanding with the patient.

Further along the continuum one finds interventions such as encouragement to elaborate or empathic validation. Both may be used extensively as a way to gather information and promote a solid therapeutic alliance. Encouragement to elaborate can be as simple as asking the patient, "Can you tell me more about that?" Empathic validation is a way to let the patient know that the therapist understands and empathizes with patient's experience. A validating comment might include, "I can certainly appreciate why you would feel that way."

At the supportive end of the continuum, one finds psychoeducational interventions and the offering of praise and advice. These interventions are much more common in supportive psychotherapy, but some patients require them during more exploratory or expressive modes of therapy. Patients may require some psychoeducation about aspects of their illness, and they may need direct advice about matters when they are about to do something self-destructive. Praise may be important to reinforce positive therapeutic behaviors or attitudes.

1.1.3 Transference

The therapeutic interventions just described may be addressed within the context of the therapeutic relationship or geared towards outside events and relationships that have nothing to do with the therapy. Another dimension of expressiveness or supportiveness involves the extent to which the interventions are focused on the transference, that is, the therapeutic relationship. This core psychodynamic concept of transference refers to patient's tendency to repeat childhood patterns of relationship with the therapist. Feelings associated with a person from patient's past, and the specific characteristics of that person, may be attributed to the therapist in the psychotherapy process. Transference is related to internal representations of self/other relationships that are embedded in neural networks from childhood. These representations exist as potentials waiting to be activated by real characteristics of the therapist who will remind the patient of a person from the past and it will serve as a basis for that internal representation (Westen and Gabbard, 2002).

The contemporary view of transference is that it always involves the interaction of the real characteristics of the therapist and internal representations of beginning therapists is to equate transference with what patients say they feel towards the therapist (Gabbard, 2004). By definition, however, transference generally refers to unconscious feelings and attributions that are outside patient's awareness until they are made more conscious by interventions in the therapy. Hence the astute psychotherapist infers transference themes through patient's nonverbal communications and actions long before they are ever verbalized. A patient who enters the office in a deferential manner and refuses to make eye contact with the therapist is imparting a good deal of transference material just from the nonverbal information conveyed in the act of entering the office. Patients who look terrified when entering the office five minutes late, expecting therapist's wrath, are also communicating transference fantasies about therapist's potential to be punitive or harsh. Patients who question all therapist's observations may be reflecting a tendency to oppose or defy authority figures that emerge in the transference relationship to the therapist.

Most beginning therapists may feel some pressure to make interpretations that involve the transference relationship in order to be more expressive or psychodynamic in their therapy. However, it is best to wait until information is close to consciousness before interpreting it, especially when it relates to the therapeutic relationship. Premature interpretations of transference may make the patient feel misunderstood and lead to the assumption that the therapist is self-absorbed and self-referential. Another useful guideline is to avoid interpreting transference until it becomes a resistance to the process.

Psychodynamic therapy involves a way of thinking, and transference is central to psychodynamic therapy. Much of the time the therapist uses transference to inform a psychodynamic understanding of the patient without making interpretations or observations about what is transpiring in the therapy. Transference is often contrasted with the therapeutic alliance, another fundamental concept which refers to how the patient is collaborating with the therapist in pursuit of common therapeutic goals and whether the patient feels help by the therapist (Gabbard, 2004). A positive therapeutic alliance is an important predictor of good outcome in psychotherapy and a necessary condition for effective interpretation. When patients are seeing their therapists as helpful collaborators and working well in the psychotherapeutic process, transference themes do not need to be addressed.

1.1.4　Countertransference

Just as the patient experiences the therapist as someone from patient's past, therapists may also experience patients as though they are figures from therapist's past. Hence countertransference is somewhat analogous to patient's transference. A young man treating an elderly woman may begin to relate to the woman as though she is his mother and be excessively deferential and polite even if the patient requires confrontation. Like transference, countertransference is initially unconscious and may only be discovered when a countertransference theme is enacted in the psychotherapy process.

Countertransference may also be induced by patient's behavior. In other words, a difficult patient with a personality disorder who infuriates his family and his friends may also infuriate the therapist. This intense feeling generated by the patient tells less about therapists past relationships and more about what is happening in the present with the patient. Hence most theoretical perspectives today view countertransference as involving a jointly created reaction in the clinician. Part of therapist's reaction is induced by patient's behavior, whereas another part of it is based on therapists past relationships brought into the present, in an analogous way to transference. Faced with a provocative and angry patient, some therapists will react differently due to their own past experiences encoded in their neural networks of representations that occurred in their childhood. Some therapists may be thoroughly enraged, whereas others might be only mildly irritated or amused.

In terms of object relations theory, countertransference involves projective identification. The patient projects a self or object representation, along with an associated affect state, into the therapist and then exerts interpersonal pressure that nudges the therapist into taking on characteristics of what is projected. Hence a patient who has internalized an interaction with an abusive parent may recreate that abusive experience through projective identification by behaving in such a provocative fashion that the therapist actually feels emotionally abusive towards the patient. Obviously, the therapist will stop short of enacting the abuse but may have to exert self-control to avoid making abrasive comments in retaliation for patient's behavior.

In some instances, simply tolerating the countertransference and serving as a durable object for the patient may be therapeutic (Carpy, 1989). In other contexts, therapists may use their countertransference experience to formulate an interpretation about what is going on with the patient. Therapists who are themselves feeling sorry for the patient as a victim might help the patient understand how the characteristic pattern of relatedness developing in the therapy illuminates what happens in outside relationships, in which other people feel sorry for the patient, leading the patient to feel validated. In some cases, judicious use of self-disclosure about countertransference feelings may be therapeutic. A therapist who is feeling depreciated by an intensely narcissistic patient said, "I note that I am feeling that you are talking down to me, and I wonder if others feel that way when they interact with you." Some countertransference feelings should not be shared with the patient because of their potential to harm the patient or the process. These include countertransference feelings of sexual arousal, boredom or hatred (Gabbard and Wilkinson, 1994).

1.1.5 Resistance

One of the defining principles of psychodynamic psychotherapy is the notion that the patient unconsciously resists psychotherapy because of ambivalence about change. Defense mechanisms that have worked for many years are heightened when the psychic equilibrium is threatened by psychotherapy. Defense mechanisms are employed to avoid unpleasant affect states. Psychotherapy is likely to produce a variety of painful feelings, and the defenses are transformed into resistances when the patient enters psychotherapy (Thoma and Kachele, 1987).

Resistance is the daily bread-and-butter work of the dynamic psychotherapist and comes in many forms. Patients fall quiet and cannot think of anything to say. They may forget appointments. They may come late because they were distracted with other matters. They may challenge everything the therapist says. They may disparage the value of psychotherapy. All of these reactions have in common an unconscious resistance to learning more about themselves—the original reason they came to psychotherapy.

Manifestations of resistance: a) keeping silent; b) forgetting appointments; c) acting out; d) challenging the therapist; e) devaluing the therapy; f) not paying the bill; g) Arriving late.

Resistance is often related to transference fantasies about the therapist. These transference resistances are often the subjects of exploration by the therapist. Patients may be terribly ashamed to reveal their secrets to the therapist because of the fantasy that the therapist will mock or criticize them. They may feel the therapist will give them the love they missed as a child and stop looking for understanding because the pursuit of love becomes more important. Astute dynamic therapists do not try to clear away resistances or bulldoze through them. Rather, they try to encourage a reflective attitude in the patient to be curious about the meaning of the resistances. In fact, resistance can be defined as a preference for nonreflective action rather than a state of divided consciousness in which one part of the patient is feeling something in the here-and-now and another part is reflecting on the meaning of that feeling (Friedman, 1991).

As this definition implies, a propensity for action might be one of the major modes of resisting therapy. If the acting occurs outside the therapy, it is often referred as acting out, where the patient channels feelings into

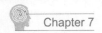
actions that may be destructive to self or others instead of reflecting on the feelings with the therapist. The action may occur in the therapy itself, and it is then referred to as acting in. The patient may come late to the session and then spend time fumbling with a Palm Pilot or a cell phone instead of talking about issues relevant to the therapy.

1.1.6   Working through and termination

Dynamic therapy often requires a considerable length of time because many patients will tenaciously hold on to self-defeating patterns and problematic object relationships. Patients must repeat the old patterns again and again to understand them in different contexts. The working-through process involves the repetitive use of interventions such as interpretation, observation, confrontation and clarification, until the patient finally begins to understand maladaptive patterns and begins to give up the old and familiar ways of thinking.

The therapist is attuned to consistent patterns of relatedness that Luborsky (1984) referred to as the core conflictual relationship theme (CCRT). The theme usually involves three components: a wish or need, a fantasy of how others will respond to this wish or need, and a subsequent response from the self (Book, 1998). A young man, for example, may want to impress others with his knowledge, mastery, and wit, but he anticipates that others will think of him as a "show-off". To resolve the conflict, he clams up and does not show his assets to others. A therapist might observe that the young man behaves this way with a girl he would like to date, with the therapist herself and with his own mother. The therapist would point out how there is a connection among a relationship from the past, the transference relationship and a current relationship outside the therapy. This triangle of insight (Menninger, 1958) is an anchoring conceptual model for the working-through process. Therapists would look for how the same relationship patterns repeat themselves in various contexts. Both fantasies and dreams may be central to the working-through process. Dreams often reveal unconscious content that lies behind person's difficulties during waking life. Dynamic psychotherapists often encourage the patient to say whatever comes to mind in reaction to a dream as a way of understanding the latent meaning of dreams. Similarly, dynamic therapists encourage patients to share their fantasies about the therapist and others as a way of decoding the fundamental relationship conflicts that stymie the patient.

At some point in the working-through process, therapist and patient begin to agree that it is time to consider termination. Ordinarily, the patient initiates the request for termination, and such requests should be explored in therapy, particularly in terms of whether they are serving a resistance function. Therapists must assess whether the patient is attempting to take flight from a difficult issue in the therapy. Those therapists will initiate an exploration of whether goals set at the beginning of the treatment have truly been accomplished. They will also want to assess whether the patient has sufficiently internalized the psychotherapeutic dialogue so that therapist's way of thinking and processing feelings can be carried out independently. Outcomes research on long-term dynamic psychotherapy suggests that changes continue well beyond termination because of patient's capacity to continue the therapeutic dialogue without the presence of the therapist (Bateman and Fonagy, 2001; Svartberg et al., 2004).

If there is a mutual assessment that goals have been accomplished and the treatment is moving towards termination, old themes from the therapy may re-emerge. Acting-out behaviors may also reappear as a way of dealing with the intense feelings brought about by the ultimate loss of the therapist. Previous losses, and difficulties mourning those losses, will also be activated by termination.

Many long-term dynamic therapies terminate in ways other than mutual agreement. Forced terminations are common because of running out of resources to pay for the therapy or because either the patient or the therapist relocates. Unilateral termination may occur when the patient feels there is no value in continuing. The therapist may also terminate unilaterally if the patient is not using the therapy and not complying with the therapeutic contract regarding such matters as excessive use of alcohol or drugs, calling the therapist before making suicidal gestures, or concealing important information from the therapist. On some occasions, the therapist may even use end-setting as a therapeutic strategy. Some patients may lack motivation to work towards goals, and they may simply come to therapy to ventilate without accomplishing much therapeutic work. At times therapists may set an arbitrary termination date as a way to attempt to motivate the patient to look at issues before time runs out.

Still other patients can never really terminate and require ongoing therapy for indefinite periods. Wallerstein (1986), in his follow-up of patients from the Menninger Psychotherapy Research Project, found that some patients had impressive outcomes when it was made clear to them that they would never have to terminate therapy. Any attempt to force termination caused their condition to deteriorate. This "therapeutic lifer" strategy can be used with a small subgroup of patients who may need to have regular contacts with the therapist at intervals of every 3 or 6 months. As long as they know the therapist will be there for another appointment, they appear to function well. This subgroup of patients is usually determined by trial and error after determining that the patient is unable to handle termination.

1.2　Technique of short-term psychodynamic psychotherapy

Definitions of short-term psychodynamic psychotherapy (STPP) vary considerably. Some authors wrote about brief therapy as a treatment in the range of 12 to 16 sessions. Davanloo, on the other hand, said that 15 to 25 sessions is a more reasonable duration for brief therapy, and he did not set a specific termination point at the beginning of treatment, unlike most therapists. Today, many practitioners view anywhere from a few meetings to approximately 24 sessions as comprising the scope of brief psychotherapy (Gabbard, 2004). If one assumes an average of about one session per week, then brief therapy is generally under 6 months in duration.

The principles outlined regarding techniques of LTTP generally apply to STPP, but the pace is markedly accelerated. In other words, constructs such as transference and resistance must be addressed early in the process rather than allowing them to develop so that a greater and more comprehensive understanding is possible. Moreover, the therapist needs to move quickly to a focus on a central hypothesis or formulation about the nature of patient's conflict. The central feature that distinguishes STPP from longer versions of psychodynamic psychotherapy is that STPP must be focal. One does not have time to look at the entire range of problems in the patient or the full extent of patient's psychopathology. Rather, the therapist and patient need to collaborate on a central focus from the first session and rapidly develop a formulation that allows them to pursue the treatment goal of dealing with the central issue or conflict in a time limited setting.

Another difference between STPP and LTTP is a more judicious use of transference interpretation. Hoglend (2003) reviewed the research literature on brief therapies and found 11 studies that identify a negative association between frequent transference interpretations and immediate or long-term outcome. Patients do not have sufficient time to develop a strong enough therapeutic alliance to withstand a great many transference interpretations. They may feel ashamed or criticized by such an approach. Most therapists would look at patterns in relationships in patient's past and in the present extra-transference settings and draw linkages between those patterns. Occasionally, a therapist might include a transference interpretation that links patient's patterns outside therapy to what is happening inside the therapeutic process. Book (1998) suggested that the use of the CCRT is a useful way to conceptualize patient's central problem so that therapist and patient can collaborate in looking for examples of it and understanding its origin.

The fact that a limit on the number of sessions is often established from the beginning of the therapy allows the therapist and the patient to link the therapy to the finiteness of time and the recognition of limits (Mann, 1973). Many patients in brief therapy come to grips with the imperfections that are inherent in life

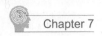

and the need to use partial answers to solve many complex problems. They also must come to terms with fantasies about an ever available therapist or parent figure and mourn the loss of unreasonable expectations about how much others can help them. Many therapists will reconsider the goals set at the outset of therapy when the patient reaches the last session, and if the patient wishes to transform the therapy into an extended or long-term process, most therapists will be open to discussion and explore the possibility with the patient.

2. Behavior therapy

Behavior therapy is a relative newcomer on the psychotherapy scene. Not until the late 1950s did it emerge as a systematic approach to the assessment and treatment of psychological disorders. In its early stages, behavior therapy was defined as the application of modern learning theory to the treatment of clinical problems. The phrase modern learning theory referred to the principles and procedures of classical and operant conditioning. Behavior therapy was seen as the logical extension of behaviorism to complex forms of human activities.

Behavior therapy has undergone significant changes in both nature and scope, and it has been responsive to advances in experimental psychology and innovations in clinical practice. It has grown more complex and sophisticated. Consequently, behavior therapy can no longer be defined simply as the clinical application of classical and operant conditioning theory.

Behavior therapy today is marked by a diversity of views. It now comprises a broad range of heterogeneous procedures with different theoretical rationales and open debate about conceptual bases, methodological requirements, and evidence of efficacy. As behavior therapy expands, it increasingly overlaps with other psychotherapeutic approaches. Nevertheless, the basic concepts that characterize the behavioral approach are clear, and its commonalities with and differences from non-behavioral therapeutic systems can be readily identified.

Behavior therapy offers a wide range of different treatment methods and attempts to tailor the principles of social-cognitive theory to each individual's unique problem. In selecting treatment techniques, the behavior therapist relies heavily on empirical evidence about the efficacy of that technique when it is applied to the particular problem. In many cases the empirical evidence is unclear or largely nonexistent. Here the therapist is influenced by accepted clinical practice and by the basic logic and philosophy of a social-cognitive approach to human behavior and its modification. In the process, the therapist must often use intuitive skills and clinical judgments to select appropriate treatment methods and determine the best time to implement specific techniques. Both science and art influence clinical practice, and the most effective therapists are aware of the advantages and limitations of each method.

Two historical events stand out as foundations for behavior therapy. The first was the rise of behaviorism in the early 1900s. The key figure in the United States was J. B. Watson, who criticized the subjectivity and mentalism of the psychology of the time and advocated behaviorism as the basis for the objective study of behavior. Watson's emphasis on the importance of environmental events, his rejection of covert aspects of the individual, and his claim that all behavior could be understood as a result of learning became the formal bases of behaviorism.

Watson's position has been widely rejected by behavior therapists, and more refined versions of behaviorism have been developed by theorists such as B. F. Skinner, whose radical behaviorism has had a significant impact not only on behavior therapy but also on psychology in general. Like Watson, Skinner insisted that overt behavior is the only acceptable subject of scientific investigation.

The second event was experimental research on the psychology of learning. In Russia, around the turn of the twentieth century, Ivan Pavlov, a Nobel laureate in physiology, established the foundations of classical conditioning. About the same time in the United States, pioneering research on animal learning by E. L. Thorndike showed the influence of consequences (rewarding and punishing events) on behavior.

Research on conditioning and learning principles, conducted largely in the animal laboratory, became a dominant part of experimental psychology in the United States following World War II. Workers in this area, in the traditions of Pavlov and Skinner, were committed to the scientific analysis of behavior using the laboratory rat and pigeon as their prototypic subjects. Among the early applications of conditioning principles to the treatment of clinical problems were two particularly notable studies. In 1924, Mary Cover Jones described different behavioral procedures for overcoming children's fears. In 1938, O. Hobart Mowrer and E. Mowrer extended conditioning principles to the treatment of enuresis. The treatment they developed is now an effective and widely used approach (Ross, 1981). These isolated and sporadic efforts had scant impact on psychotherapy at the time, partly because conditioning principles, demonstrated with animals, were rejected as too simplistic for treating complex human problems. Conditioning treatments were rejected as superficial, mechanistic, and naive. In addition, a schism existed between academic-experimental and clinical psychologists. The former were trained in scientific methods, with an emphasis on controlled experimentation and quantitative measurement. The latter concerned themselves with the "soft" side of psychology, including uncontrolled case studies, speculative hypotheses, and psychodynamic hypotheses. Some efforts were made to integrate conditioning principles with psychodynamic theories of abnormal behavior, but these formulations only obscured crucial differences between behavioral and psychodynamic approaches.

The advent of behavior therapy was marked by its challenge to the status quo through the presentation of a systematic and explicitly formulated clinical alternative that attempted to bridge the gap between the laboratory and the clinic.

For more detailed information about behavior therapy please see Chapter 3.

2.1   Treatment techniques of behavior therapy

Behavior therapy offers a wide range of different treatment methods and attempts to tailor the principles of social-cognitive theory to each individual's unique problem. In selecting treatment techniques, the behavior therapist relies heavily on empirical evidence about the efficacy of that technique when it is applied to the particular problem. In many cases the empirical evidence is unclear or largely nonexistent. Here the therapist is influenced by accepted clinical practice and by the basic logic and philosophy of a social-cognitive approach to human behavior and its modification. In the process, the therapist must often use intuitive skill and clinical judgment to select appropriate treatment methods and determine the best time to implement specific techniques. Both science and art influence clinical practice, and the most effective therapists are aware of the advantages and limitations of each.

The following are some selective illustrations of the varied methods that a typical behavior therapist is likely to employ in clinical practice.

(1) Desensitization and relaxation. Training Systematic desensitization was one of the first behavioral strategies to gain wide acceptance. Systematic desensitization relies on exposure through a progressive hierarchy of fear-inducing situations. This procedure may use pairing of progressive deep muscle relaxation and visualization of the target behavior to decondition fearful responses. Systematic desensitization is useful for treatment of simple phobias, social phobia, panic attacks, and generalized anxiety. Some evidence suggests that the active ingredient of systematic desensitization is exposure to the feared situation, first in imagination and later in reality, rather than an actual counterconditioning through the relaxation response. Progressive deep muscle relaxation is also useful as a self-directed coping strategy and for treatment of sleep-onset insomnia.

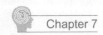

(2) Imagery-based techniques. In systematic desensitization, after isolating specific events that trigger unrealistic anxiety, the therapist constructs a stimulus hierarchy in which different situations that the patient fears are ordered along a continuum from mildly stressful to very threatening. The patient is instructed to imagine each event while he or she is deeply relaxed. Wolpe adapted Jacobson's method of progressive relaxation training as a means of producing a response incompatible with anxiety. Briefly, this consists of training patients to concentrate on systematically relaxing different muscle groups. When any item produces excessive anxiety, the patient is instructed to cease visualizing the particular item and to restore feelings of relaxation. The item is then repeated, or the hierarchy adjusted, until the patient can visualize the scene without experiencing anxiety. Only then does the therapist present the next item of the hierarchy. Real-life exposure, where possible, is even more powerful than using imagination and is the technique of choice for treating anxiety disorders.

Symbolically generated aversive reactions are used to treat diverse problems such as alcoholism and sexual disorders (e.g., exhibitionism). In this procedure the patient is asked to imagine aversive consequences associated with the problem behavior. An alcoholic might be asked to imagine experiencing nausea at the thought of a drink; an exhibitionist might be asked to imagine being apprehended by the police. This method is often referred to as covert sensitization. A hierarchy of scenes that reliably elicit the problem urge or behavior is developed, and each scene is systematically presented until the patient gains control over the problem.

(3) Exposure and flooding. The purpose of these strategies is to speed extinction of conditioned fear or anxiety responses. Behavioral theory dictates that fearfulness is reinforced by avoidance and escape behaviors. Because the basis of the fear or phobia is irrational, the optimal strategy is to increase exposure to the feared activity without aversive consequences. In obsessive-compulsive disorder, the ritualistic behavior (e.g., hand washing or checking) is hypothesized to be reinforced by the relief of the anxiety associated with the compulsion (e.g., hand washing temporarily relieves the fear of contamination). In exposure, there are at least three means of fear reduction: autonomic habituation, recognition that the fear is irrational, and explicit enhancement of morale or self-efficacy that accompanies mastering the previously dreaded activity.

In graded or progressive exposure, a hierarchy is established, ranging from least-to-most anxiety-provoking situations. The individual is taught one or more ways to cope with anxiety (e.g., relaxation or self-instruction), and with the help of the therapist, the items on the hierarchy are worked through, one item at a time. Mastery is predicated on maintaining a sufficient duration of exposure for the fear to extinguish or dissipate. In some cases, imagery (exposure "in vitro") is used before moving to exposure to the actual feared stimulus. Exposure may also be enhanced by guided support (i.e., therapist's presence during the session) or by use of coping cognitions for the duration of the exposure exercise.

Flooding, which relies on the same principles and dispatches as the hierarchical approach. The individual is exposed to the maximal level of anxiety as quickly as possible. The rationale for this accelerated approach is that it may hasten autonomic habituation. To be effective, flooding needs to be accompanied by a response prevention. In response prevention treatment of obsessive-compulsive disorder, the patient agrees not to perform the compulsion despite strong urges to do so.

(4) Cognitive Restructuring. The treatment techniques in this category are based on the assumption that emotional disorders result, at least in part, from dysfunctional thinking. The task of therapy is to alter this maladaptive thinking. Although there is some overlap with Ellis's REBT, the cognitive restructuring method most commonly used by behavior therapists is derived from Beck's cognitive therapy. An example of this method is illustrated in the following excerpt from a therapy session. Note how the therapist prompts the

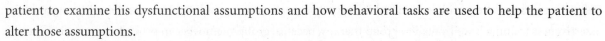

patient to examine his dysfunctional assumptions and how behavioral tasks are used to help the patient to alter those assumptions.

Patient: In the middle of a panic attack, I usually think I am going to faint or collapse.

Therapist: Have you ever fainted in an attack?

Patient: No.

Therapist: What is it then that makes you think you might faint?

Patient: I feel faint, and the feeling can be very strong.

Therapist: So, to summarize, your evidence that you are going to faint is the fact that you feel faint?

Patient: Yes.

Therapist: How can you then account for the fact that you have felt faint many hundreds of times and have not yet fainted?

Patient: So far, the attacks have always stopped just in time or I have managed to hold on to something to stop myself from collapsing.

Therapist: Right. So one explanation of the fact that you have frequently felt faint, or have the thought that you would faint, but have not actually fainted, is that you have always done something to save yourself just in time. However, an alternative explanation is that the feeling of faintness that you get in a panic attack will never lead to you collapsing, even if you do not control it.

Patient: Yes, I suppose.

Therapist: In order to decide which of these two possibilities is correct, we need to know what has to happen to your body for you to actually faint. Do you know?

Patient: No.

Therapist: Your blood pressure needs to drop. Do you know what happens to your blood pressure during a panic attack?

Patient: Well, my pulse is racing. I guess my blood pressure must be up.

Therapist: That is right. In anxiety, heart rate and blood pressure tend to go together. So, you are actually less likely to faint when you are anxious than when you are not.

Patient: That is very interesting and helpful to know. However, if it is true, why do I feel so faint?

Therapist: Your feeling of faintness is a sign that your body is reacting in a normal way to the perception of danger. Most of the bodily reactions you are experiencing when anxious were probably designed to deal with the threats experienced by primitive people, such as being approached by a hungry tiger. What would be the best thing to do in that situation?

Patient: Run away as fast as you can.

Therapist: That is right. And in order to help you run, you need the maximum amount of energy in your muscles. This is achieved by sending more of your blood to your muscles and relatively less to the brain. This means that there is a small drop in oxygen to the brain and that is why you feel faint. However, this feeling is misleading because your overall blood pressure is up, not down.

Patient: That is very clear. So next time I feel faint, I can check out whether I am going to faint by taking my pulse. If it is normal, or quicker than normal, I know I will not faint.

(5) Assertiveness and Social Skills Training. Unassertive patients often fail to express their emotions or to stand up for their rights. They are often exploited by others, feel anxious in social situations, and lack self-esteem. In behavior rehearsal, the therapist may model the appropriate assertive behavior and may ask the patient to engage repeatedly in a graduated sequence of similar actions (Alberti and Emmons, 2001). Initially, the therapist focuses on expressive behavior (e.g., body posture, voice training, and eye contact). The therapist then encourages the patient to carry out assertive actions in the real world to ensure generalization.

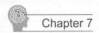

Behavior therapy is frequently conducted in a group as well as on an individual basis. Behavior rehearsal for assertiveness training is well suited to group therapy, because group members can provide more varied sources of educational feedback and can also offer a diversified range of modeling influences.

The instructional, modeling, and feedback components of behavior rehearsal facilitate a broad range of communication competencies, including active listening, giving personal feedback, and building trust through self-disclosure. These communication principles, drawn from nonbehavioral approaches but integrated within a behavioral framework, are an important ingredient of behavioral marital therapy.

(6) Self-control procedures. Behavior therapists use a number of self-control procedures. Fundamental to successful self-regulation of behavior is self-monitoring, which requires helping the patient set goals or standards that guide behavior. In the treatment of obesity, for example, daily caloric goals are mutually selected. Behavioral research has identified certain properties of goals that increase the probability of successful self-control. For example, one should set highly specific, unambiguous, and short-term goals, such as consumption of no more than 1,200 calories each day. Compare this to the goal of "cutting back" on eating for the "next week." Failure to achieve such vague goals elicits negative self-evaluative reactions by patients, whereas successful accomplishment of goals produces self-reinforcement that increases the likelihood of maintaining the new behavior.

Self-instructional training, described above, is often used as a self-control method for coping with impulsivity, stress, excessive anger, and pain. Similarly, progressive relaxation training is widely applied as a self-control method for reducing different forms of stress, including insomnia, tension headaches, and hypertension.

Biofeedback methods used to treat a variety of psychophysiological disorders also fall in the category of self-control procedures.

(7) Real-life performance-based techniques. The foregoing techniques are applied during treatment sessions, and most are routinely coupled with instructions to patients to complete homework assignments in their natural environment.

The diversity of behavioral treatment methods is seen in the application of operant conditioning principles in settings ranging from classrooms to institutions for people affected by retardation or mental illness. An excellent illustration is the use of a token economy. The main elements of a token reinforcement program are 1) carefully specified and operationally defined target behaviors, 2) backup reinforcers, 3) tokens that represent the backup reinforcers, and 4) rules of exchange that specify the number of tokens required to obtain backup reinforcers.

A token economy in a classroom might consist of the teacher, at regular intervals, making ratings indicating how well a student had behaved, both academically and socially. At the end of the day, good ratings could be exchanged for various small prizes. These procedures reduce disruptive social behavior in the classroom and can improve academic performance. In the case of psychiatric inpatients, the staff might make tokens contingent upon improvements in self-care activities, reductions in belligerent acts, and cooperative problem-solving behavior. The behavior therapist designs the token economy and monitors its implementation and efficacy. The procedures themselves are implemented in real-life settings by teachers, parents, nurses, and psychiatric aides—whoever has most direct contact with the patient. Ensuring that these psychological assistants are well trained and supervised is the responsibility of the behavior therapist.

2.2 Applications of behavior therapy

Behavior therapy can be used to treat a full range of psychological disorders in different populations. It also has broad applicability to problems in education, medicine, and community living. The following are selected examples of problems for which behavior therapy is an effective treatment: (1) anxiety disorders; (2) panic disorder; (3) obsessive-compulsive disorders; (4) depression; (5) schizophrenia.

3. Cognitive therapy

Cognitive therapy is based on a theory that maintains that people respond to life events through a combination of cognitive, affective, motivational, and behavioral responses. These responses are based on human evolution and individual learning history. The cognitive system deals with the way individuals perceive, interpret, and assign meanings to events. It interacts with other affective, motivational, and physiological systems to process information from the physical and social environments and to respond accordingly. Sometimes responses are maladaptive because of misperceptions, misinterpretations, or dysfunctional, idiosyncratic interpretations of situations.

Cognitive therapy aims to adjust information processing and initiate positive change in all systems by acting through the cognitive system. In a collaborative process, the therapist and patient examine patient's beliefs about himself or herself, other people, and the world. Patient's maladaptive conclusions are treated as testable hypotheses. Behavioral experiments and verbal procedures are used to examine alternative interpretations and to generate contradictory evidence that supports more adaptive beliefs and leads to therapeutic change.

3.1   Basic concepts

For the related basic theories please see Chapter 3.

3.2   Theory of causality

Psychological distress is ultimately caused by many innate, biological, developmental, and environmental factors interacting with one another, so there is no single "cause" of psychopathology. Depression, for instance, is characterized by predisposing factors such as hereditary susceptibility, diseases that cause persistent neurochemical abnormalities, developmental traumas leading to specific cognitive vulnerabilities, inadequate personal experiences that fail to provide appropriate coping skills, and counterproductive cognitive patterns, such as unrealistic goals, assumptions, or imperatives. Physical disease, severe and acute stress, and chronic stress are also precipitating factors.

3.2.1   Cognitive distortions

Systematic errors in reasoning called cognitive distortions are evident during psychological distress (Beck, 1967).

Arbitrary inference: Drawing a specific conclusion without supporting evidence or even in the face of contradictory evidence. An example is the working mother who concludes, after a particularly busy day, "I am a terrible mother."

Selective abstraction: Conceptualizing a situation on the basis of a detail taken out of context, ignoring other information. An example is the man who becomes jealous upon seeing his girlfriend tilt her head toward another man to hear him better at a noisy party.

Overgeneralization: Abstracting a general rule from one or a few isolated incidents and applying it too broadly and to unrelated situations. After a discouraging date, a woman concluded, "All men are alike. I will always be rejected."

Magnification and minimization: Seeing something as far more significant or less significant than it actually is. A student catastrophized, "If I appear the least bit nervous in class, it will mean disaster." Another

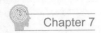

person, rather than facing the fact that his mother is terminally ill, decides that she will soon recover from her "cold."

Personalization: Attributing external events to oneself without evidence supporting a causal connection. A man waved to an acquaintance across a busy street. After not getting a greeting in return, he concluded, "I must have done something to offend him."

Dichotomous thinking: Categorizing experiences in one of two extremes; for example, as complete success or total failure. A doctoral candidate stated, "Unless I write the best exam they have ever seen, I am a failure as a student."

3.2.2　Systematic bias in psychological disorders

A bias in information processing characterizes most psychological disorders (Table 7-1). This bias is generally applied to "external" information, such as communications or threats, and may start operating at early stages of information processing. A person's orienting schema identifies a situation as posing a danger or loss, for instance, and signals the appropriate mode to respond.

Table 7-1　The cognitive profile of psychological disorders

Disorders	Systematic bias in processing information
Depression	Negative view of self, experience, and future
Hypomania	Inflated view of self and future
Anxiety disorder	Sense of physical or psychological danger
Panic disorder	Catastrophic interpretation of bodily/mental experiences
Phobia	Sense of danger in specific, avoidable situations
Paranoid state	Attribution of bias to others
Hysteria	Concept of motor or sensory abnormality
Obsession	Repeated warning or doubts about safety
Compulsion	Rituals to ward off perceived threat
Suicidal behavior	Hopelessness and deficiencies in problem solving
Anorexia nervosa	Fear of being fat
Hypochondriasis	Attribution of serious medical disorder

3.3　Process and mechanisms of cognitive therapy

3.3.1　Initial sessions

The goals of the first interview are to initiate a relationship with the patient, to elicit essential information, and to produce symptom relief. Building a relationship with the patient may begin with questions about feelings and thoughts about beginning therapy. Discussing patient's expectations helps put the patient at ease, yields information about patient's expectations, and presents an opportunity to demonstrate the relationship between cognition and affect (Beck, Rush, and colleagues, 1979). The therapist also uses the initial sessions to accustom the patient to cognitive therapy, establish a collaborative framework, and deal with any misconceptions about therapy. The types of information the therapist seeks in the initial session include diagnosis, past history, present life situation, psychological problems, attitudes about treatment, and motivation for treatment.

Problem definition and symptom relief begin in the first session. Although problem definition and collection of background information may take several sessions, it is often critical to focus on a very specific problem and provide rapid relief in the first session. For example, a suicidal patient needs direct intervention to undermine hopelessness immediately. Symptom relief can come from several sources: specific problem solving, clarifying vague or general complaints into workable goals, or gaining objectivity about a disorder (e.g., making it clear that a patient's symptoms represent anxiety and nothing worse, or that difficulty concentrating is a symptom of depression and not a sign of brain disease).

Problem definition entails both functional and cognitive analyses of the problem. A functional analysis identifies elements of the problem: how it is manifested; situations in which it occurs; its frequency, intensity, and duration; and its consequences. A cognitive analysis of the problem identifies the thoughts and images a person has when emotion is triggered. It also includes investigation of the extent to which the person feels in control of thoughts and images, what the person imagines will happen in a distressing situation, and the probability of such an outcome actually occurring.

In the early sessions, then, the cognitive therapist plays a more active role than the patient. The therapist gathers information, conceptualizes patient's problems, socializes the patient to cognitive therapy, and actively intervenes to provide symptom relief. The patient is assigned homework beginning at the first session.

Homework, at this early stage, is usually directed at recognizing the connections among thoughts, feelings, and behavior. Some patients might be asked to record their automatic thoughts when distressed. Others might practice recognizing thoughts by counting them, as they occur, on a wrist counter. Thus, the patient is trained from the outset to self-monitor thoughts and behaviors. In later sessions, the patient plays an increasingly active role in determining homework, and assignments focus on testing very specific assumptions.

During the initial sessions, a problem list is generated. The problem list may include specific symptoms, behaviors, or pervasive problems. These problems are assigned priorities as targets for intervention. Priorities are based on the relative magnitude of distress, the likelihood of making progress, the severity of symptoms, and the pervasiveness of a particular theme or topic.

If the therapist can help the patient solve a problem early in treatment, this success can motivate the patient to make further changes. As each problem is approached, the therapist chooses the appropriate cognitive or behavioral technique to apply and provides the patient with a rationale for the technique. Throughout therapy, the therapist elicits patient's reactions to various techniques to ascertain whether they are being applied correctly, whether they are successful, and how they can be incorporated into homework or practical experience outside the session.

3.3.2   Middle and later sessions

As cognitive therapy proceeds, the emphasis shifts from patient's symptoms to patient's patterns of thinking. The connections among thoughts, emotions, and behavior are chiefly demonstrated through the examination of automatic thoughts. Once the patient can challenge thoughts that interfere with functioning, he or she can consider the underlying assumptions that generate such thoughts.

There is usually a greater emphasis on cognitive than on behavioral techniques in later sessions, which focus on complex problems that involve several dysfunctional thoughts. Often these thoughts are more amenable to logical analysis than to behavioral experimentation. For example, the prophecy "I will never get what I want in life" is not easily tested. However, one can question the logic of this generalization and look at the advantages and disadvantages of maintaining it as a belief.

Often such assumptions outside patient's awareness are discovered as themes of automatic thoughts. When automatic thoughts are observed over time and across situations, assumptions appear or can be inferred. Once these assumptions and their power have been recognized, therapy aims at modifying them by examining their validity, adaptiveness, and utility for the patient.

In later sessions, the patient assumes more responsibility for identifying problems and solutions and for

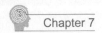

creating homework assignments. The therapist takes on the role of advisor rather than teacher as the patient becomes better able to use cognitive techniques to solve problems. The frequency of sessions decreases, as the patient becomes more self-sufficient. Therapy is terminated when goals have been reached and the patient feels able to practice his or her new skills and perspectives independently.

3.3.3   Ending treatment

Length of treatment depends primarily on the severity of patient's problems. The usual length for unipolar depression is 15 to 25 sessions at weekly intervals (Beck, Rush, and colleagues, 1979). Moderately to severely depress patients usually require sessions twice a week for 4 to 5 weeks and then weekly sessions for 10 to 15 weeks. Most cases of anxiety are treated within a comparable period of time.

Some patients find it extremely difficult to tolerate the anxiety involved in giving up old ways of thinking. For them, therapy may last several months. Still others experience early symptom relief and leave therapy early. In these cases, little structural change has occurred, and problems are likely to recur.

From the outset, the therapist and patient share the expectation that therapy is time limited. Because cognitive therapy is present-centered and time-limited, there tend to be fewer problems with termination than in longer forms of therapy. As the patient develops self-reliance, therapy sessions become less frequent.

Termination is planned for, even in the first session as the rationale for cognitive therapy is presented. Patients are told that a goal of the therapy is for them to learn to be their own therapists. The problem list makes explicit what is to be accomplished in treatment. Behavioral observation, self-monitoring, self-report, and sometimes questionnaires (e.g., the Beck Depression Inventory) measure progress toward the goals on the problem list. Feedback from the patient aids the therapist in designing experiences to foster cognitive change.

Some patients have concerns about relapse or about functioning autonomously. Some of these concerns include cognitive distortions, such as dichotomous thinking ("I am either sick or 100 percent cured") or negative prediction ("I will get depressed again and will not be able to help myself"). It may be necessary to review the goal of therapy: to teach the patient ways to handle problems more effectively, not to produce a "cure" or restructure core personality (Beck, Rush, and colleagues, 1979). Education about psychological disorders, such as acknowledging the possibility of recurrent depression, is done throughout treatment so that the patient has a realistic perspective on prognosis.

During the usual course of therapy, the patient experiences both successes and setbacks. Such problems give the patient the opportunity to practice new skills. As termination approaches, the patient can be reminded that setbacks are normal and have been handled before. The therapist might ask the patient to describe how prior specific problems were handled during treatment. Therapists can also use cognitive rehearsal prior to termination by having patients imagine future difficulties and report how they would deal with them.

Termination is usually followed by one to two booster sessions, usually 1 month and 2 months after termination. Such sessions consolidate gains and assist the patient in employing new skills.

3.3.4   Mechanisms of cognitive therapy

Several common denominators cut across effective treatments. Three mechanisms of change common to all successful forms of psychotherapy are (1) a comprehensible framework; (2) patient's emotional engagement in the problem situation, and (3) reality testing in that situation.

Cognitive therapy maintains that the modification of dysfunctional assumptions leads to effective cognitive, emotional, and behavioral change. Patients change by recognizing automatic thoughts, questioning the evidence used to support them, and modifying cognitions.

Next, the patient behaves in ways congruent with new, more adaptive ways of thinking. Change can occur only if the patient experiences a problematic situation as a real threat. According to cognitive therapy, core beliefs are linked to emotions, and with affective arousal, those beliefs become accessible and modifiable. One mechanism of change, then, focuses on making accessible those cognitive constellations that produced the maladaptive behavior or symptomatology. This mechanism is analogous to what psychoanalysts call "making the unconscious conscious."

Simply arousing emotions and the accompanying cognitions are not sufficient to cause lasting change. People express emotion, sometimes explosively, throughout their lives without benefit. However, the therapeutic milieu allows the patient to experience emotional arousal and reality testing simultaneously. For a variety of psychotherapies, what is therapeutic is patient's ability to be engaged in a problem situation and yet respond to it adaptively. In terms of cognitive therapy, this means to experience the cognitions and to test them within the therapeutic framework.

3.4   Treatment of technique therapy

Cognitive therapy consists of highly specific learning experiences designed to teach patients (1) to monitor their negative, automatic thoughts (cognitions); (2) to recognize the connections among cognition, affect, and behavior; (3) to examine the evidence for and against distorted automatic thoughts; (4) to substitute more reality-oriented interpretations for these biased cognitions, and (5) to learn to identify and alter the beliefs that predispose them to distort their experiences.

Verbal techniques are used to elicit patient's automatic thoughts, to analyze the logic behind the thoughts, to identify maladaptive assumptions, and examine the validity of those assumptions. Automatic thoughts are elicited by questioning the patient about those thoughts that occur during upsetting situations. If the patient has difficulty recalling thoughts, imagery or role playing can be used. Automatic thoughts are most accurately reported when they occur in real-life situations. Such "hot" cognitions are accessible, powerful, and habitual. The patient is taught to recognize and identify thoughts and to record them when upset.

Cognitive therapists do not interpret patient's automatic thoughts but, rather, explore their meanings, particularly when a patient reports fairly neutral thoughts yet displays strong emotions. In such cases, the therapist asks what those thoughts mean to the patient. For example, after an initial visit, an anxious patient called his therapist in great distress. He had just read an article about drug treatments for anxiety. His automatic thought was "Drug therapy is helpful for anxiety." The meaning he ascribed to this was "Cognitive therapy cannot possibly help me. I am doomed to failure again."

Automatic thoughts are tested by direct evidence or by logical analysis. Evidence can be derived from past and present circumstances, but, true to scientific inquiry, it must be as close to the facts as possible. Data can also be gathered in behavioral experiments. For example, if a man believes he cannot carry on a conversation, he might try to initiate brief exchanges with three people. The empirical nature of behavioral experiments allows patients to think in a more objective way.

Examination of patient's thoughts can also lead to cognitive change. Questioning may uncover logical inconsistencies, contradictions, and other errors in thinking. Identifying and labeling cognitive distortions are in themselves helpful, for patients then have specific errors to correct.

Maladaptive assumptions are usually much less accessible to patients than automatic thoughts. Some patients are able to articulate their assumptions, but most find it difficult. Assumptions appear as themes in automatic thoughts. The therapist may ask the patient to abstract rules underlying specific thoughts. The therapist might also make assumptions from these data and present these assumptions to the patient for verification. A patient who had trouble identifying her assumptions broke into tears upon reading an assumption inferred by her therapist—an indication of the salience of that assumption. Patients always have the right to disagree with the therapist and find more accurate statements of their beliefs.

Once an assumption has been identified, it is open to modification. This can occur in several ways: by asking the patient whether the assumption seems reasonable, by having the patient generate reasons for and against maintaining the assumption, and by presenting evidence contrary to the assumption. Even though a particular assumption may seem reasonable in a specific situation, it may appear dysfunctional when universally applied. For example, being highly productive at work is generally reasonable, but being highly productive during recreational time may be unreasonable. A physician who believed he should work to his top capacity throughout his career may not have considered the prospect of early burnout. Thus, what may have made him successful in the short run could lead to problems in the long run. Specific cognitive techniques include decatastrophizing, reattribution, redefining, and decentering.

Decatastrophizing, also known as the "what if" technique (Beck and Emery, 1979), helps patients prepare for feared consequences. This is helpful in decreasing avoidance, particularly when combined with coping plans (Beck and Emery, 1985). If anticipated consequences are likely to happen, these techniques help to identify problem-solving strategies. Decatastrophizing is often used with a time-projection technique to widen the range of information and broaden patient's time perspective.

Reattribution techniques test automatic thoughts and assumptions by considering alternative causes of events. This is especially helpful when patients personalize or perceive themselves as the cause of events. It is unreasonable to conclude, in the absence of evidence, that another person or single factor is the sole cause of an event. Reattribution techniques encourage reality testing and appropriate assignment of responsibility by requiring examination of all the factors that impinge on a situation.

Redefining is a way to mobilize a patient who believes a problem to be beyond personal control. Burns (1985) recommends that lonely people who think, "Nobody pays any attention to me" redefine the problem as "I need to reach out to other people and be caring." Redefining a problem may include making it more concrete and specific and stating it in terms of patient's own behavior.

Decentering is used primarily in treating anxious patients who wrongly believe they are the focus of everyone's attention. After they examine the logic behind the conviction that others would stare at them and be able to read their minds, behavioral experiments are designed to test these particular beliefs. For example, one student who was reluctant to speak in class believed his classmates watched him constantly and noticed his anxiety. By observing them instead of focusing on his own discomfort, he saw some students taking notes, some looking at the professor, and some daydreaming. He concluded that his classmates had other concerns.

The cognitive domain comprises thoughts and images. For some patients, pictorial images are more accessible and easier to report than thoughts. This is often the case with anxious patients. Ninety percent of anxious patients in one study reported visual images before and during episodes of anxiety (Beck et al., 1974). Gathering information about imagery, then, is another way to understand conceptual systems. Spontaneous images provide data on patient's perceptions and interpretations of events. Other specific imagery procedures used to modify distorted cognitions are discussed by Beck and Emery (1979, 1985).

In some cases, imagery is modified for its own sake. Intrusive imagery, such as imagery related to trauma, can be directly modified to reduce its impact. Patients can change aspects of an image by "rewriting the script" of what happened, making an attacker shrink in size to the point of powerlessness or empowering themselves in the image. The point of restructuring such images is not to deny what actually happened but to reduce the ability of the image to disrupt daily functioning. Imagery is also used in role-plays because of its ability to access emotions. Experiential techniques, such as dialogues between one's healthy self and one's negative thoughts, are used to mobilize affects and help patients both believe and feel that they have the right to be free of harmful and self-defeating patterns.

3.5   Cognitive-behavioral techniques

Cognitive-behavioral therapy uses behavioral techniques to modify automatic thoughts and assumptions. It employs behavioral experiments designed to challenge specific maladaptive beliefs and promote new learning. In a behavioral experiment, for example, a patient may predict an outcome based on personal automatic thoughts, carry out the agreed-upon behavior, and then evaluate the evidence in light of the new experience.

Behavioral techniques are also used to expand patient's response repertoires (skills training), to relax them (progressive relaxation) or make them active (activity scheduling), to prepare them for avoided situations (behavioral rehearsal), or to expose them to feared stimuli (exposure therapy). Because behavioral techniques are used to foster cognitive change, it is crucial to know patient's perceptions, thoughts, and conclusions after each behavioral experiment.

Homework gives patients the opportunity to apply cognitive principles between sessions. Typical homework assignments focus on self-observation and self-monitoring, structuring time effectively, and implementing procedures for dealing with concrete situations. Self-monitoring is applied to patient's automatic thoughts and reactions in various situations. New skills, such as challenging automatic thoughts, are also practiced as homework.

Hypothesis testing has both cognitive and behavioral components. In framing a "hypothesis," it is necessary to make it specific and concrete. A resident who insisted, "I am not a good doctor," was asked to list what was needed to arrive at that conclusion. The therapist contributed other criteria as well, for the physician had overlooked such factors as rapport with patients and the ability to make decisions under pressure. The resident then monitored his behavior and sought feedback from colleagues and supervisors to test his hypothesis, coming to the conclusion "I am a good doctor for my level of training and experience."

Exposure therapy serves to provide data on the thoughts, images, physiological symptoms, and self-reported level of tension experienced by the anxious patient. Specific thoughts and images can be examined for distortions, and specific coping skills can be taught. By dealing directly with a patient's idiosyncratic thoughts, cognitive therapy is able to focus on that patient's particular needs. Patients learn that their predictions are not always accurate, and they then have the data to challenge anxious thoughts in the future.

Behavioral rehearsal and role-playing are used to practice skills or techniques that are later applied in real life. Modeling is also used in skills training. Often role-playing is videotaped so that an objective source of information is available with which to evaluate performance.

Diversion techniques, which are used to reduce strong emotions and to decrease negative thinking, include physical activity, social contact, work, play, and visual imagery. Activity scheduling provides structure and encourages involvement. Rating (on a scale of 0 to 10) the degree of mastery and pleasure experienced during each activity of the day achieves several things: Patients who believe their depression is at a constant level see mood fluctuations; those who believe they cannot accomplish or enjoy anything are contradicted by the evidence; and those who believe they are inactive because of an inherent defect are shown that activity involves some planning and is reinforcing in itself.

Graded task assignment calls for the patient to initiate an activity at a nonthreatening level while the therapist gradually increases the difficulty of assigned tasks. For example, someone who has difficulty socializing might begin interacting with one other person, interact with a small group of acquaintances, or socialize with people for just a brief period of time. Step by step, the patient comes to increase the time spent with others.

Therapists work in a variety of settings. Patients are referred by physicians, schools and universities, and

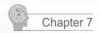

other therapists who believe that cognitive therapy would be especially helpful. Many patients are self-referred. The academy of cognitive therapy maintains an international referral list of therapists on its website (www. academyofct.org).

Therapists generally adhere to 45-minute sessions. Because of the structure of cognitive therapy, much can be accomplished in this time. Patients are frequently asked to complete questionnaires before the start of each session. Most sessions take place in therapist's office. However, real-life work with anxious patients occurs outside therapist's office. A therapist might take public transportation with an agoraphobic, go to a pet store with a rodent phobic, or travel in an airplane with someone afraid of flying.

Confidentiality is always maintained, and the therapist obtains informed consent for audiotaping and videotaping. Such recording is used in skills training or as a way to present evidence contradicting patient's assumptions. For example, a patient who believes she looks nervous whenever she converses might be videotaped in conversation to test this assumption. Her appearance on camera may convince her that her assumption was in error or help her to identify specific behaviors to improve. Occasionally, patients take audiotaped sessions home to review content material between sessions.

Sessions are usually conducted on a weekly basis, with severely disturbed patients seen more frequently in the beginning. Therapists give their patients phone numbers at which they can be reached in the event of an emergency.

Whenever possible, and with patient's permission, significant others, such as friends and family members, are included in a therapy session to review the treatment goals and to explore ways in which the significant others might be helpful. This is especially important when family members misunderstand the nature of the illness, are overly solicitous, or are behaving in counterproductive ways. Significant others can be of great assistance in therapy, helping to sustain behavioral improvements by encouraging homework and assisting the patient with reality testing.

Problems may arise in the practice of the therapy. For example, patients may misunderstand what the therapist says, and this may result in anger, dissatisfaction, or hopelessness. When the therapist perceives such a reaction, he or she elicits patient's thoughts, just as with any other automatic thoughts. Together the therapist and patient look for alternative interpretations. The therapist who has made an error accepts responsibility and corrects the mistake.

Problems sometimes result from unrealistic expectations about how quickly behaviors should change, from the incorrect or inflexible application of a technique, or from lack of attention to central issues. Problems in therapy require that the therapist attend to his or her own automatic thoughts and look for distortions in logic that create strong affect or prevent adequate problem solving.

Beck and colleagues (1979) provide guidelines for working with difficult patients and those who have histories of unsuccessful therapy: (1) avoid stereotyping the patient as being the problem rather than having the problem; (2) remain optimistic; (3) identify and deal with your own dysfunctional cognitions; (4) remain focused on the task instead of blaming the patient; and (5) maintain a problem-solving attitude. By following these guidelines, the therapist is able to be more resourceful with difficult patients. The therapist also can serve as a model for the patient, demonstrating that frustration does not automatically lead to anger and despair.

3.6 Summary

Cognitive therapy has grown quickly because of its empirical basis and demonstrated efficacy. Borrowing some of its concepts from cognitive theorists and a number of techniques from behavior therapy and patient-oriented psychotherapy, cognitive therapy consists of a broad theoretical structure of personality and psychopathology, a set of well-defined therapeutic strategies, and a wide variety of therapeutic techniques.

Similar in many ways to rational emotive behavior therapy, which is preceded but developed parallel to cognitive therapy, this system of psychotherapy has acquired strong empirical support for its theoretical foundations. A number of outcome studies have demonstrated its efficacy, especially in the treatment of depression. The related theoretical formulations of depression have been supported by more than 100 empirical studies. Other concepts, such as the cognitive triad in depression, the concept of specific cognitive profiles for specific disorders, cognitive processing, and the relationship of hopelessness to suicide, have also received strong support.

Outcome studies have investigated cognitive therapy with major depressive disorders, generalized anxiety disorder, dysthymic disorder, drug abuse, alcoholism, panic disorder, anorexia, and bulimia. In addition, cognitive therapy has been applied successfully to the treatment of obsessive-compulsive disorder, hypochondriasis, and various personality disorders. In conjunction with psychotropic medication, it has been used to treat delusional disorders and manic-depressive disorder.

Much of the popularity of cognitive therapy is attributable to strong empirical support for its theoretical framework and to the large number of outcome studies with clinical populations. In addition, there is no doubt that the intellectual atmosphere of the "cognitive revolution" has made the field of psychotherapy more receptive to this new therapy. A further attractive feature of cognitive therapy is that it is readily teachable. The various therapeutic strategies and techniques have been described and defined in such a way that one year's training is usually sufficient for a psychotherapist to attain a reasonable level of competence as a cognitive therapist.

Although cognitive therapy focuses on understanding patient's problems and applying appropriate techniques, it also attends to the nonspecific therapeutic characteristics of the therapist. Consequently, the basic qualities of empathy, acceptance, and personal regard are highly valued.

Because therapy is not conducted in a vacuum, cognitive therapists pay close attention to patient's interpersonal relations and confront patients continuously with problems they may be avoiding. Further, therapeutic change can take place only when patients are emotionally engaged with their problems. Therefore, the experience of emotion during therapy is a crucial feature. Patient's reactions to the therapist, and therapist's to the patient, are also important. Excessive and distorted responses to the therapist are elicited and evaluated just like any other type of ideational material. In the presence of the therapist, patients learn to correct their misconceptions, which were often derived from early experiences.

Cognitive therapy may offer an opportunity for a rapprochement between psychodynamic therapy and behavior therapy. In many ways it provides a common ground for these two disciplines. At the present time, the number of cognitive therapists within the behavior therapy movement is growing. In fact, many behavior therapists view themselves as cognitive-behavior therapists.

Looking to the future, it is anticipated that the boundaries of the theoretical background of cognitive therapy will gradually expand to encompass or penetrate the fields of cognitive psychology and social psychology. There is already an enormous amount of interest in social psychology, which provides the theoretical background of cognitive therapy.

In an era of cost containment, this short-term approach will prove to be increasingly attractive to third-party payers as well as to patients. Future empirical studies of its processes and effectiveness will undoubtedly be conducted to determine whether cognitive therapy can fulfill its promise.

（苏朝霞　朱　屹）

Chapter 8

Contemporary Psychotherapeutic Techniques

Besides all the therapies we have learned in Chapter three, there are also some rising psychotherapeutic techniques, such as the group psychotherapy, family psychotherapy, art psychotherapy, etc. These therapies differ widely from traditional psychotherapies and have unique styles and advantages. In this chapter we will take a glance over the most common contemporary psychotherapeutic techniques.

1. Group psychotherapy

Group psychotherapy or group therapy is a form of psychotherapy in which one or more therapists treat a small number of patients together as a group. The broader concept of group therapy can be taken to include any psychological help and guidance that takes place in group situation, including support groups, skills training groups (such as anger management, mindfulness, relaxation training or social skillstraining), and psychoeducation groups. Other, more specialized forms of group therapy would include non-verbal expressive therapies such as art therapy, dance therapy, or music therapy.

The term Group psychotherapy can legitimately refer to any form of psychotherapy when delivered in a group format, including cognitive behavioural therapy or interpersonal therapy, but it is usually applied to psychodynamic group therapy where the group context and group process is explicitly utilized as a mechanism of change by developing, exploring and examining interpersonal relationships within the group.

1.1 History

Group psychotherapy is a huge theoretical system, and it contains a number of aspects, such as research, assessment, treatment or intervention, application and so on. Lots of key figures and their ideas contributed to group phenomenon.

In 1905, American physician Joseph Pratt published his study of treating tuberculosis patients in a group setting, using "thought control classes," which likely gave the written history of group research a beginning point. Pratt was considered the pioneer or forerunner of a variety of group therapy methods. He is the earliest founder of group therapy in the world.

Trigant Burrow and Paul Schilder are also considered as the founders of group psychotherapy, and were active and working at the East Coast in the first half of the 20th century. After World War II, group psychotherapy was further developed by Jacob L. Moreno, Samuel Slavson, Hyman Spotnitz, Irvin Yalom, and Lou Ormont. Yalom's approach to group therapy has been very influential not only in the USA but across the world.

An early development in group therapy was the training group (sometimes also referred to as sensitivity-training group, human relations training group or encounter group), a form of group psychotherapy where participants (typically, between eight and 15 people) learn about themselves (and about small group processes in general) through their interaction with each other. They use feedback, problem solving, and role-play to gain insights into themselves, others, and groups.

Moreno developed a specific and highly structured form of group therapy known as psychodrama (although the entry on psychodrama claims it is not a form of group therapy). Another recent development in the theory and method of group psychotherapy based on an integration of systems thinking is Yvonne Agazarian's systems-centered therapy (SCT), which sees groups functioning within the principles of system dynamics. Her method of "functional subgrouping" introduces a method of organizing group communication so it is less likely to react counterproductively to differences. SCT also emphasizes the need to recognize the phases of group development and the defenses related to each phase in order to best make sense and influence group dynamics.

S. H. Foulkes and Wilfred Bion used group therapy as an approach to treating combat fatigue in the Second World War. Foulkes and Bion were psychoanalysts and incorporated psychoanalysis into group therapy by recognizing that transference can arise not only between group members and the therapist but also among group members. Furthermore, the psychoanalytic concept of the unconscious was extended with recognition of a group unconscious, in which the unconscious processes of group members could be acted out in the form of irrational processes in-group sessions. Foulkes developed the model known as group analysis and the Institute of Group Analysis, while Bion was influential in the development of group therapy at the Tavistock Clinic.

Bion's approach is comparable to social therapy, first developed in the United States in the late 1970s by Lois Holzman and Fred Newman, which is a group therapy in which practitioners relate to the group, not its individuals, as the fundamental unit of development. The task of the group is to "build the group" rather than focus on problem solving or "fixing" individuals.

1.2   Theories

It is no surprise that the group is a powerful healing setting, which is based on many theoretical foundations. All theories of psychopathology assert a central causal role of learning in the development of affective and behavior disorders and, in turn, posit that everyone who gains from therapeutic interventions has learned something.

1.2.1   Learning unites group theories

Learning is a change in behavior resulting from experience. The group is a therapeutic setting in which each member learns from experience with others in relationships significantly distinct from their relationships in the everyday world. Social learning theory incorporates many subsets of theoretical thinking, the group dynamics these subsets explain, the activities they involve during group counseling, and the therapeutic factors of group work. Four branches of social learning theory form the inner circle of the diagram: interpersonal learning theory, social cognitive theory, cognitive-behavioral theory, and social influence theory.

1.2.2   Interpersonal learning theory

Kurt Lewin coined the term group dynamics to describe all the things that go on in a group, both obvious and subtle. These include how people act toward each other, who has power over whom, what topics are discussed and what topics suppressed, the overall emotional tone, the pace and flow of talk, how people take turns and how long they hold the floor, and who talks and who is silent.

Group members, over time, come to act and react in the group in ways similar to how they act and interact in the world, and in turn, the group influences how members act and react in the world. Yalom and Leszcz describe this process where in the group becomes a social microcosm, in which maladaptive patterns in the world are mirrored in transactions within the group.

1.2.3   Social cognitive theory

Bandura changed the general name, social learning theory, to social cognitive theory, to emphasize the mental activities involved in social learning. This perspective on what happens in social learning focuses on observational learning—what group members discover through observing other members and the group leader. Modeling can involve imitating what one has learned through observational means: for example, groups sometimes purposely include two leaders who do not always agree, allowing the participants to observe a model of how the leaders manage disagreements in a constructive way. If the learning situation is enhanced, participants will try out this model, first in-group and then in everyday life.

Bandura emphasized that learning is enhanced in several different ways, all of which are apparent in group counseling situations. Learning is boosted under seven certain conditions: (1) if you are paying attention; (2) if you are able to remember it; (3) if you have some motivation to learn it; (4) if you believe you are capable of learning it; (5) if you have some reason to believe you will benefit from learning it; (6) if you admire a person serving as a model; (7) if you perceive the model as someone similar to you.

Observational learning, modeling, and vicarious learning augment the effectiveness of all group therapies, though they are most closely identified with social cognitive theory.

1.2.4   Cognitive-behavioral theory

An emphasis on how thoughts, emotions, and behavior change through conscious analysis and practice is the hallmark of cognitive-behavioral theory. Albert Ellis and Aaron Beck believed that most psychological distress stemmed from faulty or damaging mental processing of experience. Counseling groups devote careful attention to analysis of members" presenting problems, creation of potential alternatives in thought and action, and practice of these alternatives within the group and in the outside world.

1.2.5   Social influence theory

Social influence theory deals with aspects of group process that depend on persuasion, the reevaluation of attitudes, and the effects of in-group identity. Since therapy is basically a persuasive encounter, understanding the group dynamics that affect persuasion is critical. Goal setting, a major aim of early stages of group counseling, takes on a new twist in the light of social influence theory. Research shows that when a group is working toward a goal, members who personally accept this goal will remember specific tasks along the way, even when there is an interruption. Members who are not privately committed to the goal tend to forget the specific tasks they are supposed to engage in, to the detriment of the group's progress. If one or more members are unwilling to conform, at least outwardly, the group risks having dropouts and having stable subgroups form. Group leaders must be vigilant for signs of over conformity, stable subgroups, and undue persuasive power. They can use tactical maneuvers (such as talk tokens to equalize verbal contributions), structural changes (altering the seating pattern to mix up subgroups), and open discussions of topics like pressure to conform to the ideas of the group or the leader.

1.3   Therapeutic principles

Group psychotherapy presents itself as a complex and dynamic endeavor designed to aid those who are in chronic or acute psychological distress. Over the past fifty years, researchers and clinicians have focused on the dynamics of this complexity; specifically in terms of understanding its effectiveness—Does group counseling and psychotherapy work?—and its operations—What are the core therapeutic processes?

Yalom and Leszcz contend that 11 therapeutic factors provide an exclusive and comprehensive list of the operations and mechanisms that lead to therapeutic change in groups. Those 11 therapeutic factors has been the predominant paradigm for understanding therapeutic actions in group therapy, and serve as important organizing heuristic for group therapy theory and research. Those 11 therapeutic factors are explanted as below:

(1) Universality. The recognition of shared experiences and feelings among group members and that these may be widespread or universal human concerns, serves to remove a group member's sense of isolation, validate their experiences, and raise self-esteem.

(2) Altruism. The group is a place where members can help each other, and the experience of being able to give something to another person can lift the member's self-esteem and help develop more adaptive coping styles and interpersonal skills.

(3) Instillation of hope. In a mixed group that has members at various stages of development or recovery, a member can be inspired and encouraged by another member who has overcome the problems with which they are still struggling.

(4) Imparting information. While this is not strictly speaking a psychotherapeutic process, members often report that it has been very helpful to learn factual information from other members in the group, for example, about their treatment or about access to services.

(5) Corrective recapitulation of the primary family experience. Members often unconsciously identify the group therapist and other group members with their own parents and siblings in a process that is a form of transference specific to group psychotherapy. Therapist's interpretations can help group members gain understanding of the impact of childhood experiences on their personality, and they may learn to avoid unconsciously repeating unhelpful past interactive patterns in present-day relationships.

(6) Development of socializing techniques. The group setting provides a safe and supportive environment for members to take risks by extending their repertoire of interpersonal behavior and improving their social skills

(7) Imitative behavior. One way in which group members can develop social skills is through a modeling process, observing and imitating the therapist and other group members, for example, sharing personal feelings, showing concern, and supporting others.

(8) Cohesiveness. It has been suggested that this is the primary therapeutic factor from which all others flow. Humans are herd animals with an instinctive need to belong to groups, and personal development can only take place in an interpersonal context. A cohesive group is one in which all members feel a sense of belonging, acceptance, and validation.

(9) Existential factors. Learning that one has to take responsibility for one's own life and the consequences of one's decisions.

(10) Catharsis. Catharsis is the experience of relief from emotional distress through the free and uninhibited expression of emotion. When members tell their story to a supportive audience, they can obtain relief from chronic feelings of shame and guilt.

(11) Interpersonal learning. Group members achieve a greater level of self-awareness through the process of interacting with others in the group, who give feedback on the member's behavior and impact on others.

(12) Self-understanding. This factor overlaps with interpersonal learning but refers to the achievement of greater levels of insight into the genesis of one's problems and the unconscious motivations that underlie one's behavior.

In a classic study of therapeutic factors, Yalom, Tinklenberg, and Gilula developed a 60-item therapeutic

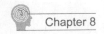

factor Q-sort for the factors. Twenty successfully treated group therapy adult patients ranked the 60 therapeutic factors Q-sort items from most to least important therapeutic factors: 1) interpersonal learning (input); 2) catharsis; 3) cohesiveness; 4) self-understanding; 5) interpersonal learning (output); 6) existential factors; 7) universality; 8) instillation of hope; 9) altruism; 10) family reenactment; 11) guidance; and 12) identification.

Several recommendations for future research in this area: 1) use therapeutic factors instruments that have well established construct validity; 2) examine therapeutic factors over time; 3) use statistical analyses that take into account the nested structure of group data; 4) do more therapeutic factors studies that examine the links between therapeutic factors and other group process or between therapeutic factors and group member outcome, 5) use statistical analyses that begin to capture the complexities of group processes; 6) move beyond correlational designs in therapeutic factors research.

Several recommendations for using Therapeutic factors in group counseling and group therapy: 1) decide which Therapeutic factors you want to emphasize in your group; 2) emphasize therapeutic factors that are related to group member outcome; 3) manipulate your leadership style, the group climate and the group structure or both to emphasize the desired therapeutic factors.

1.4 Settings

Group therapy can form part of the therapeutic milieu of a psychiatric in-patient unit or ambulatory psychiatric partial hospitalization (also known as Day Hospital treatment). In addition to classical "talking" therapy, group therapy in an institutional setting can also include group-based expressive therapies such as drama therapy, psychodrama, art therapy, and non-verbal types of therapy such as music therapy and dance/movement therapy.

Groups can be used to many special topics, such as depression and anxiety disorders, interpersonal violence (spouse abuse, domestic violence, intimate partner violence), complicated grief, addictive behaviors, attachment disorders, survivors of childhood sexual abuse, eating disorders and disturbances, and bullying.

Groups are being increasingly utilized in many settings as a counseling modality due to both recognition of their efficacy and also cost-effectiveness. The settings that groups can be used including community mental health settings, schools, colleges and university counseling centers, behavioral health settings, the department of veterans affairs.

Diversity and multicultural issues are inherent in groups. Much has changed in the field of multicultural counseling, and specifically, multicultural groups in the last ten years. Multicultural group work is a helping process that includes screening, assessing, and diagnosing dynamics of group social systems, members, and leadership for the purpose of establishing goals, outcomes, processes, and interventions that are informed by multicultural counseling knowledge, skills, and abilities. Effective groups help members understand themselves and others as individuals within the context of their culture. Multicultural counseling competencies suggest that group leaders choose interventions and methods of change based on the interplay between individuals and their worldviews.

2. Family therapy

Family therapy, also referred to as couple and family therapy, marriage and family therapy, family systems therapy, and family counseling, is a branch of psychotherapy that works with families and couples in intimate relationships to nurture change and development. It tends to view change in terms of the systems of interaction between family members, and emphasizes family relationships as an important factor in psychological health.

In the process of growing up, family members develop individual identities but nevertheless remain attached to the family group, which in turn maintains an evolving identity or collective image of its own. These family members do not live in isolation, but rather are dependent on one another—not merely for money, food, clothing, and shelter but also for love, affection, mutual commitment, companionship, socialization, the expectation of long-lasting relationships, and fulfillment of other nontangible needs. Family therapy, although has different schools, has common belief that, regardless of the origin of the problem, and regardless of whether the patients consider it an "individual" or "family" issue, involving families in solutions often benefits patients. This involvement of families is commonly accomplished by their direct participation in the therapy session. The skills of the family therapist thus include the ability to influence conversations in a way that catalyses the strengths, wisdom, and support of the wider system.

Traditionally, entrance into a family system has been seen to occur only through birth, adoption, or marriage. Today's outlook, however, makes room for other committed family households beyond legally married heterosexual couples and their children. As the field has evolved, In general, an inclusive twenty-first-century definition of family must go beyond traditional thinking to include people who choose to spend their lives together in a kinship relationship despite the lack of legal sanctions or bloodlines.

The conceptual frameworks developed by family therapists, especially those of family systems theorists, have been applied to a wide range of human behavior, including organisational dynamics and the study of greatness.

2.1   History and theoretical frameworks

Formal interventions with families to help individuals and families experiencing various kinds of problems have been a part of many cultures, probably throughout history. These interventions have sometimes involved formal procedures or rituals, and often included the extended family as well as non-kin members of the community. Following the emergence of specialization in various societies, these interventions were often conducted by particular members of a community—for example, a chief, priest, physician, and so on-usually as an ancillary function.

Family therapy as a distinct professional practice within Western cultures can be argued to have had its origins in the social work movements of the 19th century in the United Kingdom and the United States. As a branch of psychotherapy, its roots can be traced somewhat later to the early 20th century with the emergence of the child guidance movement and marriage counseling. The formal development of family therapy dates to the 1940s and early 1950s with the founding in 1942 of the American Association of Marriage Counselors, and through the work of various independent clinicians and groups-in the United Kingdom (John Bowlby at the Tavistock Clinic), the United States (Donald deAvila Jackson, John Elderkin Bell, Nathan Ackerman, Christian Midelfort, Theodore Lidz, Lyman Wynne, Murray Bowen, Carl Whitaker, Virginia Satir), and Hungary (D.L.P. Liebermann)-who began seeing family members together for observation or therapy sessions. There was initially a strong influence from psychoanalysis (most of the early founders of the field had psychoanalytic backgrounds) and social psychiatry, and later from learning theory and behavior therapy-and significantly, these clinicians began to articulate various theories about the nature and functioning of the family as an entity that was more than a mere aggregation of individuals.

The movement received an important boost starting in the early 1950s through the work of anthropologist Gregory Bateson and colleagues—Jay Haley, Donald D. Jackson, John Weakland, William Fry, and later, Virginia Satir, Paul Watzlawick and others—at Palo Alto in the United States, who introduced ideas from cybernetics and general systems theory into social psychology and psychotherapy, focusing in particular on the role of communication. This approach eschewed the traditional focus on individual psychology and historical factors-

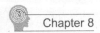

that involve so—called linear causation and content—and emphasized instead feedback and homeostatic mechanisms and "rules" in here-and-now interactions—so-called circular causation and process—that were thought to maintain or exacerbate problems, whatever the original cause. This group was also influenced significantly by the work of US psychiatrist, hypnotherapist, and brief therapist, Milton H. Erickson-especially his innovative use of strategies for change, such as paradoxical directives. The members of the Bateson Project had a particular interest in the possible psychosocial causes and treatment of schizophrenia, especially in terms of the putative "meaning" and "function" of signs and symptoms within the family system. The research of psychiatrists and psychoanalysts Lyman Wynne and Theodore Lidz on communication deviance and roles in families of schizophrenics also became influential with systems-communications-oriented theorists and therapists. A related theme, applying to dysfunction and psychopathology more generally, was that of the "identified patient" or "presenting problem" as a manifestation of or surrogate for the family, or even society, problems.

By the mid-1960s, a number of distinct schools of family therapy had emerged. From those groups that were most strongly influenced by cybernetics and systems theory, there came the Structural Family Therapy and the Milan systems model. Partly in reaction to some aspects of these systemic models, came the experiential approaches of Virginia Satir and Carl Whitaker, which downplayed theoretical constructs, and emphasized subjective experience and unexpressed feelings (including the subconscious), authentic communication, spontaneity, creativity, total therapist engagement, and often included the extended family. Concurrently and somewhat independently, there emerged the various intergenerational therapies of Murray Bowen, Ivan Böszörményi-Nagy, James Framo, and Norman Paul, which present different theories about the intergenerational transmission of health and dysfunction, but which all deal usually with at least three generations of a family (in person or conceptually), either directly in therapy sessions, or via "homework", "journeys home", etc. Psychodynamic family therapy-which, more than any other school of family therapy, deals directly with individual psychology and the unconscious in the context of current relationships-continued to develop through a number of groups that were influenced by the ideas and methods of Nathan Ackerman, and also by the British School of Object Relations and John Bowlby's work on attachment. Multiple-family group therapy, a precursor of psychoeducational family intervention, emerged, in part, as a pragmatic alternative form of intervention-especially as an adjunct to the treatment of serious mental disorders with a significant biological basis, such as schizophrenia-and represented something of a conceptual challenge to some of the "systemic" (and thus potentially "family-blaming") paradigms of pathogenesis that were implicit in many of the dominant models of family therapy. The late-1960s and early-1970s saw the development of network therapy by Ross Speck and Carolyn Attneave, and the emergence of behavioral marital therapy and behavioral family therapy as models in their own right.

By the late-1970s, the weight of clinical experience-especially in relation to the treatment of serious mental disorders-had led to some revision of a number of the original models and a moderation of some of the earlier stridency and theoretical purism. There were the beginnings of a general softening of the strict demarcations between schools, with moves toward rapprochement, integration, and eclecticism—although there was, nevertheless, some hardening of positions within some schools. These trends were reflected in and influenced by lively debates within the field and critiques from various sources, including feminism and post-modernism, that reflected in part the cultural and political tenor of the times, and which foreshadowed the emergence of the various "post-systems" constructivist and social constructionist approaches. While there was still debate within the field about whether, or to what degree, the systemic-constructivist and medical-biological paradigms were necessarily antithetical to each other. There was a growing willingness and tendency on the part of family therapists to work in multi-modal clinical partnerships with other members of the helping and medical professions.

From the mid-1980s to the present, the field has been marked by a diversity of approaches that partly reflect the original schools, but which also draw on other theories and methods from individual psychotherapy and elsewhere—these approaches and sources include: brief therapy, structural therapy, constructivist approaches, solution-focused therapy, narrative therapy, a range of cognitive and behavioral approaches, psychodynamic and object relations approaches, attachment and emotionally, intergenerational approaches, network therapy, and multisystemic therapy. Multicultural, intercultural, and integrative approaches are being developed. Many practitioners claim to be "eclectic," using techniques from several areas, depending upon their own inclinations and the needs or both of the patient(s), and there is a growing movement toward a single "generic" family therapy that seeks to incorporate the best of the accumulated knowledge in the field and which can be adapted to many different contexts; however, there are still a significant number of therapists who adhere more or less strictly to a particular, or limited number of, approach.

Ideas and methods from family therapy have been influential in psychotherapy generally: a survey of over 2,500 US therapists in 2006 revealed that of the 10 most influential therapists of the previous quarter-century, three were prominent family therapists and that the marital and family systems model was the second most utilized model after cognitive-behavioral therapy.

2.2   Classic theories and therapeutic techniques of family therapy

Different schools of family therapy make different assumptions about human nature, have different goals, and use different criteria for evaluating what constitutes a successful outcome. A therapist's theory helps organize what information to seek and how to go about seeking it, how to formulate a therapeutic plan, make interventions, and understand what transpires. In learning to do family therapy, it helps to begin by following the theory and techniques of a specific model. Patterson argues that a clear theoretical position provides the structural underpinnings for assessment and treatment planning to occur. Here are seven classical approaches to family theory and clinical practice.

2.2.1   Psychodynamic models

Psychoanalysis, both as a collection of theories and a form of practice, deserves recognition for playing the central role in establishing and defining the nature of psychotherapy. Traditionally, psychoanalysis was focused on treating neurotic individuals by examining and reconstructing childhood conflicts generated by the colliding forces of inner drives and external experiences. Shortly before World War II, a large number of European clinicians and theorists, psychoanalytic in their orientation (including Erik Erikson, Heinz Kohut, and Erich Fromm), came to the United States to escape the Nazi regime. With the arrival of these psychoanalysts, psychoanalysis began to gain greater acceptance among medical specialists, academicians, and clinicians in the American psychology community, as well as among sociologists and psychiatric social workers. Indeed, many of family therapys pioneers—Ackerman, Bowen, Lidz, Jackson, Minuchin, Wynne, Boszormenyi-Nagy—(all men, incidentally), were psychoanalytically trained. Some, such as Jackson and Minuchin, moved far from their psychoanalytic roots in favor of systems thinking, while others continued to produce theories that reflected some of their original training.

Psychodynamic models emphasize insight, motivation, unconscious conflict, early infant-caregiver attachments, unconscious intrapsychic object relations and, more recently, actual relationships and their impact on inner experience. Five psychoanalytic perspectives on therapy were rooted in psychodynamic concepts and clinical practices: the classical psychoanalytic drive theories, first introduced by Sigmund Freud; Object relations theory, a revision of earlier psychoanalytic formulations with an emphasis on the human

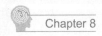

motivation to be in relationships; the self psychology theory of Heinz Kohut, which rejects classical drive theory and replaces it with a relational conceptualization of personality formation, especially through its core concepts of the self object, mirroring, and empathy; the theory of intersubjectivity, which posits that psychological phenomena occur within an intersubjective field constituted of the subjective worlds of child and caregiver or of patient and analyst; the relational psychoanalytic theory, a contemporary approach to psychoanalysis that links the influence on personality development of internalized object relations, self-states, and interpersonal or social relations.

2.2.2　Transgenerational models

Transgenerational approaches offer a psychoanalytically influenced historical perspective to current family living problems by attending specifically to family relational patterns over decades. It accents how current family patterns, alliances, and boundaries are embedded in unresolved issues from the families of origin. Advocates of this view believe current family patterns are embedded in unresolved issues in the families of origin. And it tends to remain unsettled and thus persist and repeat in patterns that span generations. How today's family members form attachments, manage intimacy, deal with power, resolve conflict, and so on, may mirror earlier family patterns. Unresolved issues in families of origin may show up in symptomatic behavior patterns in later generations. Murray Bowen, Ivan Boszormenyi-Nagy, James Framo, and Carl Whitaker incorporated generational issues in their work with families, and were considered as pioneering family therapists. Here we focus on two multigenerational views, Murray Bowen's family systems theory and Ivan Boszormenyi-Nagy's contextual therapy.

Murray Bowen, the developer and the key figure of family systems theory, conceptualized the family as an emotional unit, a network of interlocking relationships. He believed that the driving force underlying all human behavior came from the submerged ebb and flow of family life, the simultaneous push and pull between family members for both distance and togetherness. And the problems come from an unbalanced emotional unit made up of members unable to separate or successfully differentiate themselves from one another. And family systems therapy, no matter the nature of the presenting clinical problem, is always governed by two basic goals: (1) management of anxiety and relief from symptoms, and (2) an increase in each participant's level of differentiation in order to improve adaptiveness. Ivan Boszormenyi-Nagy was the primary pioneer of contextual therapy. Contextual therapy is added an ethical perspective—trust, loyalty, transgenerational indebtedness and entitlements, as well as fairness in relationships between family members. What also demands attention, in his view, is the impact of both intrapsychic and intergenerational issues within families, especially each member's subjective sense of claims, rights, and obligations in relation to one another.

2.2.3　Experiential-Humanistic models

Experiential-Humanistic models address emotional engagement, self-growth, and self-determination through present-day experience, encounter, confrontation, intuition, spontaneity, and action. Experiential family therapists tend to minimize theory (and especially theorizing) as a therapeutic hindrance and argue that change resides in a nonrational therapeutic experience that establishes the conditions for personal growth and unblocks family interaction. Experiential family therapy is an outgrowth of the phenomenological techniques. Phenomenological psychotherapy is concerned with the experience or the study of subjectivity, that is of an individual's (or family's) unique experience. Expanding experiences, unblocking suppressed impulses and feelings, developing greater sensitivity, gaining greater access to one's self, learning to recognize and express emotions, achieving intimacy with a partner—these are some of the phenomenologically understood humanistic goals for champions of this viewpoint.

Advocates, Carl Whitaker, Virginia Satir, Johnson and Greenberg aimed at nothing less than personal fulfillment, and focused attention on "in the moment" emotionality. All though have different models, such as symbolic-experiential family therapy, gestalt family therapy, the human validation process model, and colleagues, all of experiential family therapists strive to behave as real, authentic people. By having direct encounters with patients, they attempt to expand their own experiences, often having to deal with their own vulnerabilities in the process (which, when appropriate, they are likely to share with patients). Their therapeutic interventions attempt to be spontaneous, challenging, and, since personalized, often idiosyncratic, as they attempt to help patients gain self-awareness (of their thoughts, feelings, body messages), self-responsibility, and personal growth. The experiential family therapist takes on the task of enriching a family's experiences and enlarging the possibilities for each family member to realize his or her unique and extraordinary potential.

2.2.4 Structural models

Structural models focus on the active, organized wholeness of the family unit and the ways in which the family organizes itself through its transactional patterns. In particular, the family's subsystems, boundaries, alignments, and coalitions are studied in an effort to understand its structure. Dysfunctional structures point to the covert rules governing family transactions that have become inoperative or in need of renegotiation. Structural family therapy is geared to present day transactions and gives higher priority to action than to insight or understanding. All behavior, including symptoms in the identified patient, is viewed within the context of family structure. Structural interventions are active, carefully calculated, even manipulative efforts to alter rigid, outmoded, or unworkable structures. To achieve such changes, families are helped to renegotiate outmoded rules and to seek greater boundary clarity.

The structural approach in family therapy is primarily associated with Salvador Minuchin and his colleagues. They suggested that by joining the family and accommodating to its style, structuralists gain a foothold to assess the members' way of dealing with problems and with each other, ultimately helping them to change dysfunctional sets and rearrange or realign the family organization. Enactments, boundary making, unbalancing, and reframing are therapeutic techniques frequently used. The ultimate goal is to restructure the family's transactional rules by developing more appropriate boundaries between subsystems and strengthening the family's hierarchical order.

2.2.5 Strategic models

Strategic models offer active and straightforward therapeutic interventions, therapeutic double binds or paradoxical techniques, aimed at reducing or eliminating the presenting family problems or behavioral symptoms. Less focused on the meaning of the symptom or its origins, strategists typically issue a series of directives or tasks to the family. These are directed at changing repetitive interactive sequences that lead to cross-generational conflict. Two strengths of strategic family therapy are its insistent attention to removing the disturbing symptom or dysfunctional behavioral sequence by continuously tracking family's patterns of interpersonal exchanges, and its use of assignments of tasks to achieve therapeutic ends. Strategic models view families in non-pathological terms. The family receives help for what they came for, without the therapist speculating on whether other, as yet unidentified, problem areas might still exist or that further therapy perhaps is called for.

Strategic therapies derive from the work of the Palo Alto research group projects on family communication. And four perspectives on the strategic model developed in history: (1) the original mental research institute interactional view; (2) the brief therapy principles and therapeutic procedures that characterize current mental research institute activities; (3) the strategic therapy refinements advanced primarily by Jay Haley and Cloé Madanes, and (4) the strategic-related efforts developed in Milan, Italy, by Mara Selvini-Palazzoli and her associates. Efficiency and technical parsimony are the hallmark of all these models. Feedback loops, the redundancy principle, double binds, family rules, marital quid pro quo, and family homeostasis are all a part of this theoretical model. Strategic therapies view themselves as observer is part of what is being observed, which redefines the therapist as someone who, like the other participants, has a particular perspective but not a truly objective view of the family or what is best for it. One consequence of this thinking is to take "truth" away from the therapist and make goal setting a participatory process that therapist and family members engage in together.

2.2.6   Behavioral and cognitive models

Behavioral and cognitive models view personal functioning to be the result of continuous, reciprocal interaction between behavior and its controlling social conditions. Cognitive-behavioral therapy attempts to modify thoughts and actions by influencing an individual's conscious patterns of thoughts. The unique contribution of this approach, lies in its insistence on a rigorous, data-based set of procedures and a regularly monitored scientific methodology. Most cognitive-behavioral family therapists view family interactions as maintained by environmental events preceding and following each member's behavior. These events or contingencies, together with mediating cognitions, are what determine the form as well as the frequency of each family member's behavior.

Usually, behavioral family therapists strive for precisions in identifying a problem, employ quantify calculation to measure change, and conduct further research to validate their results. They design programs that emphasize a careful assessment of the presenting problem (a behavioral analysis of the family's difficulties) and include some direct and pragmatic treatment techniques to alleviate symptoms and teach the family how to improve its skills in communication and self-management. Currently, cognitive and behavioral approaches are having a significant impact in four distinct areas: behavioral couples therapy, behavioral parent training, functional family therapy, and the conjoint treatment of sexual dysfunction. Nowadays, an expansion of cognitive therapy has led some clinicians to incorporate a constructivist perspective in their work. Patients who have experienced trauma or abuse are coached to construct new "stories" to explain their conditions or situations, unfreezing hampering beliefs and thereby creating more options in their behavior.

2.3   New directions in family therapy

2.3.1   Social construction models I: Solution-focused therapy and collaborative therapy

With rapidly changing social and political awareness of multiple lifestyles and perceptions that began to gain prominence at the close of the twentieth century, some postmodern trends emerged. New directions in family therapy based on the postmodern social construction therapies; focus on the subjective perceptions of the truth or reality that each patient presents. Those therapists reject the modern scientific assumption that truth is waiting to be uncovered by careful, objective observations and measurements, postmodernists in family therapy, beginning in the 1980s, contended that multiple views of reality exist and that absolute truth can never be known. This challenge to taken-for-granted assumptions represented a deconstruction of fixed ways of thinking, leading to exploration of new assumptions and development of new constructions. From a postmodern perspective, everything is open to challenge, including postmodernism itself. In professional terms, the number of marriage and family therapists practicing this type of therapy over the last several years has grown significantly. According to one survey, it stands with behavioral and Bowen family systems among the approaches most often practiced in North America.

Postmodern-oriented therapists attempt to collaborate with family members as self-creating, independent participants. There is an assumption of a shared expertise among all participants. The therapist is no longer a detached, powerful outside observer or sole expert but rather a partaker, with his or her own set of prior beliefs, ready to play a role with family members in constructing the reality being observed. No longer needed to give directives as sole expert, the therapist works with the patients to retell and relive stories and to co-construct possible alternative stories or new outcomes. The therapist engages in a dialogue with family members, helping them shake loose from a set or fixed account of their lives (a story from which they often see no escape) so that they might consider alternatives offering greater promise.

Here are two social constructionist therapeutic approaches in which the language and meaning given events take precedence for the therapist over attending to behavioral sequences or family interactive patterns: (1) solution-focused therapy, emphasizes aiding patients in seeking solutions rather than searching for explanations about their miseries. Miracle questions, exception-finding questions, and scaling questions are commonly employed techniques; (2) solution oriented therapy, helps patients use their inherent skills to explore possibilities and develop solutions without imposing therapist explanations or solutions on the problem.

The collaborative approach pays particular attention to meanings generated between people. Therapists and patients become conversational partners engaged in a shared inquiry aimed at dissolving problems by co-creating stories that open up new possibilities.

The reflecting team technique employs two-way mirrors, so that professionals and families can reverse roles and observe one another offering differing perspectives or tentative speculations on family issues. This opening up of the therapeutic process breaks down professional-patient barriers and helps all participants communicate with one another using a shared "public language."

2.3.2   Social construction models Ⅱ: Narrative therapy

Narrative therapists focus attention on helping patients gain access to preferred story lines about their lives and identities, in place of previous negative, self-defeating, dead-ended narratives about themselves. With the therapist influential but decentered, the patients are helped to create and internalize new dominant stories, draw new assumptions about themselves, and open themselves up to future possibilities by re-authoring their stories.

The model, fast gaining major prominence in the field, is based on post structural thinking that challenges the need for a deep search for underlying "truths" and the need to repair underlying structures. Deconstructing old notions and replacing them with multistoried possibilities help reduce the power of dominating, problem-saturated stories. The therapeutic process calls for attending to and overcoming restrictive self-narratives as well as institutionalized cultural narratives.

To narrative therapists, the patient is not the problem; the problem is the problem. Thus therapeutic conversations typically begin by externalizing the problem. In some cases the problem is given a name, further identifying it as an outside force. Helping families reclaim their lives from the problem, narrative therapy takes the form of questions, often of a deconstructing kind, as the therapist helps patients achieve "thick" descriptions of an alternate story line about their future. Unique outcomes are searched for as possible entryways to developing alternate stories. As patients gain a history of the problem-saturated stories that have dominated their lives, they begin to develop a sense of other options involving more open-ended and feasible stories. Change calls for creating alternative narratives; the process is facilitated by various means for "thickening" or enriching the new story line and connecting to it in future options.

Definitional ceremonies, using reflecting teams or outside witness groups, help tell and retell the story, helping patients authenticate preferred stories. Therapeutic letters help extend the therapeutic sessions and keep patients connected to the emerging alternative stories. Community-based leagues, such as the Anti-Anorexia/Anti-Bulimia League, represent citizens who band together to offer mutual support, build upon each other's skills, and attempt to act as a political action group to change destructive media portrayals of their problems.

Narrative therapies have been paired with other approaches, including psych educational and attachment practices with successful outcomes in a range of problems from learning difficulties and development issues in children to abusive behavior and anger management in adult men.

2.4　Research on family assessment and therapeutic outcomes

Research in family therapy preceded the development of therapeutic intervention techniques, but beginning in the 1960s priorities changed, and the proliferation of techniques outdistanced research. That situation has now begun to even out, and a renewed family research-therapy connection is beginning to be reestablished. Some practitioners, likely in the past to dismiss research findings as not relevant to their everyday needs and experiences, have found qualitative research methodologies more appealing and germane than the more formal, traditional experimental methodologies based on quantitative methods.

Various research attempts to classify and assess families exist, employing either a self-report or an observational format. Most noteworthy among the former are the attempts by Olson and his associates to construct their circumflex model of family functioning based on the family properties of flexibility. And cohesion, and work by Moos to construct his Family Environment Scale. Observational measures, usually in the form of rating scales by outside observers, have been designed by Beavers to depict degrees of family competence and by Epstein, Bishop, and Baldwin to classify family coping skills according to the McMaster Model.

Both the process and outcome of family therapy interventions have been studied with increased interest in recent years. The former, involved with what mechanisms in the therapist-patient encounter produce patient changes, requires the higher priority because identifying the processes that facilitate change helps ensure greater therapeutic effectiveness. Outcome research, including both efficacy and effectiveness studies, having established that marital and family therapy are beneficial, has turned its attention to evidence-based practices—what specific interventions work most effectively with what patient populations. Of particular interest today is the search for the relative advantages and disadvantages of alternative therapeutic approaches for individuals and families with different sets of relational difficulties. Evidence-based family therapy is likely to become increasingly prevalent as efforts are under way to make healthcare delivery more effective and cost-efficient.

3. Art therapy

There are many forms of art therapy, and the most widely used one is the fine art therapy, which includes drawing, painting, collage, or simple sculpture and similar modalities. It provided a visual way to communicate and establish a relationship between the doctors and patients. Art therapy is based on the idea that the creative process of art making is healing and life enhancing and is a form of nonverbal communication of thoughts and feelings. Art is a powerful tool in therapy and it can be useful in so many aspects of evaluation and treatment. The notion that artworks in some way reflect the psychic experience of the artist is a fundamental concept in art therapy, and art expression is a way to visually communicate thoughts and feelings that are hard to be expressed in words. Art therapy has often been used to express emotional experiences, and it is also used to assist in emotional reparation, to encourage personal growth, and to increase self-understanding. It is a modality that can help patients of all ages to find relief from overwhelming emotions or trauma, to resolve conflicts and problems, to enrich daily life, and to achieve an increased sense of well-being. Art therapy has been employed in a wide variety of settings with children, adults, families, and groups, and it can be a primary way of treatment and it can be used as an adjunct to treatment, to enhance verbal therapy through working with the patient to increase self-understanding and insight. Artwork also gave us a way to express what words could not during moments when our thoughts became disorganized and inarticulate.

Art therapy is increasingly used by art therapists, psychologists, counselors, social workers, psychiatrists, and even physicians. Art therapy puts more attention on the drawing process instead of the product, or the product is less important than the therapeutic process involved. Therapist's focus is on the therapeutic needs of the person to express, not specifically on the aesthetic merits of art making. That is, what is important is person's involvement in the work, such as choosing and facilitating art activities that are helpful to the person, helping the person to find meaning in the creative process, and facilitating the sharing of the experience of image making with the therapist. Art did help the patients find a release from their illness, overcome their often-severe depression, and discover and nurture a sense of well-being.

Art therapy permits expression of emotions, thoughts and feelings in a way that is often less frightening than strictly verbal means, there is a level of comfort and a sense of safety sometimes not found through traditional therapy alone. Patients" experiences and feelings are transformed into concrete images, allowing both the therapists and patients to obtain a fresh view of conflicts, problems, directions, and potentials. Many therapists find art expression helps people to quickly communicate relevant issues and problems, especially during the brief forms of therapy. For this reason alone, helping professionals are increasingly using drawings and similar expressive art tasks in the therapeutic intervention.

3.1　A brief history of art therapy

Psychology is an innate characteristic of art. MacGregor presents a history of the interplay of art and psychology spanning the last 300 years in his book, The Discovery of the Art of the Insane. This book covers biographies of "mad" artists, depictions of madness by artists, theories of genius and insanity. He made various attempts to reach a conclusion that art is as an aid to mental health treatment and diagnosis. In 1922, a book named The Artistry of the Mentally Ill was published by a German psychiatrist Hans Prinzhorn, which described the artistic productions of patients in insane asylums in Europe. Freud, Kris, and others contributed to art therapy by theorizing that the production of fantasy is due to the unique inner world of the maker. And later on, many writers began to examine how a specific sort of creative product—art—could be understood as an illustration of mental health or disturbance, according to Freud's theory. And many authors began recognizing the potential art has as a tool within treatment. Soon enough, the term "art therapy" began to be used to describe a form of psychotherapy that placed art practices and interventions alongside talk as the central modality of treatment.

In addition to therapy for patients with mental illness with psychoanalysis approach, one of the strongest trends to emerge within modern psychology has been the focus on standardized methods of diagnostic assessment and research. Kris argues that the fine arts is the expression of the inner experience, an inner image to the outside world. This method of projection became conceptual foundation for the so-called projective drawing assessments that have evolved in psychology. These simple tests with paper-and-pencil, with their standardized methods of interpretation, formalized procedures, have been widely used in the evaluation and diagnosis of patients and are still used today (though often with revamped purpose and procedure).

3.1.1 Classical period (1940s to 1980s)

In the middle of the 20th century many more therapist began to use the term "art therapy" in their writings. Because there was no formal art therapy training from school, these writers often were trained in other fields and mentored by analysts, psychiatrists or psychologists. Among them, there were four leading writers, who were universally recognized for their contributions in the field of art therapy: Margaret Naumburg, Edith Kramer, Hanna Kwiatkowska, and Elinor Ulman. Their writings continue to be used in contemporary art therapy literature, which suggests the lasting impact of their original works on the field. More than any other authors, Naumburg is frequently referred to as the "Mother of Art Therapy", and is seen as the primary founder of American art therapy. Similar to the ideas of Freud and Jung, Naumburg conceived "dynamically oriented art therapy". She proposed that the patients' art productions were symbolic communication of unconscious material in a direct, uncensored way. While Naumburg borrowed her ideas heavily from psychoanalytic practice, Kramer took a different approach by adapting concepts from Freud's personality theory to explain art therapy process. Her "art therapy" approach emphasizes the central role of sublimation and the intrinsic therapeutic potential in the art-making process.

Ulman's contributes to the field of art therapy mostly through her work as an editor and writer. She founded The Bulletin of Art Therapy in 1961 (The American Journal of Art Therapy after 1970) when no other publication of its kind existed. In addition, Ulman published the first book of collected essays on art therapy that served as one of the few texts in the field for many years. Her gift as a writer was to precisely synthesize and articulate complex ideas. In her essay "Art Therapy: Problems of Definition," Ulman compares and contrasts Naumburg's "art psychotherapy" and Kramer's "art as therapy" models so clearly that it continues to be the definitive presentation of this core theoretical continuum. The last of these four remarkable women, Kwiatkowska, made her major contributions in the areas of research and family art therapy. She brought together her experiences in various psychiatric settings in a book that became the foundation for working with families through art.

Finally, it is important to remember other early pioneers working in other parts of the country, such as Mary Huntoon at the Menninger Clinic, who made contributions to the developing profession as well. The 1970s through the mid-1980s saw the emergence of an increasing number of publications that presented a broader range of applications and conceptual perspectives, although psychoanalysis remained a dominant influence. The development of the literature was also enriched during this period with the introduction of two new journals: Art Psychotherapy in 1973 (called The Arts in Psychotherapy after 1980) and Art Therapy: Journal of the American Art Therapy Association, in 1983. The increasing number of publications, along with the founding of the American Art Therapy Association in 1969, evolved the professional identity of the art therapist, credentials, and the role of art therapist's vis-à-vis related professionals. It was also during this period that the first formal programs with degrees in art therapy were offered.

3.1.2 Contemporary art therapy theories (1980s to present)

In a landmark book, Approaches to Art Therapy published in 1987, Rubin brought together essays by authors representing the diversity of theoretical positions within the field. Rubin (1999) noted that there were only 12 books written by art therapists. This pace began to increase in the 1980s. Rubin speculated that an art therapist was more comfortable with an intuitive approach than other mental health practitioners, because as artists they "pride themselves on their innate sensitivities, and tend to be anti-authoritarian and anti-theoretical". Recently, approximately 21% of art therapists surveyed by the American Art Therapy Association described their primary theoretical orientation as "eclectic". The next five most frequently reported models:

psychodynamic (10.1%), Jungian (5.4%), object relations (4.6%), art therapy (4.5%), and psychoanalytic (3.0%). The ideas of Freud and his followers have been part of art therapy since the earliest days, although contemporary writers are more likely to apply terms such as "transference" and "the defense mechanisms" to articulate a position rather than employ classic psychoanalytic techniques with any degree of orthodoxy. Kramer, Rubin, Ulman, and Wilson and Levick all use psychoanalytic language and concepts. Interpretations of the newer developments in psychoanalysis such as the theories of Klein, self-psychology (Lachman-Chapin) and object relations theory (Robbins) can also be found in the art therapy literature. With his emphasis on images from the unconscious, it was natural for Jung's concepts of analytical and archetypal psychology to cross over into art therapy. Works by Edwards and Wallace, McConeghey, and Schaverian all reflect this emphasis.

3.2   Mechanisms for art therapy

3.2.1   Image itself

Images do have an impact on how we feel and react. For example, just imagining biting into a lemon may cause one's mouth to pucker and seeing a favorite food may cause one to salivate. Images can create sensations of pleasure, fear, anxiety, or calm and there is evidence that they can alter mood and even induce psychoanalytic analytic theory psychoanalytic analytic theory of well-being. There is solid evidence that images have a significant impact on our bodies. Simple experiments have provided evidence that even exposure to the images of nature from a hospital room window can decrease the length of stay and increase feelings of well-being in patients. Art therapist Vija Lusebrink observes that images are "a bridge between body and mind, or between the conscious levels of information processing and the physiological changes in the body". Guided imagery, an experiential process in which an individual is directed through relaxation followed by suggestions to imagine specific images, has been used to reduce symptoms, change mood, and harness body's healing capacities. Art therapists and others have applied principles of mental imagery and guided imagery to work with individuals in a variety of settings. For example, Baron employed guided imagery as a part of art therapy in the treatment of individuals with cancer. Until relatively recently, researchers have only been able to speculate about how guided imagery works. Neuroscience is rapidly increasing the understanding of mental imagery, image formation, and the regions of the brain involved in image creation. For example, research shows that imagery we see or we imagine activate the visual cortex of the brain in similar ways. In other words, according to Damasio, our bodies respond to mental images as if they are reality. He also notes that images are not just visual and include all sensory modalities—auditory, olfactory, gustatory, and somatosensory (touch, muscular, temperature, pain, visceral, and vestibular senses). Images are not stored in any one part of the brain; rather, many regions of the brain are part of image formation, storage, and retrieval. The increasing understanding of the brain's hemispheres and their interactions has also contributed to the understanding of mental images and art making. In the past, it was believed that the right and left brain generally had two different functions; the right brain was the center of intuition, creativity, while the left brain was thought to be engaged in logical thought and language. Some claimed art therapy's value was due to its ability to tap right brain functions, observing that art making is a "right-brained" activity (Virshup, 1978). In reality, the brain's left hemisphere (where language is located) is also involved in making art. Gardner (1984), Ramachandran (1999), and others have demonstrated that both hemispheres of the brain are necessary for art expression and evidence can be seen in the drawings of people with damage to specific areas of the brain. Researchers have also discovered connections between language and certain movements in drawing. For example, in a study using positron emission tomography scan, brain activity of individuals drawing forms in space was recorded.

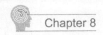

The results indicate that even simple drawing involves complex interactions between many parts of the brain. Images and image formation, whether mental images or those drawn on paper, are important in all art therapy practice because through art making patients are invited to reframe how they feel, respond to an event or experience, and work on emotional and behavioral change. In contrast to mental images, however, art making allows an individual to actively try out, experiment with, or rehearse a desired change through a drawing, painting, or collage; that is, it involves a tangible object that can be physically altered.

3.2.2   The physiology of emotion

It is well-known that the body is often a mirror of an individual's emotions. When we are anxious, our palms sweat or our faces may be ashen, or we may turn red when embarrassed. Images affect our emotions and different parts of the brain may become active when we look at sad faces or happy faces or mentally image a happy or sad event or relationship. There are also a variety of hormonal fluctuations as well as cardiovascular and neurological effects. In fact, the physiology of emotions is so complex that the brain knows more than the conscious mind can itself reveal. That is, one can actually display an emotion without being conscious of what induced the emotion. Trauma has received increasing attention in neuroscience because it is now believed to be both a psychological and physiological experience. There is general agreement that traumatic events take a toll on the body as well as the mind and, thus, posttraumatic stress disorder is defined through both psychological and physiological symptoms. Many have pointed to the true core of trauma as being physiological, and, as van der Kolk metaphorically notes, "the body keeps the score" of the emotional experience. Although many parts of the brain are important in trauma, the limbic system, the seat of survival instincts and reflexes, has been given considerable attention. It includes the hypothalamus, the hippocampus, and the amygdala, which is also pertinent to understanding traumatic memory. Though the function of the limbic system will not be covered in detail here, recent findings indicate its role in the sensory memories of stressful events and trauma. These findings are revealing why art expression is a useful part of therapy, trauma debriefing, and psychological recovery. Because the core of traumatic experiences is physiological, the expression and processing of sensory memories of the traumatic event are essential to successful intervention and resolution. Art is a natural sensory mode of expression because it involves touch, smell, and other senses within the experience. Drawing and other art activities mobilize the expression of sensory memories in a way that verbal interviews and interventions cannot. Highly charged emotional experiences, such as trauma, are encoded by the limbic system as a form of sensory reality. For a person's experience of trauma to be successfully ameliorated, it must be processed through sensory means. The capacity of art making to tap sensory material (i.e., the limbic system's sensory memory of the event) makes it a potent tool in trauma intervention. Specific drawing tasks, such as "draw what happened" and other related directives are proving to be effective in tapping sensory memories as well as generating narratives that can be altered through cognitive reframing techniques to reduce long-term sequelae of posttraumatic stress. The way in which memory is stored is also shedding light on why art therapy may be helpful to those who are traumatized. There are two types of memory: explicit memory is conscious and is composed of facts, concepts, and ideas and implicit memory is sensory and emotional and is related to body's memories. Riding a bicycle is good example of implicit memory; narrating the chronological details of an event is an example of explicit memory. Currently, there is some speculation that posttraumatic stress disorder, in part, may be caused when memory of trauma is excluded from explicit storage. Problems also result from traumatic memories when implicit memories are not linked to explicit memories; that is, an individual may not have access to the context in which the emotions or sensations arose. Art expression may help to bridge the implicit and explicit memories of a stressful event by facilitating the creation of a narrative through which the person can explore the memories and why they are so upsetting. Art activities, in this sense, may help the traumatized individual to think and feel concurrently, while making meaning for troubling experiences. Finally, art therapy can be used to tap the body's relaxation response. Drawing, for example, is hypothesized to facilitate children's verbal reports of emotionally laden events in several ways: reduction of anxiety, helping the child feel comfortable with the therapist, increasing memory retrieval, organizing narratives, and prompting the child to tell more details than in a solely verbal interview. Malchiodi observed in working with children from violent homes that art activity had a soothing, hypnotic influence and that traumatized children were naturally attracted to this quality when anxious or suffering from posttraumatic stress. Someday, through the use of brain scans and other technology, we may have a clearer understanding of exactly how to use art therapy to tap the relaxation response for patients of all ages who have undergone intense stress.

3.2.3   Psychoanalytic theory

Even though art therapy used a variety of theoretical models and followed multiple paths—art, psychology, medicine, and education, art therapy first appeared as a form of psychotherapy in the mid-20th century. The idea of art expression as a reflection of the art maker's unconsciousness was the central concepts of psychoanalytic analytic theory that stressed the importance of individual's internal world. Sigmund Freud's views are the foundation for most theories of psychotherapy and undoubtedly have been a major influence on the development of art therapy in the 20th century. Freud's theory of the unconscious influenced the development of psychoanalytic approach to art therapy as well as the development of projective drawing techniques that emphasized the emergence of unconscious material through images. Freud's theory of ego defense mechanisms, particularly sublimation which has been related to artistic expression, also influenced the course of the psychoanalytic approach to art therapy. Freud's daughter, Anna, also had an impact on art therapy. Although her father did not direct his patients to draw, Anna used art and other expressive activity in her work and recognized art expression as an aid in treatment because children could not engage in adult free association.

Carl Jung had different ideas about the symbolic role of images. In contrast to Freud, he used art as a method of self-analysis. Jung believed that if a patient relied on the therapist to interpret a dream or fantasy, the patient would remain in a state of dependence on the analyst. Jung invited his patients to paint, noting "the aim of this method of expression is to make unconscious content accessible and so bring it closer to patient's understanding". Jung's ideas about treatment developed partially from his belief that one must establish a dialogue between the conscious and unconscious in order to achieve psychic equilibrium. He believed one way this balance could be achieved was through tapping the transcendent qualities of symbols such as those in art and dreams. Jung considered symbols to be unifiers of opposites within a single entity and as natural attempts by the psyche to reconcile inner conflicts and to achieve individuation. He endeavored to work with an individual's images to reveal hidden possibilities and thereby help the person find meaning and wholeness in life.

There are several ways of mechanisms for unconsciousness to be expressed in arts, for example transference. Transference is considered to be an important part of psychoanalysis and, in Freudian theory, the examination of transference is regarded as the basis of treatment. Simply defined, transference is patient's unconscious projection of feelings onto the therapist. These projections, which originate in repressed or unfinished situations of one's life, are thought to be the essence of therapy, and the success of treatment is dependent on their accurate analysis.

Psychoanalytic and analytic approaches to art therapy are strongly linked to the idea that spontaneous art expression provides access to the unconscious. Spontaneous art expression is any image making which is nondirective; that is, the person is simply requested to make a drawing, painting, or sculpture of anything he or she wants to and may also be invited to choose freely whatever materials he or she wishes to use. The purpose of spontaneous expression, like free association, is to help patients express what troubles them as freely as possible. In the psychoanalytic approach, as well as many other approaches to art therapy, therapist's role is to facilitate an interpersonal relationship that encourages the individual to create spontaneous images and to discover personal meaning in one's expressions. While image making may be spontaneous, the therapist is expected to explain art media (such as how to use drawing or painting materials) to individuals who are inexperienced in art expression. This might even include a brief demonstration of how to use a chalk pastel or paintbrush, or even a technique such as the "scribble" (described in more detail later). Emphasis, however, is on art expression as symbolic communication rather than necessarily an aesthetic product, which promotes the idea that all expression is acceptable and is intended to encourage more free communication of conflicts and emotions. While therapists working from a psychoanalytic.

Amplification is strictly an analytic approach. It was originally a method of dream interpretation developed by Jung in which a dream image or motif is enlarged, clarified, and given a meaningful context by comparing it with similar images from mythology, folklore, and comparative religion. According to this process, an image cannot be interpreted by its content alone; it also must be considered in terms of what the content might symbolize and the symbol itself must be given a meaningful context. Jung believed that amplification established the collective context of a dream, enabling it to be seen not only in its personal aspect but also in general archetypal terms that were common to all humanity. In amplification, the person would be encouraged to stay with the original image of the shoe, perhaps saying "shoe, foot, shoe, sandal, shoe, stocking," remaining as close to the original image as possible. In general, there are two different approaches to amplification: subjective and objective. In objective amplification, the analyst collects themes from mythology, religion, and other sources to illuminate the symbol. In other words, if a person related a dream about a poor relationship with her mother and meeting a man in an underground place, the analyst might relate the myth of Demeter and Persephone's descent into the underworld, a story that reflects a similar theme. In subjective amplification, the individual uses the technique of "active imagination" to find associations to the symbol. Active imagination is a method described by Jung as a way to release creativity within the individual by using fantasy and dreams as the primary mode of healing. It is the dynamic production of inward images in which the individual is encouraged to observe those images. While making art is believed by art therapists to be one form of active imagination, it can also be the creation of mental images.

3.2.4   Attachment theory

Attachment theory has been used as a theoretical base for psychotherapy for many years but has more recently become a major interest among therapists. Siegel explains attachment as follows: "Attachment is an inborn system in the brain that evolves in ways that influence and organize motivational, emotional, and memory processes with respect to significant caregiving figures". Schore offers a neurological model for the importance of infant attachment throughout life. He notes that soon after birth the caretaker and infant develop interactions that are important to the process of affect regulation. Face-to-face contact and soothing touch are examples of ways the infant learns to respond to stimulation from people and experiences. Perry, Pollard, Blakley, Baker, and Vigilante propose that successful attachment is critical to optimal development of specific parts of the brain. He believes that a healthy attachment between infant and caretaker sets the stage for the individual to develop the capacity to "self-regulate" stimulating experiences. Early childhood bonding is imprinted on the brain, laying a foundation for relationship patterns later in life; when trauma is present, brain imprinting is changed, but may be corrected with appropriate intervention. Research in neuroscience is demonstrating that infancy is not the only chance a person has for healthy attachment and there seem to be ways to reshape and repair some early experiences. Art therapy is one way being explored to reestablish healthy attachments, both through therapist and patient, and through encouraging healthy interactions between parent and child. Riley cites how art activities are being used in early childhood attachment programs and how simple drawing exercises can be used to resolve relational problems and strengthen parent-child bonds. She explains that the nonverbal dimensions of art activities tap early relational states before words are dominant, possibly allowing the brain to establish new, and more productive patterns. Siegel and Schore believe that interactions between baby and caretaker are right-brain mediated because during infancy the right cortex is developing more quickly than the left. Siegel also observes that just as the left hemisphere requires exposure to language to grow, the right hemisphere requires emotional stimulation to develop properly. He goes on to say that the output of the right brain is expressed in "non-word-based ways" such as drawing a picture or using a picture to describe feelings or events. According to this idea, art therapy may be an important modality in working with attachment issues, among other emotionally related disorders or experiences.

4. Music therapy

Music has been a medium of therapy for centuries, and there are numerous examples of the curative or healing powers of music in the historical records of different cultures. Over the last fifty years, music therapy has developed as a clinically applied treatment administered by trained professionals in countries. In some countries, music therapy is officially recognized by political, clinical and academic institutions or organizations, and also by employment agencies. In Europe, music therapy traditions have developed on the foundations of more psychodynamic and psychotherapeutically orientated approaches. Frequently one finds the therapist is actively using music-making through the medium of clinical improvisation in order to establish a musical relationship with the patients through which he or she will be able to help them understand the nature of their problem. This active form of music therapy has involved the development of music therapy training programs, which require, at entry level, highly trained musicians in order to develop their skills in the therapeutic field. Therapists require knowledge of the potential in therapy of the various elements of music for helping the patient, together with a theoretical framework of therapeutic intervention. With this kind of therapy, and with certain clinical populations (patients), music therapy has been found to be effective and beneficial. For example, there is much documented material on the efficacy of music therapy intervention to improve and develop communication and relationship-building with patients with autistic disability, and in assessing communication disorder. Behavioral approaches in music therapy have emerged mainly in the United States of America and they have frequently developed the use of music as a stimulant, a relaxant or a reward. In addition, the structure and properties of music have been applied and manipulated to achieve development, growth and improvement in patients. In this sense, the therapeutic process does not involve a dynamic and responsive interaction with the patient, but the music is structured in order to help the patient overcome emotional, physical or psychological problem.

4.1 History of music therapy

Since antiquity, music has been used as a therapeutic tool, and ancient healing rituals including sound and music have survived in many cultures. It was still a tradition in Western cultures to maintain that music and health (physiological as well as psychological) were closely related. This tradition goes back to the legendary Greek philosopher Pythagoras (circa 500 BC) and early Greek medical science of his time. It was the eighteenth and nineteenth century that witnessed the development of modern natural and medical science, based on

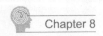

empirical and statistical principles, and saw the break between music and health. Recently—after nearly 250 years of separation—medicine, health psychology and music therapy are approaching each other again, realizing that man is not a "machine", but a complex, bio-psycho-social being. Or man is a unity of body, mind and spirit placed into a social order, and music has comprehensive effects and meaning on all levels.

Pythagoras realized this 2500 years ago, he was both a mystic and a serious scientist, who also worked empirically. He studied the surrounding world with his senses and thought deeply about the implications of his discoveries for man and culture. One of his working tools was a so-called monochord—a measure and music "instrument" with only one string. On this instrument he could experiment with notes and intervals, with the proportions of two or more notes—and their relationship to human consciousness. The discoveries of Pythagoras are still relevant. In a famous paragraph of Plato's The State (Book III) we are informed about the influence of music on the human mind. In his dialogue with Glaucon, Socrates praises the use of certain rhythms and modes that encourage man to a harmonic and brave life.

In the development of natural science, anatomy and empirically informed medicine after Renaissance, music gradually receded into the background. A few doctors were still experimenting with music and wrote treatises or reports. It was not until the 1960s and 1970s, that the classical themes and doctrines were revived.

Music therapy is a profession which has emerged over the last fifty years from a variety of professional disciplines in different countries. Or music therapy is the use of music in clinical, educational and social situations to treat patients or patients with medical, educational, social or psychological needs. In order to establish a more generic and all-embracing definition of music therapy in 1996, the World Federation of Music Therapy produced the following definition: Music therapy is the use of music and musical elements or both (sound, rhythm, melody and harmony) by a qualified music therapist with a patient or group, in a process designed to facilitate and promote communication, relationships, learning, mobilization, expression, organization and other relevant therapeutic objectives, in order to meet physical, emotional, mental, social and cognitive needs. Music therapy aims to develop potentials and restore functions or both of the individual so that he or she can achieve better intra-and interpersonal integration and, consequently, a better quality life through prevention, rehabilitation or treatment.

4.2　Mechanism of music therapy

Music can be experienced, understood and analyzed in many different ways. As music history has fostered many different theories on the essence of music, the history of music therapy has embraced many different concepts of music and its meaning. Theories of music aesthetics reflect the ever-changing historical, cultural and social framework of music production and reception, and the changing concepts of music in the history of music therapy also reflect the changing ideas of music and healing in medical theory. This can be seen when different aspects of music philosophy are observed from a historical point of view. The idea of the inherent meaning of number and proportions in music is related to the philosophical idea of harmonic proportions in the relationship of body and soul in Greek philosophy. The idea of "ethos" ("how to live a good life") is connected to humoral medicine (or theory of humors: the classic philosophy of how biological processes (health and disease) are related to the internal balance of the four body fluids: blood, phlegm, yellow bite and black bile).

Many music therapists—especially therapists working within a psychodynamic or humanistic-existential framework—reject the idea of music as an autonomous aesthetic object and maintain that music is a representation and expression of the psychological world of their patients. Music is often considered a symbolic language allowing the therapist to explore its meaning for the patient in improvisations followed by verbal therapeutic dialogue and hermeneutic ("morphological") interpretation or both. The specific musical expression of the patient and musical interaction in dyads or groups may also be interpreted as an analogy to the expression and interrelationships of the patient in general.

Music therapy has been significantly and diversely influenced by the historical development of therapy, where therapy is defined as a form of treatment administered by a therapist. Over the years, three main therapeutic schools have emerged for the treatment of mental illness, emotional disturbance and psychological disorders: (1) Psychoanalytic/psychotherapeutic: this model of therapy incorporates a wide variety of approaches which place the "unconscious" as the source of emotional disturbance. Therefore, exploring and understanding hidden or "unconscious" drives and feelings provides the main focus for therapeutic intervention; (2) behavior therapy: this approach generally regards only obvious behavior as significant, and therapeutic approaches tend to focus on the treatment and modification of behavior; (3) traditional neuropsychiatry: this approach considers physiological or chemical disorders to be the primary cause of emotional disturbance and as a consequence uses medication or primarily physiological methods as the therapeutic intervention.

In the development of music therapy, the first two models have formed the primary, therapeutic foundation for the development of music therapy theory and music therapy practice. The early development of music therapy in the USA was predominantly linked with theories of behaviorism and behavior therapy although, in recent times in certain areas, particularly the East Coast, psychotherapeutic and psychoanalytic approaches are also common. However, the main foundation for many therapists trained in the American school of music therapy is behavioral. In Europe, psychotherapeutic and psychoanalytic approaches have become more dominant. There is not a clear division, and therapists are significantly influenced by both their teachers and the forms of therapy that they have experienced. On music therapy courses, it is valuable for students to have a clear understanding of different models of therapeutic approach, based on the theory of therapy, even though they are typically being trained in a particular style of work. In addition to that, psychotherapy is a very "broad church" ranging from a spectrum of cognitive behavior therapy through to analytical, existential and person-centered therapy.

4.3　Early development

Some traditions in music therapy are based on early mother-baby interaction, and the therapeutic relationship can be perceived as involving elements of vocal and gestural behavior from this early stage. Our early experiences of sound are very formative. For example, singers find that their unborn babies are quieter when they are singing, and mothers who play instruments notice that their unborn children become more active while they are playing. There is an increase in body tension in crying babies, and while low frequencies seem to have pleasant associations, high frequencies have unpleasant ones. It has also been suggested that one attraction of "beat", pop or very rhythmic music is the emotional link with the security of the mother's womb. Tapes have been produced of the sounds of the womb, including the sound of the placenta and the blood movement in the pulses from the umbilical cord. They were used with newborn infants prone to long periods of crying to try and calm them. Babies only react to about a third of the available acoustic stimuli in their first hours of life, but this rapidly increases, and the first six months is the period of "learning to hear". After 11 to 12 weeks babies prefer human voices to other noise. At 12 to 14 weeks they can discriminate between their mother's voice and a stranger's, and between 14 to 16 weeks they can stop crying when they hear their mother's footsteps.

Helmut Moog wrote a lot about the early development of musical responses, noting the attention of infants to music at four to six months, and the beginnings of repetitive movements to music after six months. He described the emergence of "musical babbling" after speech babble has started, but that children sing their

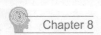

first "babble song" before they say their first word. In tests on babies of six months, he found that rhythmic tests attracted little attention, whereas songs and instrumental music attracted the most active attention and movements. Babbling songs of 12- month children begin to show aspects of musical organization with pitched glissandi, downward melodic lines and four note figures.

For music therapists it is important to have some awareness of these early stages of development in music. For example, when working with people who are mentally handicapped, despite the fact that their chronological age may be anything between 10 and 80, if their mental age is at a pre-school, even pre-verbal level, one has to adapt expectations of their skills and abilities in producing or creating melody and rhythm. In interpreting musical engagement from the point of view of the therapeutic relationship, the fact that a person may perseverate or lose attention to maintaining a steady pulse or rhythm may not be due to emotional or interactive negativity, but is perhaps more linked to their musical stage of development.

4.4   Attachment need

Daniel Stern is an American psychologist, psychoanalyst and researcher, who, in 1985, presented a theory describing the development of the interpersonal world of the infant. Stern's work is considered an essential contribution to the on-going debate in the field of developmental psychology. Based on empirically grounded research, he has revised the psychoanalytic view on development. Stern's most significant contribution is a coherent theory describing how the infant from birth actively builds and develops its sense of self. The sense of self is based on the experience of actual interactions and incidents. This means that the development of a sense of self is seen more as a product of real experiences than of unconscious drives and fantasies. There is a focus on the relational aspects of development and on the mechanisms that characterize early interaction between mother and infant.

The development of child's sense of self consists of five levels: the first three are pre-verbal and the last two are verbal. The new element in Stern's theory is that these developmental levels are seen as "layers" of maturation and experience that exist side by side (and not phases the child moves through, as in traditional psychoanalysis). These layers of development are related to different senses of the self, and to different ways of experiencing "how-to-be-with-another". This means that the experiences and knowledge that the child attains pre-verbally are different from knowledge based on words and symbols. Stern uses the terms "implicit" and "explicit" knowledge. Implicit knowledge is subconscious, action based and "tacit/silent knowledge", while explicit knowledge is conscious, and can be expressed potentially in symbolic or verbal form.

Stern describes psychological development as follows: (1) the child already actively interacts with its surroundings from birth; (2) Development is characterized by different senses of self and different ways of being with another; (3) The child builds a fundament of implicit knowledge about the world before language is developed; (4) The emergence of language makes more precise communication possible but at the same time it inhibits access to the pre-verbal sense of self. This theory has contributed greatly to the understanding of relational processes in psychotherapy. Stern's theory about pre-verbal interaction has especially contributed to the understanding of what happens in the therapist/patient relationship. Stern describes how the child builds an implicit and procedural knowledge of his/her ability to act, to have feelings, to have a coherent sense of the body and a sense of time. These sensations re-emerge in the therapeutic situation, where patients, for example, can feel unable to act, have difficulty recognizing emotions, experience a "dissolving" of body's boundaries or lose their sense of time. In other words, their difficulties lie in the domain of the sense of self that Stern calls "the core self ". Stern also describes how children develop the ability of "inter-subjectivity", and how they learn which emotions can be shared with others and which cannot. This process has great significance for the way in which the person later in life is able to share his/her inner world with others.

In therapy, the process of showing and sharing emotions can often cause great problems and, because of this, the patient has a limited capacity for inter-subjectivity. These problems are related to the sense of the self that Stern refers to as the "subjective self ". From the point of view of music therapy, Stern is especially interesting, because he describes basic pre-verbal interaction as containing many of the same elements as music. For example, he states that elements of communication such as tempo, rhythm, tone, phrasing, form and intensity are necessary for the child, in order to "decode" and organize sensory experiences of interaction into generalized mental structures. Stern describes how the child forms Representations of Interactions that have been generalized—mental structures also referred to as "schemas". In this process, according to Stern, the child obtains implicit schematic knowledge of "how-to-be-with-another". In other words, Stern's theory seems to support the view that interaction, communication and music are fundamentally made up of the same elements. This supports, therefore, the assumption that musical improvisation and music listening can reflect and activate relational patterns and the senses of self-connected to these. The aim of psychotherapy and music therapy is exploring, working through and changing dysfunctional relational patterns. Therefore it is obvious that Stern's theory is important in understanding the origin of these patterns and their dynamics in the "here and now" therapy situation. Since he presented his developmental theory, Stern has attempted to integrate the developmental aspect of his theory with the therapeutic aspect, especially in two areas. One of these areas has to do with theories on motherhood and mother/child therapy. Here Stern translates his developmental theory and his understanding of the relational dynamics between the child and its surroundings directly into therapy with dysfunctional families.

The second area concerns a theory on the meaning of the non-interpretative mechanisms in psychotherapy that Stern proposed with a group of researchers. This proposal is considered important, because it focuses on implicit experiences in therapy. Experiences that cannot be verbalized, but only felt, are found to be central to the development of patient's ability to know, recognize and share emotions. In the therapy setting this means that the therapist and patients share experiences without verbalizing them in the situation. The reason for this is that language, in the therapeutic situation as well as in a developmental context, often creates a distance to the pre-verbal sense of the self. Music in music therapy often unfolds in a non-verbal context. Clinical experience shows that musical improvisation can enhance the implicit dimension of an experience. Musical interaction is therefore considered a means of making clear the fundamental elements of interaction and thereby the basic ways of relating. The resemblance between pre-verbal relationships and transference patterns in musical interaction has been supported by recently conducted research. In this case, transference is seen as patient's repetition and re-experiencing of emotions that originate in experiences with significant others. This repetition and re-experience can be observed in relational patterns in the musical interaction. The study shows that Stern's theories on pre-verbal relationships can be used to describe relational themes in both the verbal and the musical context with adult patients, and that these relational themes and patterns have the quality of transference. Stern is less direct in his description of clinical concepts such as transference, countertransference, defence and repetition compulsion, but he argues that the unconscious, implicit level of the therapeutic relationship is related to these psychoanalytic concepts. Stern's theories have greatly influenced our understanding of how we relate and interact. His theories confirm that relational patterns, which are the focus of the therapy process, contain non-verbal knowledge about relationships, and that this knowledge seems to be expressed in the musical interaction.

4.5   Emotional effects of music

Inherent in any approach or theory of music therapy is the concept of the emotional effect of music. Although music has the power to cause mental, physical, emotional and spiritual responses in us, beyond a few generalizations we do not completely understand how and in what way different types of music will affect us. Most research shows that the effects of music are greater when the music has more meaning for the listener. Emotional reactions are often due to associations, memories and past experiences that may have been good or bad. The English psychologist John Sloboda found that people's memories of their early experiences of music could be unpleasant—such as being told they cannot sing by the school music teacher—or nice—the first time they heard Mozart's Clarinet Concerto and fell in love with the sound of the clarinet. Music often has special significance between people when they fall in love, and songs or pieces hold treasured memories—what Sloboda described as the "Darling, they are playing our tune again" phenomenon. In music therapy work with the elderly, they may often ask for children's songs, or Christmas carols. When played, tears of sadness or happy memories come, allowing the person to remember events in their life—happy or sad—and work through their feelings of loss as they come to the end of their life.

Whereas emotions result from responses to specific objects, situations whereas emotions result from responses to specific objects, situations or persons, Hevner's "Mood Wheel" was a design to see how we can move through a sequence of moods to get, for example, from solemnity to excitement. The process of moving from one emotion to another is part of the skill of the musician, composer, and certainly the music therapist. The mood of the music often needs to reflect the emotional state or mood of the patient to begin with before a subtle process of movement can occur. You cannot suddenly change the emotion in a depressed person by introducing light, fast, syncopated and amusing music into the improvisation. Contrary to popular belief, music cannot express emotions with any degree of success, but rather creates mood to which we respond at an emotional level. This is mainly referring to instrumental music, because songs do express emotions, but do so primarily through the lyrics. Stravinsky once said "music is, by its very nature, essentially powerless to express anything at all, whether a feeling, attitude of mind, psychological mood, or phenomenon of nature". However, Mendelssohn suggested the opposite view that "the thoughts which are expressed to me by a piece of music which I love are not too indefinite to be put into words, but on the contrary are too definite". Music essentially expresses mood qualities upon which we project a specific emotional meaning.

4.6   Application of music therapy

Music therapists working within the health system frequently establish collaborative professional relationships with doctors, nurses, paramedical professionals including physiotherapists, occupational therapists, speech and language therapists and others, and psychologists. Working in health systems, music therapists frequently find that their approach and treatment objectives are directed towards improving the general health of the patient, working with specific pathological problems and disorders, and maintaining quality of life and stability in the more chronic population. Work is undertaken in collaboration with the multidisciplinary team, and the music therapists find that they are approaching patients within the context of an overall plan for patient's treatment.

Music therapists also work in the field of special education and in schools. Here, music therapists are often standing alongside music teachers and music pedagogues and there can be some confusion over the different roles involved. Generally, music teaching is a process which involves teaching children to acquire skills in the use of instruments and knowledge of music. This generally involves performance, composition and abilities to analyses music. The objectives for music teachers are frequently to work with students towards the achievement of skills in music, either at instrumental performance, singing or knowledge of music. The music therapist, on the other hand, is primarily working with the non-musical needs of the patient at the centre of the treatment or remedial program, their therapeutic needs. In special education, children present with a variety of learning difficulties, behavioral problems, social problems and psychological disabilities. The music therapist takes these problems as the primary focus for intervention and the function of the music is to act as a medium for meeting the needs of the patient. Therefore, the acquisition of musical skill is not a primary objective, nor is it a requirement for the child to respond to therapy that they have achieved musical skill or even an aptitude for music. The music is a tool by which therapy occurs.

Nevertheless there is a grey area between the music therapist orientated within an educational setting and a music teacher who has adapted his/her working practice for children with special needs and has included remedial therapy objectives within his/her work. The main difference remains that a music teacher primarily focuses on promoting the development of musical skills, while a music therapist is focused on meeting therapeutic needs which nevertheless still need to be linked with the school's educational programs, and the individual educational program of each child.

5. Sandbox

A young child walks into your office, hiding behind the legs of his parent. He is terrified, and has been abused. You know that he needs to process the pain of his experience, and that the counseling process may be slow. He refuses to talk. Where do you begin? Many counselors might meet these situations, and want the patients to talk about what has happened to them and what they are currently experiencing, hope that they can verbalize their frustrations. However, the children do not communicate the way adults do with verbal communication, instead, they communicate with play. Just as Landreth suggested: Children's play can be more fully appreciated when recognized as their natural medium of communication; for children to play out their experiences and feelings is the most naturally dynamic and self-healing process where children can engage. Additionally, developmental psychology supports the use of play as a means for communicating with children. Since children do not possess the developmental or intellectual sophistication to participate in adult verbally bases therapies, it may be concluded that the very nature of childhood is fundamentally incompatible with the formal operations of adult counseling. Therefore, sandbox is a good way in treating children. Sandbox is the effective treatment modality for children. The psychotherapeutic technique known as Sandplay has experienced a major growth in popularity within the past five to ten years, as witnessed by the publication of numerous articles and several books devoted to this topic. Sandplay has been enthusiastically adopted by play therapists and art therapists, as well as by Jungian psychotherapists in their search for creative ways to assist young patients and their families.

In all, there are a myriad of techniques used and advocated in the mental health profession. Sandplay is more than just another treatment modality, because sandplay seeks and maintains the inner emotion, and they experience emotional healing when they encounter someone and when they encounter self. Just as Spare wrote, "As with every aspect of clinical practice, meaningful use of sandplay is a function of our own human hearts, and of the ever ongoing interplay between our own centers and the centers, hearts, and needs of those we are privileged to see in psychotherapy".

5.1　History of sand play

Sandplay as a therapeutic modality has been in existence since 1929, when Margaret Lowenfeld first devised a method known as the World Technique. Dr. Lowenfeld was a child psychiatrist in London, where she established the Institute for Child Psychology. Many clinicians felt her influence, and the technique took different forms as her trainees adapted their methods to their own theoretical orientations. In the comprehensive study published by Rie Rogers Mitchell and Harriet Friedman, Lowenfeld's influence is described as quite far-reaching. Many of the practitioners who met with Lowenfeld adapted their own

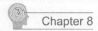

orientations to her teachings. Erik Erikson, Gudrun Seitz in Sweden, and Dora Kalff in Switzerland were among those whom Lowenfeld influenced.

5.2　Lowenfeld's contribution

Lowenfeld had an interesting history. She was born in England and spent her early years in both Poland and England. Her father was Polish and had become successful in business dealings. Margaret had one older sister who was quite gifted and successful. Margaret, on the other hand, "described herself as an unhappy and delicate child. She spent a large part of her childhood ill in bed, enduring long periods of solitude". When Margaret was 13, her parents divorced, causing her a great deal of anguish. She and her sister remained with their mother, who had progressive ideas regarding her daughters' education, in contrast to the views held by their father. He believed they should become traditional young Englishwomen and devote themselves to home and family. Both sisters, however, became physicians. Because of her early childhood experiences with illness and divorce, Lowenfeld sensed intuitively that children often did not possess the necessary language to convey their deepest feelings. For this reason she sought, through her work, to find methods that would enable a child to show her, rather than tell her, what the problem want.

Lowenfeld herself did not take credit for the initial development of sandplay into a therapeutic technique. Instead, she said that it was the children who developed the process while she only provided a sand box and toys for them to use. She described herself as the observer who took note of what the children produced in the sand, and then asked them to tell her about the scene. In addition to Lowenfeld's major studies on child's use of sand and miniatures, she also developed another diagnostic instrument, known as the Mosaic Test. This test involves the construction of a picture using plastic tiles of different shapes, sizes, and colors. When Lowenfeld analyzed these mosaics and then compared them to a child's sand World constructions, she was able to clearly conceptualize a child's inner state. Lowenfeld was also quite interested in the arts and literature, and compared some of the ideas from the arts to themes she had observed in a child's therapy, especially Chagall's technique in which different images are contained within a single larger image. Her concept of clusters grew out of this observation. She illustrates how several experiences of a child can be superimposed upon each other, causing an emotional reaction. One example might be a child who, at one period of life, suffers from a serious asthma attack that ends in hospitalization and, at a later period, is attacked by a vicious dog. Each of these incidents causes panic reactions for the child. Later, through "sand/world play," both experiences might be depicted in disguised form. She referred to this process (showing two or three traumatic incidents at the same time) as clusters.

5.2.1　Carl Jung's work

Jung's influence in Sandplay is very significant. Dr. Jung is credited with an early form of play therapy, which is described in his autobiography Memories, Dreams, Reflections. Following his break from Freud, Jung attempted to integrate this devastating experience and found that play techniques were extremely useful. He kept thinking about how he had played as a child, and of the comfort he had received from this play. He realized that he needed to find a way back to this period of his life for any resolution of his conflict to occur. So in 1912, Jung began to construct a miniature village that he made from rocks and stones that he gathered from the lake shore at his summer home in Bollingen. This activity led him to a stream of fantasies, which he later wrote down. The experience was a direct contribution to his work on active imagination, as well as to other theories that he was in the process of developing. Especially relevant to the work of Sandplay is Jung's description of the archetype of the child: The "child" is all that is abandoned and exposed and at the same time divinely powerful; the insignificant, dubious beginning, and the triumphal end. The "eternal child" in man

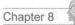

is an indescribable experience, an incongruity, a handicap, and a divine prerogative; an imponderable that determines the ultimate worth or worthlessness of a personality.

At an international psychoanalytic conference in 1937, Jung heard Dr. Lowenfeld's lecture on the World Technique. He was struck by the similarities to the experience he had had of building his miniature village. Jung was quite impressed by Lowenfeld's presentation, especially since he could see the possibility of contacting the archetypal level of the psyche in this way. This insight was incorporated some time later, through the work of Frau Kalff. Jung's archetypal theories are what differentiate this method from other applications of sandplay. The ability to understand the archetypal level of the psyche through Jungian Sandplay enables deeper healing to occur than is possible when other theoretical bases are employed. This is not meant to imply that other theories do not have their place in treatment. It does suggest, however, that there is the possibility of reaching the soul-level through contacting and mediating with the archetypes. Marion Woodman, Canadian Jungian analyst, says, "Psychological work is soul work. Psychology is the science of the soul. By soul, I mean the eternal part of us that wants to create timeless objects like art".

5.2.2   Dora Kalff's work

Lowenfeld's World Technique was incorporated into Jungian work through the efforts of Dora Kalff. During her training period at the Jung Institute in the early' 50s, Kalff attended one of Dr. Lowenfeld's lectures. She was quite intrigued by the World Technique and discussed it with Dr. Jung. Jung remembered the positive impression that this technique had made upon him some years before, so he encouraged Frau Kalff to go to London to study with Dr. Lowenfeld, which she did in 1952.

From the beginning, Jung was a strong supporter of Kalff's work with children, as he had had the opportunity to observe her abilities first-hand. Kalff's children and Jung's grandchildren used to play together and he had noticed how happy his grandchildren seemed to be after they had visited the Kalff family. He had, in fact, commented to others about this. When Kalff began her analytic training, Jung encouraged her to work with children. Kalff's personal analysis during her training was with Emma Jung, Jung's wife. After Kalff's studies with Lowenfeld in England, she returned to Switzerland and began to practice the Lowenfeld method while integrating it within her Jungian orientation. This was the first attempt at such a combination. She began to observe that there were certain developmental stages that were visible to her in the sand and she saw that the children she treated seemed to make rapid adjustments to whatever their presenting problems were. She felt that it was "almost as if an autonomous process was occurring with little or no interpretation being given by her". Kalff began her work with the Jungian postulate that there is a drive towards wholeness and healing in the human psyche, just as there is in the body. She saw the need for a free space in which this could happen, and she always referred to the sand tray as the "free and protected space," the temenos or place of healing. Kalff made no judgments about what she observed and used primarily a nonverbal approach, being careful to say nothing that might interfere with child's process of psychological development. For this quiet, accepting attitude, she drew on her study of Zen Buddhism, which holds that a seeker is never to be given a direct answer to his most searching question. Instead, each person is encouraged to turn back to his own inner resource in order to discover his own authentic answer to whatever question is being explored.

Kalff believed that the unspoken understanding, the feeling connection, in other words the transference and countertransference dynamics, that develops between the analyst and the child is the ultimate healing factor. There is some controversy among Sandplay therapists about this issue, as there are those who hold that the transference is not to the person of the therapist but to the tray. In fact, Lowenfeld went to great lengths to discourage this phenomenon and was known to switch a child's therapist from time to time in order to ensure that the transference would be to the equipment rather than to the therapist.

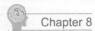

Until the last ten or fifteen years, it had been quite difficult for therapists in this country to obtain Sandplay training and supervision. During Kalff's lifetime, she provided some training in California, under the aegis and support of the San Francisco Jung Institute. This organization was instrumental in introducing Kalff to this country and in bringing her here periodically. As a result, many Sandplay practitioners were trained by Kalff on the West Coast, and that is why so many Sandplay practitioners are located there. Today there are various training opportunities for interested therapists to pursue. One source is the International Society of Sandplay Therapists (ISST). This was founded by Kalff shortly before her death, along with several influential Sandplay therapists in the United States and Europe.

In all, sandplay as practiced today was developed by Dora Kalff, who based her work upon Margaret Lowenfeld's World Technique and then combined it with the theories of Carl Jung. For this reason, Sandplay has been heavily influenced by the Lowenfeld and Jung approaches to which Frau Kalff added her interest in Zen Buddhism as well as her own creative talents. Lowenfeld wrote: Toys to children are like culinary implements to the kitchen; every kitchen has them and has also the elements of food. It is what the cook does with the implements and elements that determine the dish.

5.3   The theory of sand play

5.3.1   The benefit of sand play

Sand is a basic elemental compound, one of the most simple and common on earth. The choice to use sand as the foundation for sandplay was not an accidental, but rather a natural phenomenon. There are several unique attributes about the process of sand play: (1) sand play gives expression to nonverbalized emotion issue; (2) sand play has a unique kinesthetic quality; (3) sand play creates a therapeutic distance for patients; (4) sand play increases involvement and interest; and (5) sand play encourages the development of self. Sand play has increased in its utilization, and has demonstrated its efficacy. Sand play therapy involves more than the application of traditional talk therapy accompanied by some type of play media. Children and families yearn for a place in which to express and process their pain. For many of them, the prospect of psychotherapy is enormously daunting. To verbalize issues means to confront fearful emotions. Even the most cooperative patient must deal with the difficulties this confrontation presents. Sandplay provides a safe place for this often intimidating process to occur. Since play is the language of childhood, as well as a language for a patient of any age who is unable or unwilling to verbalize, the sand tray provides a safe medium for expression. The self-directed sandplay process allows patients to be fully themselves. Through the process of sandplay, which includes a caring and accepting relationship, children and families can express their total personalities. Sandplay is, therefore, more than a symbolization of the psyche-it is a forum for full self-expression and self-exploration.

Therapeutic connection and the processing of rooted emotional turmoil are not merely assisted by the use of sand. It is the sand that creates the path. Eichoff suggested that sand was the "means of which gross feelings can be expressed, for it can be thrown, tossed, molded, plastered, dug and smoothed; and on this base concrete symbols can be placed" Sand is more than a therapeutic medium. It is a means of expressing the very core of who we are. Indeed, as Dora Kalff so succinctly stated, "The act of playing in the sand allows the patient to come near his own totality".

Both family therapy and play therapy place heavy emphasis on the use of metaphor: children express themselves through the metaphor of play rather than verbally confronting their parents, which is much more intimidating. Their drawings, doll play, and such reveal to the therapist just what the problem is, and the family play therapist must be able to think and speak in metaphors to be fully effective. For example, when a child has chosen dolls to enact a drama in a doll house, the therapist must be careful to speak about the dolls in the language of the child. If the doll character is a mother, it is always referred to as the mother in the drama and not as child's actual mother. By exploring the feelings of the child doll in the given situation, one can be sure there is a relationship to the actual child. This technique allows the child to express herself in a safer way rather than to talk about problems being experienced with the actual mother.

5.3.2   How to play

The sandplay therapist should facilitate, rather than direct, the therapeutic experience. Children and families enter into the therapy process already feeling disempowered and out of control. As the sandplay therapist facilitates rather than choreographs the process, patients will experience healing through a growing sense of self-control, empowerment, and safety. Siegelman described this facilitation process well: "To be a participant-observer at the moment when a frightened or constricted patient feels securely enough to take her first step into the realm of symbolic play-this is being a midwife to the birth of the capacity for meaning". This facilitation creates the opportunity for the patient to fully express and explore self. Self-expression and self-exploration are crucial in the counseling process, and are foundational in sandplay. Kalff stressed this exploration of self: "the patient, through the sandplay, penetrates to that which we can recognize as an expression of self".

Sandplay should involve a dynamic interpersonal relationship. Regardless of the specific therapeutic and theoretical approach one takes to the sandplay process, the evolution and development of a dynamic interpersonal relationship is crucial. Kalff stressed the importance of the therapist creating a "free and protected space," noting that it is the love of the therapist that creates this space. The sandplay therapist should be trained in sandplay therapy procedures. Appropriate training and supervised experience, as well as personal sandplay exposure, is crucial for the therapist interested in doing sandplay.

Sandplay has enjoyed increasing popularity among psychotherapists seeking expressive interventions with their patients. There are several ways for the sand play. The therapist needs to understand child development, family stages, and individual, family, and group processes in order to be an effective healer. It is important for him to be able to join, to observe, to model, and to set limits when that becomes necessary. Most of all, the therapist must be sensitive, creative, spontaneous, directive when necessary, and always in charge of the process. This covers a large territory but these are skills and qualities that most therapists manage to acquire with experience. It is essential for the family play therapist to have training and experience with both family and play therapy techniques before attempting to combine the two. The major requirement, however, is a willingness to experiment with a new technique and to use oneself as creatively as possible. One needs to realize that perfection (whatever that might be) is not the goal, but that sincerity and openness to what each family is trying to resolve become the keys to success.

When a family is being treated in sandplay, the members are frequently quite amazed by the nonverbal aspect of what has been produced in their sand pictures. Their observations at the conclusion of the session often refer to their sense of astonishment. Especially revealing the decision-making process, the alliances that are established, the choices that are made, and the family interactions. When the family has completed the picture, there may be much oohing and aahing over what has been produced and the family members may discuss their visceral reactions. The internally felt power that results from the construction of a sand picture is quite moving to the family and the therapist alike.

5.3.3   The testing with sand play

Lowenfeld designed the World apparatus, and she asserts that "the qualities of the World apparatus from which its power of expression derives" are its "multi-dimensional nature, the dynamic possibilities it offers, the power of the apparatus to present states of mind hitherto unknown, and its independence of skill". Ruth Bowyer, Charlotte Buhler, and Liselotte Fischer all studied and verified the World apparatus, and their research is of special interest in documenting the types of cases suitable for therapy through use of the World apparatus. Charlotte Buhler recognized the potential of using miniatures as a diagnostic and research instrument. She created the World Test, which was later called the Toy World Test, in order to differentiate it from Lowenfeld's World Technique.

Lowenfeld found that emotionally disturbed children often fenced in large parts of the World, or placed wild animals where they did not belong, or placed objects in unusual surroundings. They also used the same objects repeatedly. These observations of Lowenfeld were confirmed by Buhler's studies. Buhler identified three signs which she felt had relevance to the World Test. These were defined in a monograph and are summarized below.

(1) Aggressive world signs (A-sign): These were indicated by soldiers fighting, animals biting, or other forms of aggression. She found some aggression to be normal in children, most often manifested in creations that followed the construction of the initial sand world. When A-signs were seen in the initial tray this suggested to her the possibility of a more intense aggressiveness than is usual. She also found that accidents were depicted more frequently in the sand trays of children who were disturbed, and when a number of accidents were portrayed it suggested to her the need for therapy. There were times, however, when instruments of aggression could be seen in the positive role of protection and defense.

(2) Empty world signs (E-sign): These occurred when there were fewer than fifty toys used, when the toys that were selected came from only a few categories, when major groups of people were omitted (e.g., no adults, or only children, or only soldiers and police). Buhler said that the sand tray worlds of children under 8 are normally quite empty. The empty world suggested to her an interior emptiness, or feelings of loneliness, or a need to be alone. E-signs could also suggest resistance to the task, an emotional fixation on certain objects, or blocked creativity. Complete omission of people could have a double meaning: either the desire to escape from people or else to defy them.

(3) Closed, rigid and disorganized worlds (CRDW-signs). This type of world is partially or completely fenced in, there are unrealistic rows of animals, people, or things lined up in a fixed, stiff manner, or there are disorganized worlds in chaotic form. Buhler noted that CRDW-signs were more significant symptoms of emotional disturbance than either of the other two types. CRDW-signs could also indicate an unusual need for security or protection. They might also signal rigidity or confusion. If a patient set up fences before any other materials were used, it indicated to her an unusual need for protection. This phenomenon has been observed in initial sessions with some highly anxious children. Rigid worlds can also indicate varying degrees of compulsive orderliness, perfectionism, and excessive fear. Disorganized worlds did not necessarily indicate deep emotional disturbance for young children but, for older children or adults, they could indicate varying degrees of confusion and dissolution of the personality structure. Buhler did not indicate what ages she was referring to when she spoke of young children. As part of Buhler's studies, she found that retarded individuals had significantly more empty and distorted worlds than others. She also noted that in some cases the memory of a traumatic experience, triggered by the handling of the miniatures, could be so overwhelming that no construction at all took place.

Laura Ruth Bowyer was another researcher of the Lowenfeld technique. Her studies confirmed those of Buhler and incorporated the developmental stages of the child to the overall evaluation of the Worlds. For example, it is common for a young child of 2 or 3 to engage in burying toys and then finding them in the sand, which symbolically represents child's search for object constancy. When this activity is performed by a child of

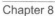

8 or 9, it can be interpreted as a regression to an earlier stage of development. These early researchers explored the relationship between child developmental stages and stages of development as they were revealed in sand productions. They hoped to learn if there were common threads among different age groups and studied themes that were common to various age groups in order to distinguish the "normal" from the "pathological." This work continues today, as there is a continuing need for refining the standardization and verification of norms in Sandplay.

6. Conclusion

Both art therapy and sand play are considered creative art experiences, and the dynamics seen in one are often seen in the other. Landgarten has written, "The value of the art task is threefold: the process as a diagnostic, interactional, and rehearsal tool; the contents as a means of portraying unconscious and conscious communication; and the product as lasting evidence of the group's dynamics". These apply directly to family sandplay as well as to family art therapy. The content area in art therapy is the medium used and includes the size of the paper, pencils, markers, crayons, and so on. It might also include clay or pictures for collages. In sandplay, the content area is patient's choice between wet and dry sand and the miniatures to be used. The process of family art therapy and family sandplay therapy are almost identical; the dynamics are revealed in the way the individuals go about building the scene together. The product or end result is the picture made or the scene produced. In sandplay, a photograph is taken to preserve the product, while in art therapy the picture itself is the product.

（刘　伟　顾思梦）

Chapter 9

Patient Psychology and Doctor-Patient Relationships

Hippocrates said that to know who have disease is more important than what disease he has. The somatic disease and mental state of a patient mutually influences each other. Hence, being familiar with the psychological characteristics of patients can help not only establish harmonious doctor-patient relationship, but also increase the rehabilitation and improve the wellbeing of patients.

1. Patient psychology (basic concepts)

1.1 Patient

According to the traditional bio-medical model, only those who have biological lesions and health-seeking behaviors, or are receiving a medical therapy can be seen as patients. But from the modern perspective of the bio-psycho-social model, "health is a state of complete physical, mental and social well-being and not merely the absence of disease or infirmity." Therefore, besides organic lesions and functional impairments in tissues and organs, subjective sick-experience and abnormal psychological or social functioning should all be included in the definition of disease. Hence, a more comprehensive understanding of "patient" should be: individual with any physical or mental disorder, whether they seek medical service or not.

1.1.1 The role

The word "role" refers to a person acting on stage. The American psychologist Mead GH, first introduced this drama term into social psychology in 1920's. He used this term to illustrate interacted behavior model in expected interpersonal relationship. Social role refers to the behavior model, mental status, and corresponding rights and obligations that are consistent with the individual's social status and identity. Any specific role should have its corresponding rights and obligations, for example, patients have not only the rights to obtain health education and treatment, but also the obligations to cooperate with medical stuff.

Two terms are especially emphasized for a social role: the role expectation and role play. The role expectation refers to a series of expectations on mental and behavioral characteristics given by the society. If the activity of the individual doesn't meet the requirement of role expectation, it will be viewed as inadequate. For example, teacher as a social role is expected to teach new knowledge, answer questions, and be a model for students. Their behaviors should meet the requirement made for that role. Physicians are expected to help the sick or the wounded. Their behaviors should meet these requirements. Another term is role play, which means that an individual actually adopted the behaviors that meet the social expectations for that role. Role reversal on the other hand, refers to the case in which various roles are taken simultaneously by an individual and she/he should adjust her/his behavior according to different requirements of different role. For instance, someone being a leader at work can also be a husband or a father at home, or a patient in the hospital. Role conflict refers to the inner experience when an individual's behavior of one role doesn't meet the expectation of other roles. Multiple roles taken by one individual can sometimes be contradicted with each other.

1.1.2　Role of patient

The patient role, also known as patient identity, is a special social role which is in a state of illness, and with treatment- and medical-seeking behaviors. Patient identity often leads to changes in the mind and behavior. Patient role expectation includes behaviors that can help alleviate symptoms and recover, such as following doctor's advice to take medicine, stay in bed, etc.

People have the need of treatment and rehabilitation when tormented by painful disease. In such case, they need to transform themselves from other social roles to patient role. People observed the interaction between patients and other people, and proposed four elements for the patient role: (1) Patients can relieve themselves from duties required by conventional social roles. (2) Patients are not responsibility for their state of being because illness is a state beyond the control of an individual. (3) Patients are responsible for the recovery. (4) Patients are responsible for seeking medical assistance.

1.1.3　Rights and obligations of the patient role

Scholars have summarized the following rights and obligations for the patient role:

Rights of the patient role: (1) be entitled to the right of medical service; (2) be entitled to the right of being respected and understood; (3) be entitled to the right of informed consent on disease treatment; (4) be entitled to the right of keeping personal privacy; (5) be entitled to the right of supervision on his/her medical rights; (6) be entitled to the right of exempting social responsibility taken on before the disease.

Obligations to the patient role: (1) to seek medical service in time, and strive for rehabilitation as soon as possible; (2) to seek effective medical help and follow the doctor's guidance; (3) to obey all the rules and regulations of medical service department, and pay medical fees; (4) to cooperation with doctors and nurses in their coordination for diagnose and medical care.

1.1.4　Transition and adaptation of patient role

Anyone may take the patient role for some time in our life and some may even take it for a lifetime. The more similarities between an individual's original social role and the patient role, the easier transition s/he may experience to be in the patient role. There are two types of results when one switches from her/his former social role to a patient role: role adaption and role maladjustment.

Role adaption refers to that the patient's behaviors are in accordance with the expectations of the patient role. While role maladjustment refers to that the patient fails to accomplish the transition of roles, which may result in a series of negative emotions, such as fear, anxiety, depression, etc. Role maladjustment includes:

(1) Role denial. Some patients may refuse the patient role by denying their own sickness, even though they were made clear about the diagnosis and the evidence based on which the diagnosis was made. Illness often means declination in social functioning, which is related to problems such as reduced income, failure in education, work or marriage. These are often the reasons that make some people refuse the patient role, and use the defend mechanism, denial, to avoid the problems.

(2) Role conflict. On taking up the patient role, one might perceive discordance between the new role and various other roles one has been holding before the illness. The conflict may result in anxiety, anger, worry, sadness, etc. For instance, a department manager with a quick tempo and extensive interpersonal relationship may find it hard to adapt to the patient role when s/he is sick. S/he may find it impossible to stop the work s/he usually does to do nothing but rest and take prescribed medicine.

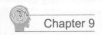

(3) Role reduction. One that has been in the patient role may for some reason take up temporarily or permanently another role. For instance, an inpatient mother may give up her own patient role and be engaged in taking care of her sick daughter.

(4) Role intensification. Sometimes patients may refuse to go back to their ordinary social roles on recovery. Some may feel upset or fear to do so because it means they will leave the environment that they are familiar with and feel pleasant. But it also can be a result of some psychological needs, such as need for other's care, or simply attention.

(5) Role abnormality. This is a special form of role maladjustment that can be presented as intensified frustration, anger or other emotions. Patients may feel bored, pessimistic and may choose to relieve themselves from these conditions using alcohol or drugs and some may commit suicide or be engaged in violence.

1.1.5   Factors that affect role adaption

Many factors may affect the adaptation to the patient role, including age, cultural background, post-experience as a patient, etc. But the most direct influence is from the nature of the disease. Patients are more likely to seek medical help in time when there are obvious symptoms.

Medical staff should assist patients to accomplish the transition from their ordinary social roles to the patient role. It is often helpful to familiarize them with the medical environment that they are new to, and talk about their worries, and all these can be done to establish a harmonious doctor-patient relationship. When the patient's condition is good enough to be relieved from their patient role, medical stuff can also do something to facilitate the transition from the patient role to ordinary social role.

1.2   Care-seeking behavior and compliant behavior of patient

1.2.1   Care-seeking behavior

(1) Types of care-seeking behaviors

Possible reactions of an individual when s/he feels sick include, neglect, denial, self-treatment, and seeking care from others. Care-seeking behavior refers to the behavior of seeking medical help when an individual feels sick. It can be classified into three types: active care-seeking behavior, passive care-seeking behavior, and mandatory care-seeking behavior. Active care-seeking behavior is the most common type, which means actively seeking medical help. Passive care-seeking behavior is the kind of behavior in which patients is not willing or unable to implement care-seeking behavior on their own. It often happens when patients are unconscious or conscious but unable to conduct the behaviors, such as when the patient is an infant. Mandatory care-seeking behavior often means that the behavior is against the will of the patients. It is primarily for patients with infectious diseases or posing threats to themselves or others.

(2) Cause of care-seeking behavior

Whether an individual will seek medical help depends on sicknesses associated with many physical, mental and social factors he perceives. For instance:

1) Physical reasons

Subjective feelings of discomfort and pain are very important physical reasons that push an individual to seek medical care.

2) Psychological reasons

Some people may seek medical care to get relieved from negative psychological conditions such as overwhelming stress, negative emotions, etc.

3) Social reasons

Some people may seek medical care for conditions that not only cause discomfort, pain or even death to themselves but also pose threats to others, such as those with infectious diseases who may be isolated during treatment.

(3) Factor associated with care-seeking behavior

Care-seeking behavior is a complicated behavior which is influenced by many factors. For instance:

1) Age

Generally speaking, care-seeking behavior happens relatively more in infancy and childhood, because these are the phases of life that receives more protection. It happens relatively less in young adults, while thereafter, the occurrence increases with aging.

2) Severity of the disease

One may not seek help for an ordinary cold, but may see a doctor immediately when bitten by a snake or dog. The ruling factor in these two cases is the severity of the disease.

3) Personality

People who are sensitive, suspicious or dependent are more likely to see doctors than those independent or self-confident.

4) Educational level

Compared with those with relatively low level of education, people with higher level of education are more likely to see doctors, because they may be better equipped with knowledge of the conditions and possible dangers of the disease.

5) Socioeconomic status

People with stable income and of higher social status are more likely to see doctors, because they tend to take more concern of their own health. By contrast, those with lower socioeconomic status tend to have passive care-seeking behavior.

1.2.2 Compliance

Compliance means that the patient should follow the guidance of doctors and nurses. Specifically, they should cooperate with them in medical examinations, take drugs on time and in the right dose, do regular exercise as recommended, etc. Compliance is to some extent a determinant factor on therapeutic effect and prognosis.

Factors associated with compliance. For instance, compliance is influenced by various factors:

1) Confidence in the doctor. Compliance is very much decided by how much confidence a patient lays on the doctor. This is influenced both by the characteristic of the patient and the doctor's reputation.

2) Severity of the disease, and care-seeking method. Chronic patients and out-patients are less likely to compliant prescriptions, while emergency patients, critical ill patients, and inpatients generally show more compliance.

3) Patient's expectation of treatment. Patients may show less compliance if they were not treated in ways they wanted.

1.3 Psychological needs of patients

People can actively pursue the fulfillment of their needs when they are in good health; however, it may become much more difficult when they are sick. On the other hand, new needs may emerge when people get sick. Medical stuff should provide assistance to help patients get their needs, including psychological needs to be fulfilled.

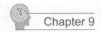

1.3.1 Existence needs

The existence needs, including eating, breathing, excretion, sleep, etc., are easy to meet when a person is in health, but they may become much more difficult in illness. Fulfillment of the existence needs can be influenced by the category and severity of the disease. For example, deglutition disorders will make it difficult to meet the need for food.

1.3.2 Safety needs

Disease itself can be a threat to the safety needs. During an illness, a patient's daily life is disturbed, and the security is lost. They may feel afraid to be alone and eagerly need other's care and assistance.

1.3.3 Need of social connection and association

Patients need care and acceptance. They particularly need concern, sympathy, and understanding from doctors, nurses, and relatives, when they were hospitalized and separated from their family. Meanwhile, in patients who have gone through changes in their routines and everyday life, need to be accepted by group, communicate with other patients. In addition, patients need to be socially connected and associated, specifically, with medical staff and other patients.

1.3.4 Esteem needs

Patients often feel themselves being a burden or cumbersome to others. Their needs for respect is often much stronger that healthy people due to their decreased self-esteem. They need to be respected for their personality and privacy. Respect can be embodied in many ways, for example, offering the information of diagnosis and treatment of their disease, giving informed consent, etc. Patients need assistance and adequate information to be adapted to new environment after hospitalized. The information may include hospital rules, knowledge of their disease, treatment plan, operation effects, skill level of their doctor and responsible nurses etc. It can help enhance patient's compliance to cooperate with medical staff, eventually benefit the treatment and rehabilitation.

1.3.5 Self-actualization needs

Self-actualization needs include the sense of power and achievement. People with disability may be frustrated and the need for self-actualization may be the strongest. In any way, it is very important to encourage patients to build up their confidence and fight with disease.

Patient's psychological needs can be shown in various ways. Doctors and nurses with better knowledge and understanding of these psychological needs would guide and help the patients more specifically.

2. Patient's psychology (clinical characteristics) and intervention

The patient will have different psychological reactions distinct from healthy people when they are in illness. The psychological activity of healthy people mainly focuses on adapting to social life. The psychological activity of patients is mainly focused on the disease that affects their lives. The psychological characteristic of patient was different due to age, gender, and the type of disease. It is demonstrated that patients have following psychological characteristics during the time of sickness.

2.1   Patient's psychology: clinical characteristics

2.1.1   Patient's cognitive activities

(1) Perceptual abnormality

Patients turn their attention from outer world to inner personal experience and feelings after they take in the patient role. Their direction, selectivity, and range of perception change correspondingly. Patients' subjective sensation is enhanced as a reaction to the disease and the change of role. Patients may become more sensitive to the change of the environment, such as sound, light, and temperature, and get nervous if something happens. Their sensitivity to body reaction may be also increased, especially to their breathing, blood pressure, heartbeat, gastrointestinal peristalsis, and position, as well as their symptoms. They may demonstrate abnormality in time and space perception, for example, inpatients often feel that time moves on too slow. Patients who always stay in bed may show abnormal space perception. They may report lying on a shaking bed.

(2) Impaired memory and thought

Some somatoform disorders are accompanied with obviously memory loss, such as some organic brain lesions, and chronic kidney failure. Most patients with cerebrovascular disease portray varying degree of cognitive impairment. Diabetics are impaired in attention, orientation, memory, and thought because of glucose fluctuations. The consequences of chronic obstructive pulmonary disease are cerebral hypoxia and respiratory failure. It was demonstrated through the Neuropsychological Tests that attention, language, visual memory, general intelligence, and mathematical problem solving abilities are to some extent damaged in severe patients.

2.1.2   Characteristics of patient emotion

Emotional instability is a common problem in patients. Patients may be irritable and disabled in emotion control. Hyperthyroid patients manifest emotional fluctuation, such that they are nervous, easy to be excited. The most common emotions in patients include anxiety, depression and anger.

(1) Anxiety

Anxiety is an emotion experienced when perceived with threat or expecting adverse consequence. Anxiety often companies with obviously physiological reaction, which primarily shows the excitability symptoms of the Sympathetic Nervous System (SNS), such as accelerated heart rate, elevated blood pressure, sweat, accelerated breathing, insomnia, and headache, etc. Anxiety can be attributed to many causes, such as worry about disease, ambiguous on the nature and outcome and prognosis of the disease, doubt on the reliability and safety of the examination and the treatment, worry and fear about the unfamiliar hospital environment, especially on witness the rescue processes or death scenes.

(2) Depression

Depression is a group of symptom that is characterized by emotional hypoactivity, including feeling down, lack of interest, etc. Patients with a depressed mood may be notably sad, anxious, or empty; they may also feel notably hopeless, helpless, dejected, or worthless. Other symptoms expressed may include senses of guilt, irritability, or anger. Further feelings expressed by these patients may include feeling ashamed or an expressed restlessness. They may notably lose interest in activities that they once considered pleasurable to family and friends or otherwise experience either a loss of appetite or overeating.

(3) Anger

Patients feel anger and distress because they think it is unfair that the disease occurs to them. Meanwhile,

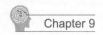

patients may feel anger when the treatment was hampered, or their conditions get worse. Anger is often accompanied with aggressive behavior, which may be extravert, such that they may vent their dissatisfaction and resentment on others, or introvert, such that they may refuse further treatment, or even commit self-harmful activity.

2.1.3   Characteristic of patient will behavior

In the progress of treatment, patients may portray regressive behaviors, which they may behave in a pattern that appears childish, and incompatible with their age and social status. For instance, some patients will moan, cry, or shout at others to get their attention or care. Some patients may become dependent on others especially.

2.1.4   Personality change of patient

Generally speaking, personality is stable and does not change with time and environment. However, it will change for some patients in case of illness. They may become increasingly dependent, passive, and obedient. Especially in the case of those who are in chronic deferment disease or disease resulted from body image. They are difficult to adapt to new behavior model. Some patients may become inferior, self-blaming; some post-stroke patients will show characteristic deterioration, isolation and withdrawal.

2.2   Basic intervention on patient psychological problems

Psychological intervention focuses on patients' cognitive activity, emotional problems, changes of behavior and personality. Meanwhile, the category of disease, psychological and physiological characteristic of patients with various ages and different genders should be taken into account. It can help patients to improve adverse symptom and enhance compliance of treatment by taking comprehensive intervention measures. It is mainly used through the following skills.

2.2.1   Supportive therapy

Doctors should know the adverse psychological factors and various stresses, understand and respect patients. They should encourage patients and listen to them about their pain and sorrow. Doctors should help patients release their negative emotions, and encourage them to cultivate positive and optimistic emotion. Doctors should help patients establish social supportive system and establish confidence to conquer disease and provide them with useful information. Guide patients to adjust their unhealthy habits, help them arrange their life scientifically to eliminate psychosocial stress.

2.2.2   Cognitive therapy

Patients' psychological reaction and its intensity are determined by patients' cognition and assessment of the disease and symptoms. What's more, cognitive model is determined by patients' personality and social-culture background. Inappropriate cognition will distort objective facts and hamper rehabilitation of the disease.

Therefore, doctors should help patients identify the problems on distressed emotion and cognition and help them change their way of thinking about the issue in concern. Ellis's Rational Emotion Therapy and Beck's Cognitive Therapy are the most commonly used skills in clinical settings to correct adverse cognition of patients.

2.2.3   Behavioral therapy

It is common that patients show various emotional problems and physiological dysfunctions. Doctors can help them relieve from these symptoms and promote rehabilitation through behavioral therapy. Behavioral therapy is a therapeutic skill that corrects emotional disorders and physiological dysfunctions through learning and training. The basic techniques include relaxation exercise, biofeedback therapy, systematic desensitization, and so forth. These methods can enhance the self-control of the patients, relieve and eliminate symptoms via learning and training. For example, biofeedback therapy can be used for treatment of anxiety. Relaxation exercise can be used for treatment of excessive anxiety, fear and emotional instability.

2.2.4 Health education and consultation

Patients' understanding of their disease and body status can be helpful in relieving anxiety, and enhancing their confidence to conquer the disease. It can be done through health education. The content of health education is extensive, which includes basic knowledge of the disease per se, common treatment, and coping strategies in emergency, etc. Patients are provided with medical knowledge concerning their disease and rehabilitation. They are guided to the possible problems in marriage and other areas during the time of illness.

Example 1

The mental problems of cancer patients and the interventions

The etiology and pathogenesis of cancer are still not very clear. Both psychological and social factors contribute to the occurrence of cancer, while negative psychological reactions and inappropriate ways of handling can further worsen the situation and shorten the life expectancy. In the process of diagnosis and treatment, most patients will show various psychological reactions including dramatic emotional and behavioral changes.

(1) Common psychological changes in cancer patients

Although modern medical diagnosis and treatment of cancer have made great progress, most of the cancers are still difficult to be cured. The side effects of cancer therapy often create strong psychological impacts on the patients, and lead to fear and pessimism. Some patients show social withdrawal symptoms, for example, they may avoid interpersonal communications. Some operations can cause image damage or functional loss which hurt patients' self-esteem. When a patient is told the result of the diagnosis of cancer, there is a process of significant psychological change, which can be roughly divided into four periods (Table 9-1).

Table 9-1 Psychological changes of cancer patient

Stage	Psychological changes	Period
I Shock-fear period	When patients first hear about themselves getting cancer, they may express their feelings of shock and fear, and often with physiological reactions, such as palpitation, dizziness and fainting, even stupor.	<1 week
II Denial-doubt period	Patients wipe off severe emotional shock to calm down, often with the aid of denying mechanism to cope with tension and pain by cancer diagnosis. Patients may doubt whether the doctor's diagnosis is correct or not.	1-2 weeks
III Anger-depression period	Patient's mood will be irritable, angry, and sometimes with attacking behaviors; Patients often feel sad, frustrated and despairing, some patients may have suicidal thoughts or commit suicide.	After 2 weeks
IV Acceptance-adaptation period	Patients eventually accept and adapt to the fact, but most patients are difficult to restore to the normal state of mind.	After 4 weeks

(2) The intervention of cancer patient psychological problems

First of all, tell patients the truth. There are different views on whether to give cancer diagnosis to patients or not, but most scholars advocate giving diagnosis and treatment information at the right time. After being

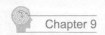

told the possible side effects and complications during the treatment, patients may have better psychological adaptation to treatment, and will benefit from the treatment. The information should be given in a way that fully considers the patient's personality, handling styles and the severity of illness, and this should be done at the right time.

Second, change the wrong conception of cancer. Many negative psychological reactions result from patients' inappropriate conception that "cancer equals death". Doctors should help the patients to have a scientific knowledge of the disease, and adapt to the new role of being a patient in time, cooperate with the doctors in the treatment.

Third, deal with patient's emotional problems. Most cancer patients have emotional problems, such as fear of death and worry of expected pain and disability. Cognitive therapy can be used to correct patient's inappropriate cognition, such as "cancer is an incurable disease", thereafter supportive psychotherapy, relaxation techniques, and music therapy treatment can also be used. Doctors can use appropriate drugs to ease patients' severe anxiety, fear and depression.

Fourth, alleviate the pain. Doctors should attach great importance to the pain which often result in fear, despair, and loneliness, and further worsen the physical situation. So the principle of treatment is to reduce the pain first, and consider psychological problems later.

Fifth, rebuild a healthy lifestyle. Help the patients to access more knowledge about healthcare, to raise the awareness of anti-cancer and set up a healthy lifestyle, and eventually eliminate the chances of cancer.

Example 2

The mental problems of terminal illness patients

When patients find out that they have got a terminal or life-threatening illness, there are massive feelings of helplessness and uncontrollable emotions. Most patients have never really thought that death should be so close to them. When there is nothing more than doctors can to treat patients, it is hard for both patients and doctors.

Every dying patient has their own way of coping and handling things but most patients do tend to go through a similar range of feelings and emotions. Elizabeth Kubler-Ross, a psychiatrist from Switzerland and a pioneer in hospice studies, spent a lot of time with dying people comforting and studying them. She published a book On Death and Dying in 1969, and proposed a perspective of five stages of grief. She described a common process of feelings and emotions that most patient with terminal illness experiences, called the Kubler-Ross Five Stage Model. It describes how patients react in each of the five stages which may last for different periods of time and may replace each other or exist side by side at times. The five stages are: Denial, Anger, Bargaining, Depression, and Acceptance; as detailed below:

(1) Denial stage. When patients know that they will probably die, they experience initial paralysis, and inevitably try to avoid the terrible situation. Patients often find it hard to believe the diagnosis, and think it will not happen to them. Denial stage is usually a temporary defense. It is a way of coping with their emotions, and gives patients time to come to terms with what is happening. This is a common feeling and emotion, and it may last quite a while in some cases. And for some patients it can last right up to the end.

(2) Anger stage. When the initial denial wears off, many patients move into anger stage. When patients realize that the situation is real, they usually turn to anger. They may feel it is not fair for them. They may get so angry and look to blame someone or something else for making this happen to them. The anger can be directed to themselves, the doctor who delivered the bad news, or those who are caring for them on a daily basis. It is often reported that they are more irritable towards colleagues or family members just for tiny things. They often have a strong sense of grief for what is lost. During the process of coming to the acceptance of what

is happening, patients tend to have sharp swings in mood.

(3) Bargaining stage. When patients move on to this stage, they attempt to postpone what is inevitable. They may beg the illness, "just let me live to see my children grown up."

Most of these bargains are secret deals with God, others, or life, when they say "If I promise to do anything, then you make the situation not happen to me, or just give me more time". Patients start bargaining in order to find a way out of the situation. Most of the patients are scared of death, while some of them are scared of the pain and symptoms of illness. Others may be afraid more of losing family and the way of life now, rather than the illness itself.

(4) Depression stage. Sadness and hopelessness are important parts of the depression stage when patients realize that bargaining is not going to work, death is inevitable. Patients despair at the recognition of their mortality. At this stage, the patient may become silent, refuse visitors and spend much of the time mournful and sullen.

(5) Acceptance stage. As patients realize that there is nothing else to be done, they move into a stage of acceptance. In this last stage, patients embrace mortality or inevitable future. Patients may start to make positive plans for their own deaths. Medical stuff can help them and make them feel more in control of what is happening. Talking with them about their feelings and emotions may be a good way to show support. The Kubler-Ross model is very useful in identifying and understanding how patients coping with the bad situations.

3. Doctor-patient relationships

Clinicians should not only constantly improve the techniques and ability, but also build mutual trust and respect with the patients, so as to provide satisfactory medical services to the patients. In the process of medical treatment, the interactions between doctors and patients compose a special kind of interpersonal relation. A good doctor-patient relationship can not only promote mutual understanding and trust in doctors and patients, but also be used as a part of the treatment process, and improve patient's disease prognosis and health outcomes. Approaching the doctor-patient relationship in a comprehensive way to get the best clinical results is one of the important goals of medical psychology.

3.1   The characteristics of the doctor-patient relationships

The doctor-patient relationship is a result of medical treatment, and always in a process of evolvement, which means it is both stable and dynamic. Compared with other types of relationships, the doctor-patient relationship has the following features:

First, oriented. The patients seek medical care from the doctors for their illness, so the doctors and patients need to establish an alliance for medical work. The goal of the doctor-patient relationship is to relieve the pain of patients, and promote a recovery. In such a relationship, patients always trust and respect their doctors, and entrust their health and even life to their doctors; on the other hand, doctors should respect and be responsible for patients' life. Therefore, the purpose of establishing good doctor-patient relationship is to facilitate the clinical medical work.

Second, professional. Although doctors and patients are equal in the relation, the patients are actually in an inferior position due to the lack of information of medicine, diagnosis and treatment. Therefore patients tend to expect a closer relationship with the doctors, while the doctors tend to avoid such interventions and activities outside of their working hours. Without professional boundaries between doctors and patients, doctors may easily develop job burnout.

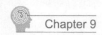

Third, time-bound. During the time when doctors provide medical services for patients, the doctor-patient relationship goes through different stages: establishment, development, effecting and ending. Compared with other types of relationships, timing is an obvious characteristic of the doctor-patient relationship, which means after the treatment, this particular doctor-patient relationship also ends.

Fourth, dynamic. In the process of medical treatment, the doctor-patient relationship will change constantly. Doctor-patient communication is an important factor that affects the relationship. Effective communication can lead to harmonious doctor-patient relationship, but ineffective ones may destroy the trust and cooperation, and even result in conflicts. The outcome of the treatment often affects the doctor-patient relationship.

3.2   Factors affecting the relationship between doctors and patients

The relationship between doctors and patients is not only the basis and prerequisite for medical practitioners to provide medical services, but also an important factor affecting the therapeutic effect and the quality of medical services. A good doctor-patient relationship can promote good communication between doctors and patients, and achieve the mutual trust, respect and understanding between doctors and patients, so that medical activities can be carried out smoothly. This relationship is affected by many factors, including doctors, patients, medical treatment and social environment, etc.

3.2.1   The influence of doctors on doctor-patient relationship

(1) Doctors' communication skills. Communication between doctors and patients is the most important factor affecting the relationship between doctors and patients. Doctors who lack communication skills may show less sympathy towards patients, may hurt patients and their families' self-esteem and dignity, and even violate the rights of patients in verbal and nonverbal communication. Failing to respect the privacy of patients or fulfill the obligation to inform patients, will seriously affect this relationship. Bad communication will also increase the risk of iatrogenic stress in patients, and bring damage to patients' mind and body.

(2) The impact of doctors' personal stress events. Doctors are both practitioners with social roles and individuals with unique personality traits. For example, changing of family relationship, or other stress events that occurs to a doctor, may affect the doctor-patient relationship. At times of this kind, some doctors may shows indifference, disgust, neglect, or irritability to patients, and some may even be affected in the medical decision-making. This is very dangerous.

(3) The influence of doctors' counter-transference on the relationship between doctors and patients. In the doctor-patient relationship, in addition to doctors' roles of treating patients, doctors' personal needs, desire, values sometimes unconsciously project to the patient. For example, when facing a very attractive patient, the rational thinking of doctors may be instantly "captured", meanwhile, they may unconsciously hope to develop more intimate doctor-patient relationship and contact with the patient, thus makes the doctor-patient relationship deviated from a professional one. However, this is something that must be avoided.

(4) The influence of doctors' professional quality and personality on doctor-patient relationship. Studies have found that the effect doctors' personality has on the relationship between doctors and patients are also very obvious. Doctor-patient relationship, as a special interpersonal relationship, reflects doctors' personality traits, such as anxiety, lacking of sense of security, etc. During a doctor-patient relationship, there will be more nervous, hesitant, avoiding responsibility in a higher occupational stress. Doctors with stable emotion, rich knowledge and professional skills, are more likely to respect patients, accept them, be meticulous and decisive, which are good for the establishment of quality and personal charisma for a good doctor-patient relationship. Humorous conversations of doctors are important components of the doctor-patient communication. For those who are filled with fear and anxiety, it is often the best "relaxant".

3.2.2　The influence of patients on the relationship between doctors and patients

(1) The impact of disease factors on the relationship between doctors and patients. Different diseases make the patients show different behaviors in the doctor-patient relationship. Severe patients with chronic diseases or psychoses often make the doctor-patient relationship different. For example, patients suffering from cancer may project their anger, sadness to the medical staff, or even refuse the treatment that is not "ideal". There are also patients who fear their medical conditions so much that they repeatedly ask doctors for assurance and comfort.

(2) Patient's empathy on the relationship between doctors and patients. The social rationality of patient's role makes some patients maintain long-term relationship with doctors in the role of patients. During a long-term relationship between doctors and patients, the relationship becomes so important to the patients, and replaces their lacked interpersonal and social support, meanwhile, the patients unconsciously project their intimate relationship and emotions of personal relationships on to the doctors, resulting in the "empathy". In the emotional relationship between doctors and patients, patients' symptoms are subject to unconscious control. This may exist for a long time. Doctors may also feel that patients' symptoms cannot be eliminated, although there are no biologically confirmed abnormalities, the treatment effect is not good, the symptoms persist and the doctors suffer a setback. In this case, the doctors need to understand the meaning of patient's symptoms, and the patients maintain their own valuable interpersonal relationships through the symptoms. If the doctors have the perceptions to this relationship, they will not feel particularly anxious and frustrated, and can introduce the patients to a psychotherapist or psychiatry department for further treatment.

(3) The influence of patient's personality on doctor-patient relationship. In clinical work, doctors often face patients with different personality traits. Some personality traits of patients bring special difficulties in communications between doctors and patients, or make the relationship between doctors and patients suffer. For example, some patients are too dependent on doctors, some have a lot of demands needing to be continuously concerned about, and some stubbornly insist on their own interpretation of the symptoms, which will obviously affect the doctor-patient relationship.

(4) The influence of patient's cultural factors on doctor-patient relationship. The age, occupation, education level, nation and beliefs of the patients affect the communication between doctors and patients. They sometimes also affect the relationship between doctors and patients. In this regard, the doctors need to know the patients' understanding of the disease and treatment expectations from different cultural perspectives.

3.2.3　The influence of medical treatment on doctor-patient relationship

(1) Medical time. The duration one patient visits the same doctor have a significant impact on the maintenance of doctor-patient relationship and dynamic changes. The longer the patients see the same doctors, the more satisfied the patients feel about this doctor-patient relationship, and the doctors are recognized by patients in terms of mutual respect, loyalty, trust and treatment effect. But those who constantly change doctors are more difficult to establish a stable and good doctor-patient relationship.

(2) Patient's experience for the medical process. In the process of medical treatment, doctors' diagnosis and treatment behavior can make the patients understand that doctors' explanation of their symptoms is in line with their own disease beliefs. Patients are more willing to look for doctors who meet their own accurate needs. In short, patients prefer to find doctors who can meet their expectations. When the patients feel that doctors do not have the characteristics they desire, they will break off the doctor-patient relationship and look for other doctors who might fulfill their own expectations. This is the reason why some doctors are so popular, even though their professional skills are only at an average level.

（辛秀红　方建群）

Chapter 10

Consultation-Liaison Psychiatry and Psychosomatic Disorders

Consultation-liaison psychiatry is a centuries-old field of medical practice and research which bridges the biological, psychological, and social domains of psychiatric and medical illnesses. Consultation-liaison psychiatry refers to the skills and knowledge utilized in evaluating and treating the emotional and behavioral conditions in patients who are referred from medical and surgical settings. Many such patients have comorbid psychiatric and medical conditions, and others have emotional and behavioral problems which result from the medical illness directly or as a reaction to it and its treatment. Psychosomatic medicine refers to the study of "mind-body" relationship in medicine. Investigators in psychosomatic medicine who were pioneer practitioners of consultation-liaison psychiatry have historically been interested in the psychosomatic aspects of medical patients. In the United States, the term psychosomatic medicine is often used interchangeably with consultation-liaison psychiatry, which is a neutral collaboration with colleagues and patients in nonpsychiatric settings, and the standard consultation is performed at the request of the primary clinician. Liaison Psychiatry expands the role of the psychiatrist to facilitate comprehensive treatment approaches within a system of care and to enhance communication among disciplines and across divisions in health care systems.

1. Introduction

1.1 History of consultation-liaison psychiatry and psychosomatic medicine

(1) Take an example

In USA, psychosomatic medicine and consultation-liaison psychiatry began in the 1920s—1930s with the development of general hospital psychiatry units and the psychosomatic medicine movement. Rockefeller Foundation grants in 1934 and 1935 aided this developmental process by establishing closer collaboration between psychiatrists and other physicians. The number of consultation-liaison psychiatry services grew, and by the 1960s—1970s, a specialty scientific literature had developed. In 1974, the Psychiatry Education Branch of the National Institute of Mental Health (NIMH) decided to support the development and expansion of consultation-liaison services throughout the United States. By 1980, NIMH supported 130 programs and contributed materially to the training of more than 300 consultation-liaison psychiatry researchers. Federal budget cuts dramatically in the 1980s. Nevertheless, consultation-liaison psychiatry continued to grow and develop during the 1980s. More recently, as primary care has expanded its scope of practice and influence, consultation-liaison psychiatrists have found themselves well suited to teach and consult with primary care physicians. The years since 2000 have seen a focus on achieving added qualifications status by the American Board of Medical Specialties. In May 2003, the American Board of Medical Subspecialties recognized the practice of consultation and liaison psychiatry in the general hospital as a discrete psychiatric subspecialty that requires advanced training and qualification by an examination conducted by the American Board of Psychiatry and Neurology. In recognition of its earliest scientific bases, the subspecialty was named Psychosomatic Medicine by the American Board of Medical Subspecialties to distinguish it from other consult practices in medical subspecialties. In June 2005, the American Board of Psychiatry and Neurology administered the first examination to certify subspecialists in Psychosomatic Medicine. Psychiatric fellowship training programs in Psychosomatic Medicine qualify physicians in the skills and techniques of consultation-liaison psychiatry within the domain of psychosomatic medicine and related research.

(2) Take another example:

Ancient civilizations

Imhotep, court physician and architect to King Djoser (2630—2611 BCE) of Egypt, built the Step Pyramid in Sakkhara, Egypt, some 4500 years ago, as a medical instrument to keep the king's body through eons until his soul returned, a truly "psychosomatic" instrument. This pyramid is the oldest pyramid still standing, and Imhotep was named as god of medicine. Ancient Chinese and Indian medicine was inherently "psychosomatic" in that the psyche and the soma were seen to be intrinsically interconnected. In Chinese medicine, excesses or deficiencies in seven emotions—joy, anger, sadness, grief, worry, fear, and fright—were commonly considered to cause disease (Rainone, 2000). In Vedic medicine, certain personality components were considered to reside in particular organs, for example, passion in the chest and ignorance in the abdomen, and powerful emotions may cause peculiar behavior. Hippocrates (470-70 BCE) was perhaps the first physician to systematize clinically the notion that psychological factors affect health and illness. In a famous case, what might now be called "forensic psychiatric" opinion, Hippocrates defended a woman who gave birth to a dark-colored baby on the grounds that her psychological impression on seeing an African was sufficient to change the color of her fetus (Zilboorg, 1941). Hippocrates was an excellent clinical observer of psychiatric manifestations of medical disease as shown by his detailed descriptions of postpartum psychosis and delirium associated with tuberculosis and malaria (Zilboorg, 1941). Hippocrates condemned the prevailing view of epilepsy as a "sacred" disease, holding that it was a disease like any other. Though his theory of the "wandering uterus" underlying hysteria lacked scientific foundation, Hippocrates' humoral theory of disease anticipated present-day neurotransmitters. His emphasis on climate, environment, and lifestyle in health and illness, together with his awareness of the role of psychological factors in physical health and his belief in biologic/physiologic explanations of pathogenesis, entitle him to the title of not only the father of medicine, but also the father of psychosomatic medicine and the biopsychosocial approach.

With the descent of the Dark Ages, a tyrannical religious monism attributing mental and physical illness to witchcraft, and divine retribution stifled scientific inquiry. A textbook for the diagnosis (torture) and treatment (execution) of witches was the Malleus Maleficarum (The Witch's Hammer, 1487) written by two Dominican monks, James Sprenger and Henry Kramer, and prefaced with a bull from Pope Innocent VIII.

(3) The mind-body philosophy through the 19th century

The Hippocratic tradition in medicine was revived with the Renaissance and nourished by the Enlightenment. The French mathematician and philosopher Rene Descartes (1596—1650) proposed that the human body was like a machine, subject to objective investigation, while the soul or mind was a separate entity that interacted with the body in the pineal gland and that it was in the domain of theology and religion. This mind-body dualism facilitated the scientific study of the body at the expense of such studies of the mind. A number of competing and complementary theories, briefly described below, have been proposed since then to attempt to explain the nature of mind and body/matter.

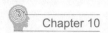

Benedictus de Spinoza (1632—1677), a Dutch lens crafter and philosopher, proposed a monism called double aspect theory, that is, the mental and physical are the two different aspects of the same substance, which in his view was God. Gottfried Wilhelm Leibniz (1646—1716) proposed psychophysical parallelism, that is, mind and body exist in parallel harmony predetermined by God from the beginning. Immaterialism, as advocated by George Berkeley (1685—1753), declared that existence is only through perception of the mind, that is, the body is in the mind. On the opposite pole is materialism, which holds that matter is fundamental and that what we call mind is a description of a physical phenomenon. Julien Offroy de la Mettrie (1709—1751) advocated that human souls were completely dependent on the states of the body and that humans were complete automata just like animals as proposed by Descartes.

Epiphenomenalism, proposed by Shadworth Holloway Hodgson (1832—1912), an English philosopher, postulated that the mind is an epiphenomenon of the workings of the nervous system. Mind and emotions, being epiphenomena, cannot affect the physical, just as a shadow cannot affect a person. Thomas Henry Huxley (1825—1895) popularized this view and placed it in an evolutionary context. Double aspect monism, proposed by George Henry Lewes (1817—1878), postulated that the same phenomenon, if seen objectively, is physical, and, if seen subjectively, is mental. William Kingdon Clifford (1845—1879) coined the term mind-stuff theory. In this theory, higher mental functions, such as consciousness, volition, and reasoning, are compounded from smaller "mind-stuff" that does not possess these qualities, and even the most basic material stuff contains some "mind-stuff" so that compounding of the material stuff would produce higher order "mind-stuff." This theory holds psychical monism-mind is the only real stuff and the material world is only an aspect in which the mind is perceived.

In spite of strong monistic trends, the major trend in medicine and psychiatry through the 19th and 20th century has remained dualistic and interactional, that is, how the mind affects the body and vice versa. Johann Christian Heinroth (1773—1843) coined the term psychosomatic in 1818 in the context of psychogenesis of physical symptoms. Psychosomatic relationship in the form of hypnosis was demonstrated and exploited by Anton Mesmer (1734—1815), though he improperly claimed it to be magnetic in nature ("animal magnetism"). Hypnosis was revived as a subject of medical investigation, diagnostics, and treatment by two competing schools, one at the Salpetriere Hospital in Paris headed by the neurologist, Jean-Martin Charcot (1825—1893), and the other at the university in Nancy, France, led by the physician, Hippolyte Bernheim (1840—1919). Charcot believed that hypnotizability was a result of brain degeneration in hysteria, while Bernheim and the Nancy school (including Ambroise-Auguste Liebeault and Pierre Janet) believed that psychological suggestion underlay the hypnotic phenomena.

(4) Modern psychosomatic medicine

Advances in molecular genetics and imaging technology have elucidated the role of genes in our constitution, brain morphology, and behavior. Psychoneuroendocrinology and psychoneuroimmunology have elucidated the mechanism by which stress affects the human organism. Health and illness is now conceptualized as a result of the interactions among genes, early environment, personality development, and later stress. This interaction is in no small measure influenced by salutary factors such as good early nurturance and current social support. It is also clear that all illnesses are the results of the interaction, where there is no subset of illness that is any more psychosomatic than others. Nevertheless, the term psychosomatic continues to be used to denote studies and knowledge that place particular emphasis on psychosocial factors in medical illness.

Some consider psychosomatic medicine to denote an interdisciplinary approach that includes physicians, oncologists, psychologists, etc., in contrast to consultation-liaison psychiatry, which is clearly a field within psychiatry.

There are a number of national and international "psychosomatic" organizations, such as the American Psychosomatic Society, Academy of Psychosomatic Medicine, European Society of Psychosomatic Medicine, and International College of Psychosomatic Medicine, and "psychosomatic" journals such as Psychosomatic Medicine, Psychosomatics, Journal of Psychosomatic Research, and Psychotherapy and Psychosomatics. General Hospital Psychiatry, International Journal of Psychiatry in Medicine, and Psychosomatics are mainly consultation-liaison psychiatry journals. Most of the organizations and journals are interdisciplinary, participated in by members of various specialties and professions. In Europe and Japan, there is often a department of psychosomatic medicine in medical schools, apart from the psychiatry department. Such psychosomatic departments mainly deal with patients with psychophysiological disorders, and may use complementary medicine techniques such as yoga and meditation.

In the United States, most CL psychiatrists practice in general hospital settings evaluating and treating psychiatric, emotional, and behavioral problems of medical patients. Research in the emotional aspects of specific medical patients gave rise to such fields as psychonephrology, psycho-oncology, and psychodermatology.

1.2   Epidemiology of psychiatric disorders in primary care

Fewer than 25% of the patients with psychiatric disorders see specialty mental health professional; most are seen in primary care settings (Regier et al., 1993). Anxiety or depressive disorders are diagnosed in 10%-15% of primary care patients (Spitzer et al., 1994; Ustun and Sartorius 1995). Half of the visits to physicians by patients with clear psychiatric diagnoses occur in primary care clinics (Schurman et al., 1985). Primary care physicians write most prescriptions for antidepressant (Simonet al., 1993) and antianxiety medications (Mellinger et al., 1984).

Medical conditions, particularly chronic illnesses, significantly increase the likelihood that a person will develop a mood disorder, an anxiety disorder, or a substance-related disorder (Hall et al., 2002).

1.3   The functions and reasons of consultation-liaison psychiatry

1.3.1   The dual roles of the consultation-liaison psychiatrist

There are two sets of dual interrelated roles that a consultation-liaison psychiatrist plays: consultation and liaison, and consultant and psychiatrist. The term consultation-liaison psychiatry encompasses two primary functions that of a psychiatric specialist providing expert advice on consultee's patient, and that of a liaison or link. The liaison function is inherent in the comprehensive approach utilized by the psychiatric consultant to the patient and the health care system. The consultation-liaison psychiatrist is both a consultant and a psychiatrist; that is, he or she has two masters—the requesting physician (consultee) and the patient. The obligation to the requesting physician often extends to serving the interests of the health care facility and of society at large. Sometimes this duality leads to an internal conflict, such as in situations when the perceived interest of the patient conflicts with the desires of the consultee, the needs of the hospital, or of society.

1.3.2   Clinical function

The consultant's primary clinical function in an acute general hospital is to facilitate the medical treatment of the patient, as the patient is in the hospital primarily for medical care. In this sense, consultation should be distinguished patient from referral, usually seen in outpatient settings and chronic care facilities. In a referral, the psychiatrist is asked to take over the psychiatric care of the patient if indicated, whereas in a consultation, the psychiatrist renders an opinion or advice to the requesting physician. In addition to such advice and opinion, the requesting physician usually, and implicitly, requests collaborative care of the patient if indicated,

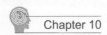

which forms the basis of the direct rendering of treatment by the CL psychiatrist. Except in emergencies and psychotherapy inherent in diagnostic interview, and facilitation of communication through meetings and phone calls with members of family and staff, direct treatment of patients including ordering medications should be done with the explicit knowledge and cooperation of the consultee so as to prevent a diffusion of responsibility for direct care.

1.3.3   Educational function

The liaison part of consultation-liaison psychiatry largely denotes its educational function. The objects of education are patients, requesting physicians, nursing staff, patient's families and friends, and the health care system. Examples of liaison education include teaching the psychological needs of patients based on their personality types, the immediate management of psychiatric conditions, the use of psychotropic drugs, and the determination of capacity to consent to procedures. Studies have clearly demonstrated that psychiatric consultation in the hospital decreases morbidity, mortality, length of stay and cost through the earlier recognition and treatment of psychiatric disorders, and improves quality of life and measures of self-care. These findings mandate psychiatric education of colleagues, case finding through psychiatric screening, and expansion of services by the consultation-liaison psychiatrist.

1.3.4   Administrative function

The administrative functions of the consultation-liaison psychiatrist are often mandated by either the government or the institution and often involved compulsive measures such as emergency hold and involuntary hospitalization of patients. Institutional rules usually mandate that an acutely suicidal or homicidal patient has to be evaluated by a psychiatrist, who will decide whether the patient should be placed on an emergency involuntary hold or be transferred to a psychiatric facility when medically stable. The consultation-liaison psychiatrist may be required to evaluate a patient with suspected dementia and apply for a conservator. The risk-management department of the health care institution relies on the consultation-liaison psychiatrist to evaluate patient's capacity to sign out against medical advice or to refuse medical/surgical procedures, and for general behavioral problems that disrupt the facility's function.

1.3.5   Research function

The consultation-liaison setting provides unique opportunities for research in the interface between psychiatry and medicine. Much of psychosomatic research in the 20th century has been done by consultation-liaison psychiatrists. The consultation-liaison setting gave rise to such subspecialty fields as psychonephrology, psycho-oncology, and psycho-obstetrics, and gynecology. The role of psychiatric intervention in medical utilization has also been a productive field of research, and has provided evidence that psychiatric intervention actually reduces the cost of health care. Numerous studies in the past decade have demonstrated that psychiatric consultation contributes to reduced costs in health care delivery, and improves access to mental health care.

Psychiatric consultation, like any other consultation, is not the primary reason for patient's hospitalization or contact with the health care system, and not a few patients may be surprised that a psychiatric consultation has been requested. Primary physicians may also be reluctant to request a psychiatric consultation because of the perceived stigma. Therefore, requesting a psychiatric consultation on a patient requires a certain amount of motivation on the part of the referring physician. This motivation is often generated by a strain in the health care unit consisting of the doctors, the nursing staff, and allied professionals. Common causes of such strain are patient's anxiety, communication difficulties, or behavioral problems, and administrative/legal requirements.

While some psychiatric consultations are generated at patient's request, most arise out of discomfort on the part of one or more health care staff members, and recognizing this discomfort or strain is an essential part of a successful consultation. It is consultant's job to ameliorate the strain so that the health care personnel can proceed to provide medical care without hamper.

1.4　The doctor-patient relationship

An effective doctor-patient relationship may be more critical to successful outcomes in psychiatry (because of the blurred boundaries between the conditions from which patients suffer and the sense of characteristics of the patients themselves) than it is in other medical specialties. In psychiatry, more than in most branches of medicine, there is a sense that when the patient is ill, there is something wrong with the person as a whole, rather than that the person has or suffers from a discrete condition. There must be time and space in the doctor-patient relationship to know the person from several perspectives: in the context of person's biological ailments and vulnerabilities; in the setting of person's current social connections, supports, and stressors; in the context of person's earlier psychological issues; and in the face of person's spirituality.

In the general hospital, the doctor-patient relationship has several unique features, including limited privacy, the interplay of medical and psychiatric illness, and the interplay of relationships among the psychiatrist, the patient, and the medical or surgical team. In psychiatry, the physician must understand and view the patient as a whole person, which requires both accurate diagnosis and formulation, blending biological, social, psychological, and spiritual perspectives. In the doctor-patient relationship, conflict can arise from many sources and can either derail the relationship or provide an opportunity to improve communication, alliance, and commitment.

For more detailed information about doctor-patient relationship please see Chapter 9.

2.　Clinical consultations

2.1　Common reasons for psychiatric consultation

The most frequent emotions, behaviors, and symptoms that patients exhibit that draw the attention of the health care professional and result in a psychiatric consultation request are the following:

(1) Anxiety and agitated behavior.

(2) Altered states of consciousness/delirium.

(3) Psychotic symptoms.

(4) Depressed affect.

(5) Suicidal behavior.

(6) Suspected psychogenic physical symptoms.

(7) Patient behavior generating strong feelings.

(8) Addiction and pain problems.

2.2　Categories of psychiatric differential diagnosis in the general hospital

The borderland between psychiatry and medicine in which consultation psychiatrists play their trade can be visualized as the area shared by two intersecting circles in a Venn diagram (Figure 10-1). As depicted in the figure and consistent with the fundamental tenet of psychosomatic medicine (i.e., that mind and body are indivisible), the likelihood that either a psychiatric or a medical condition will have no impact on the other is incredibly minute. Within the broad region of bidirectional influence (the area of overlap in the Venn diagram), the problems most commonly encountered on a CL service can be grouped into six categories (modified from Lipowski; see Figure 10-1).

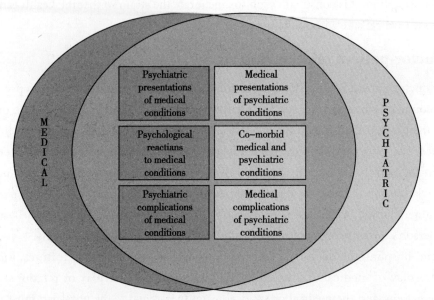

Figure 10-1　A representation of the overlap between medical and psychiatric care

2.3　The art of psychiatric consultation in the general hospital

As for any physician, his or her chief responsibility is diagnosis. The consultation-liaison psychiatrist is aided in this enterprise by identifying four key differences between general hospital psychiatry and practice in other venues: clinical approach, environment, style of interaction, and use of language.

2.3.1　Clinical approach

A senior psychiatrist at the Massachusetts General Hospital, Dr. George Murray advises his students to think in three ways when consulting on patients: physiological, existential, and "dirty". Each element of this tripartite conceptualization is no more or less important than the other, and the most accurate formulation of a patient's problem will prove elusive without attention to all three.

2.3.2　Environment

The successful psychiatric consultant must be prepared to work in an atmosphere less formal, rigid, and predictable than one typically found in an office or a clinic; flexibility and adaptability are crucial.

2.3.3　Style of interaction

The adaptability required by these environmental circumstances allows the psychiatric consultant to be more flexible in his or her relations with the patient. For example, psychiatric consultants should permit themselves to crouch at the bedside; shaking hands or otherwise laying on of hands may achieve the same end. Performance of a physical examination provides an excellent opportunity to allay anxiety and dramatically distinguishes consultation work from office-based psychiatry, where any touching of a patient-land colleagues one physical examination-is considered taboo.

2.3.4　Use of language

Allowance for flexibility also extends to psychiatrists" use of language; they can feel free than they might in other practice settings to use humor, slang expressions, and perhaps even foul language. All of these varieties of verbal expression create a temporarily jarring juxtaposition between the stereotypical image of the austere, reserved physician and the present one; defenses may be briefly disabled just long enough to connect with the truth and allow connection with the patient. For example, in a technique taught by Murray, the psychiatrist raises a clenched fist in front of an angry but anger-phobic patient and asks him, "If you had one shot, where would you put it?" In this case, the sight and sound of a "healer" in boxer's pose inquiring about placement of a "shot" creates a curious, or even humorous, incongruity that disarms patient's defenses and allows an otherwise intolerable emotion (anger) to emerge (if it is in the first place).

Lack of the formal arrangements of office-based psychiatric practice makes such techniques permissible in the general hospital, often to the delight of residents, who sometimes feel unnecessarily constrained in their interpersonal comportment and in whom even a little training unfortunately does much to limit their natural spontaneity.

2.4 Diagnostic evaluation in the general hospital

Consultations requests may have many origins and serve varied needs for the patient, team and system of care. Requests can be made by the patients, primary providers, multidisciplinary teams, and by the family members.

Requests can arise when a physician ponders the clinical status of the patient in regard to mood or affect (e.g., depressed after surgery), cognition (e.g., ability to make medical decisions), or behavior (e.g., agitated or threatening). When performing a consultation, the psychiatrist, like any other physician, is expected to provide diagnosis and treatment.

2.4.1 Receive a consultation request

Most health care institutions have formal mechanisms for requesting a consultation, such as a computerized request form or a written request, delivered by fax, email, or telephone etc. Informal requests may also be made either by telephone or in person. While informal consultations, especially when urgent, are often attended to, it is a good idea to insist on a formal consultation request as well.

2.4.2 Talk to the referring physician and clarify the consultation request

Consultation requests are often vague and sometimes misleading, usually because the consultee lacks the vocabulary of psychiatry. The consultee is aware of the discomfort of the strain caused by the illness, but has difficulty putting it into words. Thus, it is critical that the consultant interviewed the consultee, usually by phone, and ask for additional information about the consultation, particularly what help to the consultee would like to acquire from the consultant. It is a good idea to ask the referring physician to be sure to let the patient know to expect a psychiatric consultant, and, if possible, to introduce the consultant to the patient.

2.4.3 Review the current and pertinent past records

A careful review of the current medical record is indispensable to a thorough and comprehensive evaluation of the patient. The seasoned consultant is able to accomplish this task quite efficiently, knowing fruitful areas of the chart.

2.4.4 Gather collateral data

The gathering of collateral information from family, friends, and outpatient treaters is no less important in consultation work than in other psychiatric settings. For several reasons (e.g., altered mental status, denial,

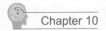

memory impairment, and malingering), patient's accounts of their history and current symptoms are often vague, various, and unreliable.

2.4.5　Interview and examine the patient

Next follows the interview of the patient and performance of a mental status examination, in addition to relevant portions of the physical and neurologic examinations. The relative merits of an open-ended interview compared with a structured clinical examination are debated. The two styles are not mutually exclusive, but both are necessary to obtain valuable longitudinal and cross-sectional information. The patient should be provided as much information as possible.

Structured examination is necessary for some historical data and for parts of the mental status examination. The consultant should at the very least review the physical examinations performed by other physicians. This does not, however, preclude doing his or her own examination of relevant systems, which, unless the patient is on the neurology service or is known to have a motor or a sensory problem, has likely been left unexamined. Vital signs are especially relevant in cases of substance withdrawal, delirium, and other causes of agitation. Formal testing for cognitive status via the Folstein Mini-Mental Status Examination provides a baseline cognitive assessment for the initial evaluation; the score is easily recognized by other specialists, and can be followed serially.

However, most information needed to make a diagnosis and a biopsychosocial formulation is obtained by simply listening. Many data are gained from patient's responses to open-ended questions, such as "What brings you into the clinic?", "How has this illness affected your life?", and "Why do you think your doctor asked the psychiatrist to see you?" Several personal and professional attributes are important to being an effective consultation-liaison psychiatrist.

The initial interview should ordinarily take not more than 30 minutes, and should identify patient's current concerns, the presence of major or minor psychiatric syndrome and its history, past history of psychiatric problems, the family history, the occupational status of the patient, and current mental status.

2.4.6　Formulate a diagnosis and management plan

To arrive at a diagnosis, laboratory testing comes after history and examination. By the time a psychiatric consultation is requested, most hospitalized patients have already undergone extensive laboratory testing, these should be reviewed. If consultations are dictated, put a brief note in the medical record immediately following the consultation with diagnostic or treatment suggestions that can be considered immediately. Differential diagnoses, diagnostic workup, symptomatic treatment and, in most cases, cognitive capacity are documented. When the consultant seeks to narrow the differential diagnosis, it should be communicated to the treatment team that further investigations such as neuroimaging or specialized laboratory investigations are required.

2.4.7　Write a note

The psychiatric consultation note should be a model of clear, concise writing with careful attention to specific, practical diagnostic and therapeutic recommendations. If the stated reason for the consultation differs from the consultee's more fundamental concern, both should be addressed in the note. If the referring physician adopts the consultant's recommendations, he or she should be able to transcribe them directly onto the order sheet or into computerized order-entry systems.

2.4.8　Provide periodic follow-up

Psychiatric consultants generally should follow up patients until they are discharged from the hospital or clinic or until the goals of the consultation are achieved. This is necessary for three reasons. First, urges to "sign off" on patients are frequently related more to negative reactions toward patients than to resolution of the presenting symptoms. Second, symptoms can recur, and a premature sign-off creates a potential loss of credibility and may lead to reconsultation. Finally, follow-up instills confidence that the CL psychiatrist is available and willing to help. Follow-up of the patient is provided in collaboration with the treatment team, and the frequency of contact determined by patient's clinical status. For example, a patient experiencing delirium while the team conducts a search for the underlying causes may require daily mental status examinations by the psychiatric consultant to monitor progress. Follow-up after the initial consultation may allow the consulting psychiatrist to determine whether there should be changes in the initial recommendations.

2.5 Treatments in consultation psychiatry

As in other practice settings, in the general hospital, psychiatric treatment proceeds along three aspects: biological, psychological, and social.

2.5.1 Biological management

The use of medication in disease requires careful attention to such conditions like all the medications a patient is currently taking, the contribution of underlying medical conditions, possible drug interactions, and possible dosage adjustments. When prescribing psychopharmaceuticals for medically patients taking other medications, the consultant must be aware of pharmacokinetic profiles, drug-drug interactions, and adverse effects. Other variables include nonadherence to prescribed medication, and polypharmacy in patients treated by different doctor.

2.5.2 Psychological management

Psychological management of the hospitalized medically patient begins—as does all competent treatment—with diagnosis, in this case, personality diagnosis. The consultant must realize that the patient may find the psychiatrist is the only outlet available to vent his or her feelings about treatment in the hospital. This is an appropriate function of the consultant—and, in fact, may be the tacit reason for the consultation.

2.5.3 Social management

Psychiatric consultants may be called on to help make decisions about end-of-life care (e.g., do-not-resuscitate and do-not-intubate orders), disposition to an appropriate living situation (e.g., home with services, assisted-living residence, skilled nursing facility, or nursing home), short-term disability, probate guardianship for a patient deemed clinically unable to make medical decisions for himself or herself, and involuntary psychiatric commitment.

2.6 Emergency consultations

A few situations need immediate attention, requiring a rapid assessment of a range of factors, including a scan of the physical situation (e.g., the patient might use medical equipment as a weapon) and the environment (e.g., multiple patient room or intensive care setting). Violent patients may be suffering from delirium or substance withdrawal. The concurrent presence of security guards allows safe assessment. The emergency use of psychotropic medication can relieve these dramatic situations. Suicidal patients become emergencies if there is an attempt at self-harm or if drugs, knives, or weapons are detected that the patient is secretly storing to use for self-harm. Following initial assessment, it is necessary to observe closely the patient who is acutely suicidal but too medically ill to be transferred to a psychiatric unit.

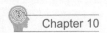

2.7 Outpatient setting consultations

Consultation-liaison psychiatry is often thought of as an inpatient clinical-specialty. Just as brief admissions have become routine in general hospitals, the way we provide psychiatric care has also changed, with a focus on treatment at home whenever possible. The spectrum of psychiatric disorders in the outpatient population differs considerably from that in hospital inpatients. The inpatient consultation-liaison psychiatrist typically is called upon to assess patients with delirium and those admitted following an overdose or self-harming behavior, whereas among outpatients the most common problems are mood disturbance and somatoform disorders. An outpatient consultation-liaison service can provide a broader range of management options and a possibility for follow-up; patients who are prescribed antidepressants, for example, can be reviewed at an appropriate time and any necessary changes made.

2.8 Liaison psychiatry

The liaison psychiatrist is a regular member of a treatment team in transplant programs, cancer centers, or dialysis units. A subspecialized focus of liaison psychiatrists on diseases states (e.g., HIV psychiatry) or medical specialty (e.g., gynecology or pediatrics) has developed in recent years.

Transplantation psychiatry is important due to the psychological stress upon patients and families who undergo lifesaving procedures or wait on a list for a limited number of available organs. The organ to be transplanted dictates the common psychiatric issues within each procedure. For related-donor kidney transplants, the psychiatric consultant may evaluate both overt and covert family pressures that the putative donor experiences and how the potential recipient feels in response. Treatment adherence is important, especially in patients with diabetes who have not followed diabetic regimens. The essential issue in liver transplantation recipients who have been substance abusers is their history of abstinence. If potential recipients are still using alcohol or other substances of abuse they need rehabilitation and abstinence before receiving a liver transplant, although candidacy is individualized and may vary according to the scarcity of the organ to be transplanted. Liaison psychiatrists may be called upon to assist with screening to identify latent psychiatric disorders, and to assist with the psychological stressors as discussed. For heart transplantation patients, ongoing support is necessary during the waiting period before an available organ is found. Such patients commonly experience anxiety and depression, and wrestle with mortality.

In oncology settings, central issues are depression in the terminally ill, delirious states due to diseases and treatments, and family reactions. In nephrology centers, patients who request termination of hemodialysis must be evaluated for delirium and dementia. The treatment of underlying depression may alter the request to cessation of hemodialysis. The role of the psychiatrist in nephrology also focuses upon patients who resist dietary and fluid limitations, often in the context of depression and dementia. The psychiatrist will have many opportunities to teach health professionals to recognize and manage psychiatric disorders in chronic illness and end-of-life care.

3. Core concepts in psychosomatic medicine

3.1 Psychiatric disorders caused by medical conditions

Psychiatric symptoms can occur as a direct consequence of an underlying medical condition. Most studies have led to the general consensus that all "potentially psychiatric" symptoms of the medical condition should be included in the diagnosis of the psychiatric disorder. In the case of depressive symptoms, for example, this strategy risks the psychiatric diagnosis of patients who do not meet full criteria of Major Depression (false positive), but avoids the failure to diagnose patients who do meet criteria (false negative).

Psychiatric symptoms caused by medical conditions have important implications, not only for diagnosis but also for evaluation, treatment and management of both medical and psychiatric conditions. Detection and diagnosis of the medical cause often relies upon the rich experiences of the primary medical clinician; however the patient with psychiatric symptoms might not present to medical care, but rather to a psychiatric setting causing a possible delay in medical diagnosis. The patient with medically-induced psychiatric symptoms who presents to medical settings may be dismissed as not medically ill. Treatment of the presenting psychiatric symptoms, without detection of the underlying medical condition, may actually exacerbate the medical condition. Consultation-liaison psychiatrists identify those patients who elude diagnosis in primary care due to the prominence of the psychiatric presentation. They educate medical and psychiatric colleagues about the medical masquerade, and may be a stalwart force toward completing the medical evaluation of a patient with psychiatric symptoms. The following section will highlight this principle by clinical examples.

3.2　The patient with cerebrovascular disease and depression

The neuropsychiatric complications of stroke include cognitive deficit, and behavioral and emotional dysregulation. Depression following stroke is a frequent and adverse neuropsychiatric sequela of stroke, yet it is undiagnosed by most nonpsychiatric physicians. Depression in the aftermath of stroke (Post-stroke Depression and Post-Stroke Pathological Affect) responds to aggressive treatment but escape detection when interpreted as an "understandable" response to the stroke.

3.3　The patient with postoperative delirium

Delirium is an acute cognitive disorder with global impairment in brain function, and fluctuating consciousness and attention. Associated features include hyperactivity, hypoactivity, and reversal of the sleep-wake cycle. Delirium is a common presentation in hospitalized elderly patients, affecting up to 30% of elderly surgical patients. The most common predisposing surgical procedures are emergency hip fracture repair, gastrointestinal surgery, coronary artery bypass grafts, and lung transplants.

3.4　Patient with depression and cardiac disease

Depression is an independent risk factor for ischemic heart disease. It predicts higher morbidity and mortality after uncomplicated myocardial infarction. For 6 months after the infarction, even up to 5 years, depression has an impact on cardiac mortality, eclipsing standard cardiac variables such as left ventricular ejection fraction. The possible mechanisms for these phenomena include a three-fold increase in medication nonadherence, shared risk factors (smoking, diabetes, and obesity), lower heart rate variability, chronic inflammation (increased biomarkers such as C-reactive protein), platelet activation, and sympathoadrenal activation due to increased physiological stress. Studies to determine the role of psychiatric treatments aimed at lowering cardiac risk have indicated an improved quality of life, but no clear reversal of increased mortality.

3.5　Psychological reactions to medical illness

Medical illness creates a crisis. The patient is faced with multiple emotional, physical and financial challenges that can create serious psychological distress. The personal aspects of illness include pain, disability, and loss of function and autonomy due to the disease and or its treatment. People react differently to the challenges before them in accordance with their coping style, environmental circumstances, and the nature of the disease and its treatment.

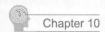

3.6　Somatic presentations of psychiatric disorders

The common presentation of somatic concerns in primary care can be related to psychiatric disorder, such as anxiety or depression is most commonly. Patients with major depression are more likely to present for care in primary care settings, to complain of somatic illness. These psychiatric illnesses are commonly under-recognized in busy outpatient settings. When the psychiatric disorder is identified and effectively treated, the somatic symptoms are alleviated correspondingly.

3.7　The demoralized patient

Demoralization does not qualify for a primary psychiatric diagnosis. It is common in medical and surgical settings in the context of a reaction to acute or chronic stress, such as the onset, treatment, or terminal of illness. The management of demoralization involves promotion of the primary physician's role in soothing patient's fears about the illness through relevant information about treatment options.

3.8　Future directions

Consultation psychiatry is the bridge between psychiatry and the rest of medicine. As medicine advances, there will be new psychological and emotional challenges for patients requiring the skills and techniques of consultation psychiatrists. Consultation psychiatry is already dividing into subspecialized areas to accommodate the expansion of medicine. Consultation-liaison psychiatrists are focusing upon HIV/AIDS, oncology and nephrology as primary interests. Concurrently, the stresses of hospital life will continue, strained by the forces of economics and health care policies. The shift from hospital-based care to outpatient settings has expanded consultation services into outpatient clinics and specialized care facilities. As new psychiatric treatments emerge, the consult psychiatrist will provide them to patients underserved in nonpsychiatric settings. Newly recognized as a discrete subspecialty, yet centuries old in practice, psychosomatic medicine has a new role in the ancient art of medicine. Graduate education programs with dedicated fellowship training in psychosomatic medicine will advance the mission to improve patient care. With increasing technologies and advances in biomedical knowledge, this subspecialty will provide the biopsychosocial elements of comprehensive patient care and clinical research to improve clinical outcome and enhance quality of life to patients.

（邹　涛）

Chapter 11

Psychiatric/Psychological Disorders

Mental illness refers to the disorders in cognition, emotion, volition and behavior of mental activity on different degree influencing by various biological, psychological and social environment factors, which cause brain function disorder. Mental illness includes psychosis, neurosis, mental retardation, personality disorders, etc. In the research and development of modern psychiatry, more and more scholars adopt the concept of psychiatric/psychological disorders to replace the concept of mental illness. Psychiatric/psychological disorders refer to any congenital or acquired mental disorder, including a series of different symptoms and behavioral disorders. These symptoms will bring individual pain in most cases, impaired social function, such as self-care ability, interpersonal communication skills, learning ability, work or housework, and abide by the norms of social behavior ability damage. The formation and development of psychiatric/psychological disorders is the interaction of biological, psychological and social factors, congenital or child will continue to exist in some disorders, such as mental retardation; social factors will exist in anxiety disorders and stress related disorders.

Hundreds of millions of people all over the world are affected by psychiatric disorders. There are 25 million people globally suffer from schizophrenia and 154 million people from depression, 24 million from Alzheimer and other neurocognitive dementias, about 877,000 people die by suicide every year are estimated by World Health Organization (WHO) in 2002. WHO's World Mental Health (WMH) surveys in 85,052 respondents (2007) found that median and inter-quartile range (IQR) of age onset are: anxiety disorders 7-14 (IQR: 8-11), mood disorders 29-43 (IQR: 35-40), impulse control disorders 7-15 (IQR: 11-12). Median and IQR of lifetime prevalence estimates are: anxiety disorders 4.8-31.0% (IQR: 9.9-16.7%), mood disorders 3.3-21.4% (IQR: 9.8-15.8%), impulse control disorders 0.3-25.0% (IQR: 3.1-5.7%).

1. Criteria for distinguishing between normal and abnormal psychologies

Mental health is a state of well-being in which every individual realizes his or her own potential, can cope with the normal stresses of life and work productively and fruitfully, and is able to make a contribution to her or his community (WHO, 2009). Mental health is used to describe either a level of cognitive or emotional well-being or an absence of a mental disorder, includes an individual's ability to enjoy life and procure a balance between life activities and efforts to achieve psychological resilience.

How to distinguish between normal and abnormal psychology?

(1) Medical criteria

This criterion deems that we can find the basis of anatomy and pathophysiological changes in the brain or the body if someone is suspected some kind of psychological or behavior disorder. The psychological or behavioral performance is seen as a symptom of the disease, and the causes are attributed to brain dysfunction.

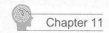

A person with mental disorders should have a pathological process. Some mental disorders that have not been able to detect significant pathological changes may be found in the future.

(2) Statistical criteria

In the general population, people's psychological characteristics obey the normal distribution in statistics. The normal or abnormal psychology of a person can be determined by the degree of deviation from the average. On the basis of statistical data, using psychological test as a tool, we may determine the boundaries between normal and abnormal psychology. The statistical criteria provides quantitative data of psychological characteristics, the operation is simple and convenient. But there are also some drawbacks in this standard, for example, highly intelligent people are very few people in the population, but are rarely considered abnormal. Therefore, the universality of statistical criteria is relative.

(3) Introspective experience criteria

This criteria contains two aspects: one is patient's introspective experience, the patients themselves feel anxiety, depression or discomfort without obvious cause, feel unable to control their behavior, and so on; the second is observer's introspective experience, the observer judge person's behavior according to their own the past experience. This criteria is very subjective, different observers have their own experience, so the criteria of evaluation behavior is not the same. However, the observer can form a similar view of the same behavior if trained in the same kind of discipline.

(4) Social adaptation criteria

People can maintain a stable state of physical and mental activity, to adapt to the environment and change the environment under normal circumstances. Therefore, the behavior of normal people accords with the social norms, social requirements and ethical standards. However, we think that the persons are suffering from mental disorders if person's ability of social behavior is not in accordance with the social recognition with the reason of organic or functional defects.

2. Etiology and pathogenesis of psychological disorders

The etiology of psychological disorders is concerned with the causes and mechanisms of various psychological diseases. Most of the psychological disorders are multifactorial diseases, which are related to many biological, psychological and social factors. We should focus on the understanding various etiological models of various psychological disorders. The exploration of this field is still a long-term task for the future.

2.1   Biological factors

2.1.1   Genetic factors

In a variety of psychological disorders, in addition to the already clear gene mutations related diseases, such as Huntington's disease and hepatolenticular degeneration, other psychological disorders such as Alzheimer's disease, schizophrenia, bipolar disorder, depressive disorder, panic disorder, obsessive-compulsive disorder, autism, attention deficit hyperactivity disorder, anorexia nervosa, showed some degree of familial aggregation, which were determined by genetic factors. Therefore, these psychological disorders have a genetic predisposition to different degrees, in some diseases there is susceptibility of gene transfer from parents to their kids.

At present, a number of interactive virulence gene lead to a form of psychological disorders, each gene has pathogenic effect, accumulation of pathogenic effect of multiple virulence genes determines the level of individual genetic susceptibility. Lifetime risk of schizophrenia in the general population is about 1%, with heritability estimated at up to 80%, the disease risk of parents, sibling, children of their own are 4.4%, 8.5%, 12.3%, respectively. At the same time, the susceptibility genes schizophrenia (such as NRG1 on chromosome 8, DTNBP1 on chromosome 6, G-72 on chromosome 13 and chromosome 3, HTR2A, DRD3 and so on) weakly associated with disease. Moreover, the cumulative effect is often not the pathogenic gene mutations, but the gene polymorphism, such as the APO gene related with Alzheimer's disease, COMT Val 158 Met gene related with schizophrenia, 5-HTT gene related with anxiety disorders, and 5-HT1d receptor gene related with obsessive-compulsive disorder. On the other hand, some polygenic variation may contribute to risk of different psychological disorders, such as schizophrenia and bipolar disorder may share the common polygenic variation of XVIIIB (MYO18B), ZNF804A, and NOTCH4.

The role of genetic factors is not sufficient to represent the vast majority of the causes of psychological disorders, genetic factors can only determine the genetic predisposition of individuals, constitute an important aspect of biological predisposition. On this basis, coupled with environmental factors (including intrauterine environment, postnatal growth environment and conditions, various physicochemical and biological stimuli, psychosocial stress), it may lead to the clinical onset of disease. Epigenetic research believes that the role of the environment may lead to changes of non-gene sequence which affect gene expression, resulting in individual disease, and this epigenetic also have certain genetic predisposition.

2.1.2   Brain structure and function

With the development and application of brain imaging techniques (CT, MRI, DTI, PET, SPECT, etc.), computer technology and related software, it has been proved that the brain structure and function of psychological disorders are abnormal. The abnormal structure of different regions may lead to different mental symptoms: frontal lobe lesions often leads to mental retardation, language disorders, personality changes; temporal lobe and frontal lobe with anatomical and functional connections, so temporal lobe lesions often lead to similar symptoms, other symptoms such as olfactory, gustatory hallucination, automatism, emotional instability often appear; spatial perception disorder is most often caused by a partial lesion, manifested as autotopagnosia entities, sensory disturbance, dressing apraxia; occipital lesions often cause visual disturbances and hallucinations; pituitary lesions will due to endocrine disorders and psychiatric symptoms, similar to performance of schizophrenia.

Schizophrenia has received the most extensive attention, in brain structure, currently found brain volume decreases, lateral ventricle and the third ventricle volume increases, cortical thinning, matter volume of frontal gray decreased, the volume of temporal lobe (superior temporal gyrus, hippocampus, amygdala) decreases,; in brain function, generally accepted findings include the hyper function in front part of the frontal lobe cortex and medial temporal lobe cortex, the former may be correlated with psychomotor inhibition (such as poverty of thought, apathy, spontaneous movement decreased), while the latter may be correlated with distorted reality symptoms (hallucinations and delusions).

Mood disorder is also widely concerned and studied. In the brain structure, patients with depressive disorder have been found to have enlarged lateral ventricles, reduced basal ganglia volume and hippocampal volume, patients with bipolar disorder was found to have the enlarged amygdala volume; in the brain function, there is evidence related to clinical manifestations of mood disorders and abnormal brain function: dysfunction of dorsolateral and dorsomedial prefrontal cortex with cognitive dysfunction, dysfunction of orbitofrontal cortex and amygdala with emotional information processing, dysfunction of the basal ganglia and psychomotor symptoms etc.

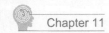

It is worth noting that, abnormal brain regions involved in a variety of psychiatric disorders are often more than one, which urges people to understand the disease mechanism from the local perspective to neural network (or neural circuits), such as fronto-limbic circuitry and fronto-thalamic-cerebellar circuits in schizophrenia, the orbitofrontal-basal-ganglia-thalamo-cortical circuits in obsessive-compulsive disorder, and the prefrontal-amygdala-hippocampus loop in post-traumatic stress disorder. However, there is no specific neuroimaging cause to various mental disorders at present.

2.1.3   Central neurotransmitter

Neurotransmitter transfers the neural communication base on the synapses, which is the basic way to realize the neuropsychological function. The basic idea of neural biochemical model of psychological disorders is abnormal level of central neurotransmitter activity and receptor distribution and function can led to a variety of psychological disorders, also become the theoretical basis for the development of new psychotropic drugs. The neurotransmitters most closed to psychological disorders include dopamine, 5-hydroxytryptamine, nor-epinephrine, acetylcholine, gamma-aminobutyric acid and glutamic acid, etc.

Dopamine (DA) participates in the process of a variety of neuropsychological, including muscle movement and coordination, curiosity and exploration, reward, emotion and behavior regulation, also involved in neuroendocrine. DA system have been associated with a variety of psychological disorders, for example, overactive of DA is associated with schizophrenia and mania; decreased DA activity is associated with depressive disorder, attention deficit hyperactivity disorder. In addition, DA is also involved in the pathogenesis of substance dependence, and may be related with anhedonia in depression and schizophrenia. 5-hydroxytryptophan (5-HT) participates in regulate mood, diet, sleep wake cycle, sexual behavior, pain, neuroendocrine activities in hypothalamic pituitary. The relationship between 5-HT and psychological disorders is more extensive, including schizophrenia, depression, bipolar disorder, generalized anxiety disorder, panic disorder, phobia, OCD, eating disorders, autism, and ADHD. Nor-epinephrine (NE) is involved in the central regulation of emotion, learning and sleep wake cycle, feeding behavior, especially in stress (keep the brain awakening and alert function). NE dysfunction has been found to be associated with schizophrenia, bipolar disorder, depression, anorexia nervosa, phobia, generalized anxiety disorder, panic disorder and stress related disorder. Acetylcholine (Ach) is involved in arousal, REM sleep, learning, memory, emotion and sports. Degeneration of the Ach system is the main neurochemical change in Alzheimer's disease. In addition, Ach and NE can balance the neurotransmitter metabolism associated with mood disorders, the former over activities can lead to depression, the later over activities can lead to mania. Amino acid neurotransmitters include the excited glutamic acid (Glu) and inhibitory gamma aminobutyric acid (GABA). Research shows that the Glu NMDA receptor in prefrontal lobe and thalamus and the number of GABA neurons activity were significantly reduced in patients with schizophrenia, which may results the negative symptoms and cognitive symptoms. In addition, GABA and mood disorders may also have some relationship, mood regulation of antiepileptic drugs (carbamazepine, valproate) may be related with the regulation of GABA in the brain.

2.1.4   Neuroendocrine

Neuroendocrine is involved in the regulation of mood and behavior, and is associated with various psychological disorders. Previous study found that the activity level of the hypothalamic pituitary adrenal axis (HPA) increased in patients with depression, the increased level promote the cortical hormone releasing hormone (CRH) and glucocorticoid. Depression is also associated with dysfunction of hypothalamic pituitary thyroid axis (HPT), hypothalamic pituitary growth hormone (HPGH) axis and hypothalamic pituitary gonadal axis (HPG).

In addition to depression, the relationship between neuroendocrine dysfunction and other psychological disorders also support in many researches, such as HPA and PTSD, anxiety disorder, anorexia nervosa, HPT and OCD, panic disorder, PTSD, as well as HPGH and schizophrenia, schizoaffective mental disorder, bipolar disorder, OCD, etc. In addition, HPG is also involved in the pathogenesis of schizophrenia. Although the relationship between psychological disorders and neuroendocrine dysfunction has been found, the results are not reproducible, so that they are not sure, and some of them are difficult to explain. The role of neuroendocrine in the pathogenesis, pathology, symptoms, treatment and prognosis of psychiatric disorders will remain a long-term research focus.

2.2   Psychological factors

From Sigmund Freud's (1856—1939) psychoanalytic theory, since the end of nineteenth century, the major progress of contemporary psychology includes the birth and development of behaviorism, humanism and cognitive theory. These theories explored the essence and regular of human psychology from different perspectives, explained the mechanism of psychological disorders and created a variety of psychological treatment.

For more detailed information about Freud's psychoanalytic theory please see Chapter 3.

2.3   Social factors

Man is a social animal. Society not only gives us protection, but also is the source of all kinds of psychological stress and pain. Therefore, people pay more and more attention to the relationship between social factors and psychological disorders. There are many social factors related to the occurrence, development and prognosis of psychological disorders, including social culture, social change, social pressure and social support.

Social environment and social culture have important effects on both physical and mental health. The occurrence of many mental disorders is closely related to the special social culture. For example, the epidemic of Koro is a special phenomenon in south China, India and Southeast Asia; "Killer" in Malaysia is also closely related with social and cultural background; in Islamic countries, alcohol dependence was significantly lower than that of other regions. Social changes have also a significant impact on the generation of psychological disorders. For example, in early 1950s, paralysis of dementia is popular in China, but in 60s gradually disappear; drug abuse was rarely happen previously, but occurred after China's reform and opening up. With the improvement of the living standard, the incidence of senile mental disorders, especially senile dementia, increases gradually. Stress factors are more important in urban environment than in rural areas, because the stress factors play an important role in the occurrence of anxiety and depression. In addition, war, racial discrimination, violent crime, political persecution, economic crisis, poverty and other social pressures, can cause serious damage to mental health.

Social support refers to the help, protection and support provided from individual's social environment. Previous researchers found that people with psychological disorders have reduced closed relationships and narrowed personal networks. Lack of social support, especially in patients with the need to support cannot be provided in time, will make the emergence of psychological disorders. Generally speaking, good social support give protection to the individual; lack of social support network often make patient's symptoms are not easy to improve. In social support system, family support is the most important, good family support not only helps to relieve the individual psychological stress, reduce the occurrence of psychological disorders, but also contribute to a better recovery of patients with psychological disorders. However, excessive social support, such as finding a variety of reasons not to restore the work of patients with schizophrenia is not conducive to the rehabilitation of the disease.

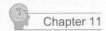

2.4　The relationship between pathogenic factors

Biological and psychosocial factors play an important role in the development of psychological disorders. However, biological factors may play a dominant role in some psychological disorders, but in other psychiatric disorders are secondary effects. A large number of clinical evidence shows that the causes of many psychological disorders are the result of a combination of various factors. Psychological and social factors play an important role in anxiety, depression and stress related disorders, and is one of the main factors in the pathogenesis. At the same time, these patients also have neurophysiological changes, for example, patients with anxiety disorder have abnormal NE system, OCD and depression have the decrease of 5-HT. On the other hand, biological factors play a leading role in schizophrenia, bipolar disorder and mental retardation, psychological and social factors tend to be predisposing factors. In schizophrenia, pathogenic factors include both the biological factors (genetic factors, neural and biochemical changes and pathological changes) as the basis of disease occurrence and development, and psychosocial factors (relatives died suddenly, trauma, romance, divorce, unemployment) as the precipitating factors.

3. Symptoms of psychological disorders

Each symptom has its own definition, and has the following characteristics: the appearance of symptoms is not controlled by patient's consciousness; once symptoms appear, transfer cannot make them disappear; the content of the symptoms does not match the surrounding environment; the symptoms will bring social function damage to patients. In the examination, we should first determine whether there are symptoms of psychological disorders, and then analyze what symptoms exist. Abnormal mental activity is a very complex process, and have individual differences. The performance of psychological disorders symptoms is affected by some factors: individual factors, involving gender, age, and physical condition and personality characteristics can make a symptom unique; environmental factors, involving personal life experience, current social status and cultural background, may affect patient's symptoms. Therefore, in the examination, we must do a specific analysis of specific circumstances considering the impact of the above factors.

3.1　Disorders of cognition

3.1.1　Disorders of sensation and perception

(1) Disorders of sensation

1) Hyperesthesia. An increased susceptibility to the general stimuli of the external, for example, the patients feel the sun is particularly dazzling, the sound is particularly harsh, the smell is unusually pungent. More commons are in neurosis, brain weak state and chronic pain disorders.

2) Hypoesthesia. A reduction in the sensitivity to the general stimuli of the outside world, for example, the patients almost cannot feel the intense pain, the environment becomes dim, and the color becomes blurred. More commons are seen in depression, stupor and disturbance of consciousness.

3) Cenesthopathy. The body is internally generated by a variety of discomfort and unbearable feelings, such as pull, squeeze, walk, ant crawling, etc. More commons are in neurosis, schizophrenia, depression.

(2) Disorders of perception

1) Illusion. It is a distorted perception, and is misperceptions of external stimuli. For example, a person misperceives a coat hanged on the door as that of a man. This symptom more often occurs when attention is not focused on the sensory modality, or when there is a strong affective state.

2) Hallucination. It is a perception experienced in the absence of external stimuli to the sense organs. A hallucination is experienced as originating in the outside world (or within one's own body) like a percept. For example, a person hears somebody sing outside the window, actually nobody sing there. Not only psychological disorders but also healthy people can experience hallucinations, especially when they are tired and stress.

According to the different sensory organs, hallucinations can be divided into auditory hallucinations, visual hallucinations, gustatory hallucinations, olfactory hallucinations, and tactile hallucinations. Auditory hallucinations is the most common symptom in clinic, may be experienced as voices, noises, or, music. Visual hallucination is another common symptom in psychological disorders. The figures in visual hallucinations do not exist in real world, may be amplificatory or shrunken figures than that in real world, or horrific scene. Olfactory and gustatory hallucinations are frequently experienced together, often as unpleasant smells or tastes, and generally accompany with the persecutory delusion. Tactile hallucinations may be experienced as sensations of being touched, pricked, or strangled, which more common seen in organic mental disorders

3) Disturbance of perceptive synthesis. Patients can perceive the nature of objective things themselves correctly, but mistakenly perceive their individual attributes. For example, patients feel the shape, size and volume of the outside world changed (metamorphopsia); the distance of surrounding changed; time goes by so slowly or rapidly, feel the development and changes of things is not restricted by time. The patients also feel the surroundings and environment change, become unreal, like a scenery show (derealization).

3.1.2　Disorders of thinking

(1) Disturbance of the form of thought.

These disorders include flight of ideas, thought slowness, thought blocking, perseveration of speech, circumstantiality, loosening of associations, symbolic thought, neologism, paralogism, etc. Flight of ideas means that person's thoughts and conversation move quickly from one topic to another so that one thought is not completed before another appears. These rapidly changing topics are always understandable, because the links between different thoughts are normal. Thought slowness is opposite to flight of ideas, which is mainly characterized as moving slowly in thoughts and conversation, has difficulty in associations. Loosening of associations means losing the normal structure of thinking, the conversation appears as muddled, illogical, and inaccurate, so it is very hard to talk with the person with loosening of associations. Neologism denotes that patient's invented and incorrect use words or phrases to describe his or her morbid experiences, common seen in schizophrenia.

(2) Disorders of the content of thought.

These disorders include delusion, obsessive ideas and overvalued ideas. Delusion is a false, distorted, pathological belief or judgment that has no basis of fact and is inconsistent with the accepted beliefs of individual's educational and cultural background. The content of delusion is absurd and illogical. For example, a person firmly believes that he has one thousand wives. Many types of delusions appear in patients with psychological disorders, such as delusion of persecution, delusion of observation, delusion of guilt, delusion of grandeur, delusion of being loved, delusion of special significance, delusion of non-consanguinity, etc. Obsessive ideas are repeated persistent thoughts, impulses, or images that enter the mind despite person's efforts to exclude them. The characteristic feature is the subjective sense of a struggle—the patient attempts to resist the obsession that occasionally intrudes into his awareness. Obsessive ideas include obsessive doubt, obsessive rumination, obsessive reminiscence and obsessive contradictory ideas. An overvalued idea is a kind of exact belief, which is directly related to the self. On the basis of patient's personality and personal experience, there is a certain factual basis for the occurrence. But overvalued ideas are too extreme, that most

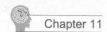

people in the same cultural background are not acceptable, so often lead to interpersonal conflict. Overvalued ideas has a strong emotion and motivation, it has a significant impact on patient's psychological activity and behavior.

3.1.3   Disorders of attention

Aprosexia is the most common attention disorder, involving damage on attention keeping, selectivity, scope and transfer. People will be easily distracted, shifting attention from one target to another in a disorganized fashion if an individual's selective attention is impaired. Disorders of attention can be seen in many kinds of psychological disorders, such as mood disorders, anxiety disorders, schizophrenia and organic mental disorders.

3.1.4   Disorders of memory

Memory is the reappearance of past events and experiences. The memory is divided into four processes: recognize, maintain, recognition, and recall. Damage on any four processes will lead to disorder of memory. Common memory disorders includes amnesia, paramnesia, confabulation and Korsakoff's syndrome. Amnesia is a failure of memory, it is the loss of memory which is experienced in a certain period or event, but not a decrease of memory capability. Anterograde amnesia is the deficits in storing new information to memory. The patients cannot retain in memory what he has experienced after his head injury, but he can recall everything before the injury. Retrograde amnesia is the deficits in memory when an individual completely or partially fails to remember events that occurred before a certain time. Paramnesia is a mistake of memory, which is the reorganization of events that have not taken place at the time and place. Confabulation is the reorganization or remembering of events that have not taken place at all. déjà vu is that the patient has an unusual familiarity with a strange scene, which are common in patients with epilepsy.

3.1.5   Disorders of intelligence

Intelligence is the ability to solve new problems and form new concept using past knowledge. Disorders of intelligence can be divided into mental retardation and dementia. Mental retardation refers to that mental development stunted or stay in a certain stage due to various pathogenic factors (heredity, infection, poisoning, head injury, etc.) because congenital or perinatal or in growth before maturity (18 years ago). The intelligence was significantly lower than that of normal children with the increase of age. Dementia is the decreased in comprehensive intelligence due to chronic or progressive brain disease, and can be damage on memory, thinking, orientation, comprehension, calculation, learning capacity, language, etc.

3.1.6   Insight

Insight is a very important concept of clinical psychiatry, refers to patient's ability to understand their own mental illness. Some patients with psychological disorders can maintain insight, such as neurosis. However, most of the patients with psychological disorders are generally lack of insight, so they do not admit that they have psychological disorders, do not take the initiative to seek medical treatment, and even refused to see a doctor. With or without as well as the degree recovery of insight is an important indicator to determine the severity of the disease and the degree of disease improvement. Both the mental symptoms disappear and insight recover means clinical recovery of psychological disorders.

3.2   Disorders of emotion

Disorders of emotion can be caused by obvious causes in person's life or without any reason, and can be divided into depression, elation, anxiety and phobia.

Disorders of emotion usually include several components other than the mood itself. For example, feelings of depression are usually accompanied by gloomy preoccupations and psychomotor slowness, anxiety are usually accompanied by autonomic over-activity and increased muscle tension.

3.2.1　Depression

Depression is an increased negative mood, characterized by extreme feelings of sadness, emptiness, despair, pain and isolation. It is always accompanied by associated changes in behavior, thinking and somatic discomfort. Patients with depression may withdraw socially, become disinterested in normal activity and feel pessimistic about the future, weight loss and sleep disorders.

3.2.2　Elation

Elation is an elevation of mood, characterized by feelings of great energy, happiness, excitement and power. It is also accompanied by changes in behavior and thinking. The individual is interested in everything and ways optimistic and worries little, but this elevation of mood is always unstable and subject to change. The individual is very distractible, moving from one idea to another. As well, the individual always have a strong reaction to trivial things (irritability). The individual need little sleep and increased sexual desire.

3.2.3　Anxiety

Anxiety is accompanied by subjective discomfort and objective abnormal performance, which is often associated with intrusive thoughts or worries and physical discomfort. Patients always worry about their health or other problems without obvious and objective evidence. It is always accompanied by autonomic arousal, such as tachycardia, sweating, dry mouth, pale skin, etc., and motor restlessness, such as tremor, muscle tension, pain, stiffness, etc.

3.2.4　Phobia

Phobia is a persistent irrational fear of and wishes to avoid a specific object, activity, or situation. The individual has insight (they think the fear is irrational), but finds it difficult to control his fear and often tries to avoid the feared objects and situation if possible. The object that provokes the fear may be a living creature such as a dog, snake, or spider, or a natural phenomenon such as darkness and thunder, avoidance also affects the social function of patients. The individual is very painful, often accompanied by symptoms of autonomic dysfunction.

3.3　Disorders of will and behavior

Will is the psychological process that people consciously set goals and overcome difficulties with their own actions to achieve their goals. The disorders of will include hypobulia, abulia, parabulia and ambivalence. Hypobulia accompany with the depression and thought slowness, the individual has no interested in everything and do not want to participate in activities. In abulia, the patient has no obvious motivation for any activity, and no plan or requirement, always be solitary and withdrawn. Abulia usually accompany with poor thinking and apathy (negative symptoms) in schizophrenia. Parabulia refers to the intention and general requirements of patients that violate or not allowed by ordinary people, it is difficult for people to understand the certain activities or behavior of patients. Ambivalence means that patients produce contradictory activities of the will on the same thing at the same time, however, the patient is not aware of this, which is one of the characteristics of schizophrenia.

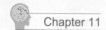

Disorders of behavior include psychomotor excitement and psychomotor inhibition, the latter includes:

(1) Mutism. Patients are silent, do not answer any questions. But sometimes the thought of the patients can be expressed using a gesture or a pen or pencil.

(2) Mannerism. The patients made strange, foolish, and childish action, posture, gait and facial expression.

(3) Stereotyped. The patients continue to repeat a monotonous action, often with the appearance of stereotyped language.

(4) Echopraxia. The patient imitates other people's movements with no aim, often with imitation of language at the same time.

(5) Tics. Symptoms are irregular repeated movements involving a group of muscles, such as sideways movement of the head or rising of one shoulder.

(6) Compulsive act. Includes forced washing, forced counting, compulsive ritual action.

(7) Impulsive and aggressive behavior. The behavior is not inhibited, cannot be suppressed. Impulsive behavior has the following characteristics: suddenly; does not match the situation or social behavior and psychological inducement; without thinking and any sense of resistance and difficult choice; difficult to understand.

3.4　Disorders of consciousness

Consciousness is awareness of the self and environment. The patient awareness of self and the cognitive ability of surrounding environment were damaged in consciousness disorder, which show the decreased in clarity of perception and attention, break down in the thinking process, slowness in motor behavior, sleep cycle disorder and disorientation. The level of consciousness can vary between the extremes of alertness and coma. Coma is the extreme form. The patient in a coma shows no external evidence of mental activity and little motor activity other than breathing, there is no response even to strong stimuli, but have pathological reflex. Sopor is an infrequently used term for a state, the person in a sopor can be aroused only by strong stimuli. Stupor refers to a condition in which the person is immobile, mute, and unresponsive but appears to be fully conscious. Confusion means inability to think clearly and occurs together with partial impairment of consciousness, illusions, hallucinations, delusions, and a mood change of anxiety or apprehension in acute organic disorder confusion.

3.5　Disorders of sleep

Sleep disorders are the disturbances in the quantity or quality of sleep that interfere with an individual's normal function such as job performance and interpersonal relationship. Sleep disorders are a common problem all over the world. Sleep can be disturbed by many factors in modern society, including problems from within the body, and external environmental factors, for example, medical disorders, drug use, stress, diet, irregular bed times, activities before bed, and artificial lights, etc. There are numerous sleep disorders as well as multiple classification systems. The most representative of which include International Classification of Sleep Disorders (ICSD), Diagnostic and Statistical Manual of Mental Disorders, 4th edition (DSM-IV), and International Classification of Diseases, 10th edition (ICD-10). The 2nd edition of the ICSD (ICSD-2) was published by the American Academy of Sleep Medicine in 2005, and was widely accepted by clinicians. This system classifies sleep disorders into eight major categories: insomnia, sleep related breathing disorders, hypersomnias, circadian rhythm sleep disorders, parasomnias, sleep related movement disorders, isolated symptoms and normal variants, and other sleep disorders. We here introduce several common sleep disorders. Insomnia is the most common sleep disorder phenomenon.

3.5.1 Insomnia

Insomnia is characterized by difficulty in falling asleep or remaining asleep throughout the night. It is very difficult for peoples with insomnia to fall asleep after going to bed, easily awaken during the night, or unable to enter the deep sleep stages. They often feel fatigued rather than refreshed in the morning. Insomnia is the severe lack of high-quality sleep, and can affect people's life in many ways. Common symptoms of insomnia also include fatigue, decreased alertness, poor concentration, decreased performance, muscle aches and other overly emotional states, such as becoming anxious and irritable. Chronic insomnia results to impaired occupational performance and affects the quality of life.

Insomnia has different forms of clinical presentation. When it is difficult to fall asleep, it is called as sleep onset insomnia; it is called as sleep maintenance insomnia when sleeper has difficulty in maintaining sleep throughout the night; another forms of insomnia presents as waking up too early in the morning and having difficulty getting back to sleep.

(1) Diagnosis of insomnia. There are many similarities in different diagnostic systems. Diagnostic criteria typically require the presence of nighttime and daytime symptoms for at least one month. In ICSD-2, the following three criteria need to be met to diagnose insomnia: 1) A complaint of difficulty initiating sleep, difficulty maintaining sleep, or early awakening, or chronically non-restorative or unqualified sleep; 2) The above sleep difficulty occurs despite adequate opportunity and circumstances for sleep; 3) The impaired sleep produces deficits in daytime function, at least one of the following forms of daytime impairment is included: fatigue; attention, concentration, or memory impairment; social dysfunction or poor school performance; mood disturbance or irritability; daytime sleepiness; motivation, energy, or initiative reduction; proneness for errors/accidents at work or while driving; tension, headaches, or gastrointestinal symptoms in response to sleep loss; and concerns or worries about sleep.

In DSM-IV criteria, individuals are required to meet two or more of the following to be considered as presenting insomnia: 1) Difficulty initiating sleep (taking 30 minutes or more to fall asleep); 2) Difficulty maintaining sleep (more than 30 minutes of awakening during the night) and a sleep efficiency (ratio of sleep to time spent in bed) of less than 85%; 3) Sleep disturbance at least 3 nights a week; 4) Significant impairment of daytime functioning (fatigue, mood disturbances) caused by the disrupted sleep.

(2) Classifications of insomnia. The magnitude and prevalence of insomnia are difficult to assess. The duration of insomnia is probably the most important guide to evaluate and treat insomnia. Insomnia can be mild to severe depending on how often it occurs and for how long it lasts. Usually, insomnia can be classified into three types: transient, short term and chronic.

Transient insomnia is when the duration of poor sleep lasts several days. It is often associated with a transient situational stress, and disruptions to circadian rhythms. For example, individuals probably experience transient insomnia before taking a big exam or other stressful conditions. Transient insomnia would usually be self-resolved after the individual is adjusted to the stressful event or the events are resolved. Changes in sleep schedule or in work shift, or sleeping in a strange place during a trip may also promote transient insomnia. Jet lag is a very common cause of insomnia in cross-country travelers.

Short-term insomnia involves sleep disturbances that lasts up to 4 weeks in duration. The reasons of short-term insomnia are often an acute illness or a serious injury, ongoing stress related to school or work, such as an impending task deadline. Especially, negative life events such as a death in the family or the loss of a job often trigger short-term insomnia.

Chronic insomnia is poor sleep that persists for more than 4 weeks, even for years. This form of insomnia is a complex disorder with many possible causes. Common reasons may include: poor sleep habits, chronic

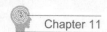

stress, medication such as antidepressants, substance abuse such as caffeine and alcohol, psychiatric disorders such as depression, anxiety disorders, and schizophrenia, and other chronic diseases such as chronic obstructive pulmonary disease, congestive heart failure, and restless legs syndrome. Sometimes, it is not easy to pinpoint the reasons for chronic insomnia, which may last for years disrupting sleep almost every night. Serious health risks are associated with chronic insomnia. Research has shown that the elderly with chronic insomnia were more likely to have ischemic heart disease.

(3) Causes of insomnia. The causes of insomnia are various, generally including medical causes, psychiatric or psychological causes, and environmental causes, as detailed below:

1) Medical causes some chronic diseases are associated with insomnia such as the chronic pain, dyspnea especially chronic obstructive pulmonary disease, cardiac conditions include ischemia and congestive heart failure, and endocrine conditions such as thyroid dysfunction.

Restless legs syndrome often leads to insomnia. Restless Legs Syndrome is characterized by a compulsory desire to move the limbs usually associated with a sensation of burning or tingling. The movement of legs can partially or temporarily relieves the symptoms.

In addition, several normal physical factors can cause sleep disorders, such as when hormones are fluctuating intensely. For example, many women report insomnia during their menstrual periods or menopausal periods. Pregnancy is also a common cause of sleeping disorders in women.

2) Psychiatric or psychological causes. Many patients with mood disorders often suffer from insomnia. Insomnia is not a special disease; it is a kind of syndrome. Insomnia is the most common manifestation in mood disorders such as depression and anxiety. Drug use or withdrawal from caffeine, tobacco, alcohol, and other substances may affect the overall quality of sleep. In addition, use of certain medication, such as -blockers, some antidepressants, amphetamines, and withdrawal from drugs such as benzodiazepine can cause insomnia.

Stress undoubtedly plays a key role in insomnia. Many studies reported that insomnia is related to stress, such as negative life events, work-related stress, extended working hours, increased demands on worker productivity, and interpersonal conflicts. It is common for individuals to experience insomnia when they lose family or a job, or suffer from severe illnesses. When individuals get involved in interpersonal conflicts and do not have effective coping strategies, insomnia and emotional problems are the most common manifestations. In particular, the studies found that psychosocial stressors were more likely to be associated with insomnia than were health problems, indicating the strong link between stressors and sleep problems.

In particular, psychological responses to the failure to sleep are the most common causes of insomnia. After not sleeping well for several days, many people become worried, frustrated, or depressed. This causes them to place added psychological pressure on themselves to sleep. This leads to increased anxiety at bedtime, which further interferes with sleep. Once this expectation of insomnia is established, a vicious sleep cycle of "failure-worry-more failure-more-worry" develops.

3) Environmental causes. The common cause of insomnia is that the circadian rhythm is disrupted. Sometimes changes may suddenly occur in one's normal life style, and the individual is unable to adjust quickly to a new sleep schedule. For example, rapidly traveling across several time zones upsets the circadian rhythm that regulates the timing of sleeping and waking, and results in individuals" failure to fall asleep in a normal day-night sleep cycle, also known as jet lag. In addition, people who work nights or rotate shifts feel sleepy when nighttime comes, and have difficulty to fall asleep when this routine is maintained for a period of time.

The cause of insomnia is also related to poor environmental conditions, including changes in the external context leading to temporary adaptation difficulties. This type of insomnia is often called the situational insomnia. Sleep is often disrupted by poor environmental conditions such as excessive hot and cold, as well as light and sound pollution.

(4) Etiology of insomnia. As mentioned above, several psychological and physiological factors contribute to the onset and maintenance of insomnia. Psychological factors are known to play a major role in the development of insomnia. Although insomnia is frequently associated with psychiatric disorders, it should be emphasized that in many cases psychopathology is subtle. In the late 1980s, Spielman proposed a model of insomnia in terms of predisposing, precipitating, and perpetuating factors, which are also known as the "3P Model" of insomnia. According to Spielman, three types of factors contribute to insomnia at different points.

Predisposing factors refer to psychological or biological characteristics which increase vulnerability to insomnia. These factors do not result in insomnia directly, but they increase the risk that an individual will develop insomnia. These factors include personality such as the susceptibility to depression, the trait of anxiety, and hyperarousal state. In other words, individuals with these factors are vulnerable to insomnia.

Precipitating factors refer to negative life events, medical situations, environmental or psychological factors that can trigger insomnia in vulnerable individuals. These factors include divorce, death of a significant other, medical conditions such as disease and injury, familial or occupational stress, and sleep schedule changes.

Perpetuating factors refer to those elements that maintain or exacerbate insomnia. They are typically recognized as cognitive and behavioral mechanisms. From this perspective, individuals with insomnia usually have some misconceptions about normal sleep requirements, and excessively worry about sleeplessness and the daytime effects of inadequate sleep. Consequently, it is very hard for them to fall asleep because these dysfunctional beliefs often produce sleep disruptive behaviors, such as sleeping in late, or becoming more agitated at bedtime.

(5) Treatment of insomnia. Insomnia is a common sleep problem. The mechanisms of insomnia have not been made clear, and the treatments of insomnia need to be tailored according to each particular individual needs. In some cases, insomnia can be improved by psychological treatments, and in other cases may need physical exercise programs to relieve stress and develop good sleeping habits. However, in some cases an individual may need to take sleeping pills for a short period of time, when alternative treatments do not have the desired effect.

3.5.2   Parasomnias

Parasomnias refer to intrusions into the sleep process creating disruptive sleep-related events. Parasomnias include nightmare disorder, sleep terror disorder, sleepwalking, and sleeptalking.

Sleep terrors refers to a sudden arousal from sleep and intense fear, and often accompanied by screaming and physiological reactions such as rapid heart rate, perspiration, and sweating. When an individual awakens from a terrified state, he or she might appear to act confused and respond poorly. Sleep terrors are fairly common in children aged 3 to 5. Strong emotional tension and the use of alcohol or both can increase the incidence of sleep terrors among adults. Sleep terrors usually occur during stages 3 and 4 sleep (deep and slow wave sleep). Individuals who have sleep terrors usually do not remember the episodes the next morning.

Nightmares are frightening dreams that abruptly awaken the sleeper and typically cause feelings of terror and anxiety. Nightmares are usually associated with REM sleep, and the individual awakening from a nightmare is able to describe the dream contents in detail. It can be caused by many factors including illness, anxiety, the loss of a loved one, or negative reactions to medicine. There are also some studies regarding the nightmare effect of on individual's waking-state activities, for instance through a structure-validated measurement, the nightmare experience questionnaire (Chen et al., 2014).

Sleepwalking occurs when an individual seems to be awake and moving around but is actually asleep. It is difficult to awaken the individual during an episode. Sleepwalkers have no memory of their actions after an

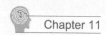

episode. They may engage in very complex activities, such as opening the door and walking down the street. They can prevent obstacles from injuries, and then return to bed to sleep. This disorder is most commonly seen in prepubertal children, aged 6 to 12. The majority of sleepwalking disappears in adulthood. It is not dangerous to wake a person who is sleepwalking, but sleepwalking itself can be dangerous because the sleepwalker is unaware of his or her surroundings and can bump into objects, or can fall down. Sleepwalking is not a serious disease, and has nothing to do with emotional problems. The exact mechanisms of sleepwalking are not clear. Sleepwalking most often occurs during slow wave sleep, stages 3 and 4 sleep early in the night rather than during REM sleep. Therefore, specialists propose that sleepwalking may have nothing to do with dreaming.

Sleeptalking refers to the utterance of speech or sounds that occurs during sleep without awareness of the event. An individual who talks during sleep typically cannot remember their actions the next morning. Sleeptalking itself is harmless, but can be disturbing to sleep partners or family members who witness it. Sleeptalking often occurs when individuals have medical conditions such as fever, or emotional stress, or other sleep disorders such as sleepwalking.

The exact causes and mechanisms of these sleep disorders are not clear. Research indicates that these sleep disorders can be associated with some medical conditions such as having a fever, heartburn, iron deficiency, and peripheral neuropathy. Many psychological factors also play an important role such as stress and emotional problems. Treatment of sleep disorders should comprise a combination of behavior modifications, counseling, and medications.

3.5.3 Narcolepsy

In spite of having a normal amount of sleep at night, individuals with narcolepsy tend to have frequent daytime sleepiness and fall asleep in totally inappropriate situations, such as on the midst of a conversation or on the job working in a plant.

Narcolepsy usually has the following symptoms: Sudden sleep attacks may occur while an individual is performing any type of activity at daytime, such as eating dinner, driving the car, or taking on a conversation; sudden loss of muscle tone, or muscle weakness may occur while an individual is awake. This muscle weakness may affect specific muscle groups or the entire body; Hallucinations may occur before a sleep attack, and sometimes emotional excitement can trigger an onset of sleep attack. This phenomenon is also known as cataplexy, which is often brought on by strong emotional reactions, such as laughing or crying.

A narcoleptic episode usually lasts from several seconds to more than several hours, and it is dangerous for the individual to fall asleep while walking, driving, or cooking. The causes of narcolepsy have not yet been made clear. Narcolepsy is often associated with brain damage or neurological disease, and studies shown that there is a genetic predisposition to narcolepsy. Research supports the finding that narcolepsy is caused by an interplay of genetic and environmental factors and appears mostly in sporadic cases. Narcolepsy is usually treated with a combination of medication, behavioral treatments, and counseling.

4. Classification and diagnostic criteria of psychological disorders

The development of the classification and diagnostic criteria of psychological disorders is one of the major advances in the field of psychiatry. It greatly promotes the mutual communication between schools and improves the diagnostic inconsistency. As structured diagnostic tool, diagnostic criteria not only for the research, also widely used in clinical practice and played an important role in the exploration pathology of the psychological mechanism of various psychological disorder, as well as new drug development, clinical

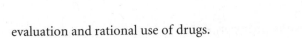

evaluation and rational use of drugs.

The classification of psychological disorders is the process of classifying complex psychological phenomena according to the established standards. The purpose of disease classification is to classify diseases into different types according to their own characteristics. Because most of the etiology and pathology of psychological disorders is unknown, the classification of the basic axis is mainly based on clinical symptoms. However, it must be pointed out that, according to the diagnosis of symptoms can only explain the state of the disease at that time, if the symptoms change, especially the main symptoms change, the diagnosis may change. What's more, the same diagnosis inevitably involves a variety of diseases with different etiologies and similar symptoms. But the symptom classification is beneficial to the current symptomatic treatment.

Classification and diagnosis systems

Three established systems are currently used in clinical practice and research for classifying psychological disorders in China. The International classification of Diseases (ICD) is published by the World Health Organization (WHO) and used internationally. The Diagnostic and Statistical Manual of Mental Disorder (DSM) system is established by the American Psychiatric Association, which has been widely used in the United States and some other countries.

4.1 The International Classification of Diseases

The International Classification of Diseases (ICD) is an international standard diagnostic classification for a wide variety of health conditions. The tenth edition of ICD (ICD-10) has been wildly used, in which mental and behavioral disorders consist of 10 main groups:

F0 Organic, including symptomatic, mental disorders

F1 Mental and behavioral disorders due to use of psychoactive substances

F2 Schizophrenia, schizotypal and delusional disorders

F3 Mood (affective) disorders

F4 Neurotic, stress-related and somatoform disorders

F5 Behavioral syndromes associated with physiological disturbances and physical factors

F6 Disorders of personality and behavior in adult persons

F7 Mental retardation

F8 Disorders of psychological development

F9 Behavioral and emotional disorders with onset usually occurring in childhood and adolescence

In addition, there is a group of "unspecified mental disorders".

4.2 Diagnostic and statistical manual of mental disorders

The first edition of the DSM was published in 1952. The fourth edition, DSM-IV, was originally published in 1994 and revised as DSM-IV-TR in 2000. The latest edition, DSM-5, published in 2013. DSM-5 is still a continuation of phenomenological classification based on the principle of the past because the etiology of most mental disorders is still unknown. The descriptive classification of DSM-5 did not follow the five axis DSM- IV-TR diagnosis methods, the new model of three-dimensional diagnosis: the diagnosis, the psychological factors and social background, the evaluation function (recommend the use of WHO Disability Rating Scale (WHODAS)). DSM-5 pays more attention to the judging the severity of psychological disorder symptoms, more emphasis on using the concept of scale and questionnaire. DSM-5 formally introduced "spectrum" than the other versions, such as autism spectrum disorders and schizophrenia spectrum. There is no classification of schizophrenia in DSM-5; bipolar disorder and depression are two separate diseases; OCD

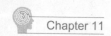

and stress related disorders were broken from the classification of anxiety disorders.

There are 22 main groups of mental and behavioral disorders in DSM-5:

(1) Neurodevelopmental disorders

(2) Schizophrenia spectrum and other psychotic disorders

(3) Bipolar and related disorders

(4) Depressive disorders

(5) Anxiety disorders.

(6) Obsessive-compulsive and related disorder

(7) Trauma- and stressor-related disorders

(8) Dissociative disorders

(9) Somatic symptom and related disorder

(10) Feeding and eating disorders

(11) Elimination disorder

(12) Sleep-Wake disorders.

(13) Sexual dysfunction

(14) Gender dysphoria

(15) Disruptive, impulse-control, and conduct disorders

(16) Substance-related and addictive disorders

(17) Neurocognitive disorders

(18) Personality disorder

(19) Paraphilic disorder

(20) Other mental disorder

(21) Medication-induced movement disorders and other adverse effects of medication

(22) Other conditions that may be a focus of clinical attention

5. Examination of psychological disorders

Clinical psychological doctors should understand patient's mental suffering in the mental examination, should not regard the mental symptoms as "strange", not to discriminate against patients. Doctors should give the patients with mental support, enhance patient's confidence to overcome the disease, must keep the confidential in psychiatric symptoms and related privacy issues (private life) of the patients.

5.1　Clinical interview

For more information regarding clinical interview, please see Chapter 4.

5.2　Physical and auxiliary examination

Patients must undergo a comprehensive physical examination and laboratory examination, outpatient patients also should be checked on the condition of physical examination, especially neurological examination.

According to the need, doctors may select a number of auxiliary examination, mainly to identify the physical disease with psychological disorders, or whether with physical disease, or drug treatment before and after some of the effects on the organ. The main auxiliary examinations mainly included renal function test, liver function test and dexamethasone suppression test (DST), Thyrotropin releasing hormone test (TRH), and electroencephalogram (EEG) examination.

In addition, polysomnography (PSG) is helpful for the diagnosis of sleep disorders, epilepsy, migraine, substance abuse, depression. Brain evoked potentials may be helpful in the diagnosis of mental retardation, ADHD, schizophrenia and depression. In recent years, it has been found that schizophrenia, affective disorder, obsessive-compulsive disorder and anorexia nervosa have signs of atrophy of the cerebral cortex and the expansion of the ventricles, which can be diagnosed by computed tomography (CT), magnetic resonance imaging (MRI). Functional magnetic resonance imaging (fMRI) is commonly used in the studies on biological basis of psychological disorders, has great application value for the study of cognitive function, and is the hotspot of psychiatric research and one of the important development direction. Positron emission computed tomography (PET) is helpful to study the physiological and biochemical metabolic processes in various parts of the body, and is used in receptor function in \mental disorders and detection of receptor binding rate of psychotropic drugs.

5.3　Psychological measurement and psychiatric symptom rating scale

Mental symptom scale can be standardized and quantified on psychiatric symptoms, to grasp the changes of symptoms, evaluation the treatment effect, severity of the disease, and has clinical significance in research work.

The commonly used scale: (1) the Clinical Global Impression Scale (CGI), is mainly to determine total disease severity and changes; (2) the Brief Psychiatric Rating Scale (BPRS), is mainly used to observe the severity and evaluating therapeutic effects in the treatment of schizophrenia; (3) the Positive Symptom Rating Scale (SAPS), the scale for the assessment of negative symptoms (SANS), mainly reflects the clinical characteristics of schizophrenia, and the prominence of the positive and negative symptoms; (4) the Zing's Self-rating Depression Scale (SDS), is mainly self-rating depressive symptoms, reflect patient's emotional experience; (5) the Self-rating Anxiety Scale (SAS), is mainly used to evaluate self-anxiety experience; (6) the Hamilton Depression Scale (HAMD), mainly by doctors to assess the severity and treatment of depressive symptoms after the symptom changes; (7) he Hamilton Anxiety Scale (HAMA), the main assessment of symptoms severity and treatment evaluation the symptoms of anxiety; (8) the Yale Brown Obsessive Compulsive Scale, the main assessment of obsessive-compulsive symptoms severity scale; (9) the Young Mania Rating Scale is mainly used in manic bipolar affective disorder, schizoaffective disorder manic state; (10) the Symptom Checklist 90 (SCL-90), the scale can reflect all kinds of symptoms, subjective symptoms in patients with accurate assessment, widely used in psychiatric and psychological counseling outpatient; (11) the Activity of Daily Living Scale (ADL), the main evaluation subject's ability of daily life.

In addition to assessment of psychiatric symptoms scale, some psychological measurement tools: (1) the Minnesota Multiphasic Personality Measurement of Personality test (MMPI), mainly for various types of mental disorders and personality assessment for clinical diagnosis. (2) the Eysenck Personality Questionnaire (EPQ), mainly reflecting personality tendency of subjects, such as internal external orientation, psychotism, neuroticism and subjects of the cover; (3) the Raven Standard Reasoning Test (SPM), mainly used for 5.5 years to adult subjects, testing the ability of abstract thinking; (4) the Wechsler Intelligence Scale, can calculate the verbal IQ, performance IQ and total IQ scores; (5) the Mini-Mental State Examination (MMSE), mainly for the screening of dementia.

The mental symptom scale and psychological measurement are generally carried out by questionnaire, homework and projection. The examination is an important part of the psychological technician and clinicians, who should be familiar with the methods of measurement, the choice of test and the analysis of the results of the commonly used scales. It is worth mentioning that the results of any evaluation scale cannot replace the clinical diagnosis of psychiatric department, and can only be used as auxiliary diagnosis or clinical reference.

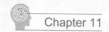

6. Types of psychological disorders

6.1　Schizophrenia

Schizophrenia is one of the most common severe psychological disorders, with many obstacles, such as thinking, emotion, behavior and disharmony between mental activities and environment. The onset of this disorder is slow, and occurs in young adults, the course of disease is chronicity, repetition and relapse, and some patients tend to mental decline. The lifetime prevalence of schizophrenia is 0.38%-0.84% worldwide, for instance, 1.3% in the United States, and 0.66% in China. Genetic factors play an important role in the pathogenesis of schizophrenia, in addition, studies have shown that dysfunction of dopamine, glutamate also involved in schizophrenia. More and more studies show that schizophrenia may be a kind of neurodevelopmental disorders and neurodegenerative diseases.

(1) The main clinical symptoms of schizophrenia.

The symptoms of schizophrenia are complex and diverse. Two concepts of acute schizophrenia and chronic schizophrenia were introduced in the textbook of psychiatry in Oxford. The main performance of the former is with hallucinations, delusions and thinking disorder (positive symptoms); the main performance of the latter is with apathy, lack of will, slow motion and social decline (negative symptoms).

1) Hallucinations. Auditory hallucinations is the main clinical symptom, patients behavior often is controlled by auditory hallucinations, automatic speaking. The content of the hallucinations is absurd and bizarre, divorced from reality.

2) Delusions. Main clinical symptom is delusion of reference, persecution, and influence. The content of the delusion is absurd, for example, the patients have a sense of control, believe that they are controlled by external forces (psychoautomatism).

3) Association disturbance of thinking. For instance, the lack of coherence and logic in the process of thinking, loose thinking, and lack of specificity and reality.

4) Affective disorder. For instance, the emotional apathy, disharmony between emotional reaction and thinking content and external stimuli.

5) Disorder of will and behavior. For instance, the obvious decline or lack in will activity, activity reduction, lack of initiative, passive behavior, retreat.

(2) Treatments for schizophrenia.

The drug therapy is the main treatment, at the same time, psychological treatment provide supplementary in the different stages of the disease. The methods of psychotherapy include cognitive behavior therapy, family therapy, individualized therapy, social skills training and supportive psychotherapy.

The doctors can choose the second generation antipsychotics such as risperidone, olanzapine, quetiapine, aripiprazole, or first generation antipsychotic drugs such as perphenazine, sulpiride etc. according to the clinical symptoms in the different stages of the disease. Drug treatment should be systematic and standardized treatment, emphasize on early, enough dose, enough courses of "the whole course of treatment". In principle, a single medication was recommend, combined medication can be used when poor efficacy in single medication. Patients accompany with depression, self-injury, suicide, refuse food, disobey, stupor, impulsive, hurt people, and cannot be tolerated with drug therapy, were recommend Electric convulsive therapy (ECT), which is safe, fast onset, but the effect is not durable longer.

Psychotherapy must be part of the treatment of schizophrenia. Psychological treatment cannot only improve patient's mental symptoms, insight, and enhance the compliance of treatment, but also improve the relationship between family members, and promote social contact with patients. Behavioral therapy helps to correct some of patient's functional deficiencies, improve interpersonal skills. Family therapy has made it possible for family members to find the problems of communication for a long time, which can help to reduce the negative emotions and simplify the communication.

Recovery and comprehensive social rehabilitation means patient's decline of energy and physical are recover, the patients achieve and maintain a good state of health, restore the original work or learning ability, rebuild the appropriate stable interpersonal relationships. Psychological and social rehabilitation should encourage the patients to participate in social activities and engage in their own work. For withdrawal manifestations of chronic schizophrenia, patients can carry out daily life ability, interpersonal skills training and labor occupation training, make the patient retain a part of social life, reduce disability as much as possible.

[Case 1]

A 23-year-old man. Personality: taciturn, less communicative, and grumpy. One year ago, he had insomnia and depression because his father died. The young man do not want do anything, say and laugh by himself, fear and agitation sometimes. His abdomen is painful, but he cannot say where it is. He always think he is guilty, often said: "I cannot live for a few days, I am guilty. The young man believes other person know the things he thought, his neighbors monitor his behavior with a tape recorder, and his brain is controlled by a died man. The young man does not care about his mother when his mother is unwell (The relationship between the mother and the young man is very good before). The young man cannot go to work now, stay at home all day with being in a daze and absent-minded, rarely communicate with other people. Once ran outside (3 days away from home, ask where to go, the patient cannot answer). Two questions are raised as follows:

(A) Is this man's behavior normal?

(B) What abnormal signs and symptoms of psychological disorder is he showing?

6.2 Bipolar disorder

Bipolar disorder is a type of affective disorder, defined as mania or hypomania, and a depressive mood disorder. The incidence of bipolar disorder is similar in men and women and across different cultures and ethnic groups. The prevalence and incidence of bipolar disorder are very similar across the world. Age-standardized prevalence per 100,000 ranged from 421.0 in South Asia to 481.7 in Africa and Europe for men and from 450.3 in Africa and Europe to 491.6 in Oceania for women (World Health Organization, 2000). However, severity may differ widely across the globe. The peak age of onset is 15 to 19 years. The first time for bipolar disorder is often depressive episodes, mania or hypomania happens after one or several times of the depression onset. Long-term repeated attacks of bipolar disorder, result in chronic diseases, personality change and social function damaged. Patient's work, study, life and communication ability are likely to damage whether in depression or manic episodes. Therefore, treatment should be positive to avoid adverse consequences once diagnosed with bipolar disorder.

(1) The main clinical symptoms of bipolar disorder.

Typical manic episodes are manic mood, irritability, jubilant, fast of speech, exaggerated and full of energy. Attention shift with the environment, the amount of sleep reduce, hyperactivity, reckless behavior. The whole experience and behavior of patients have the trait of disease, lack of insight.

The typical symptoms of depression are sad, anxiety and irritability. Patients suffering from pain, loss of speech, loss of attention, indecision, reduced interest in daily activities, social withdrawal, helplessness and despair, and recurrent thoughts of death and suicide.

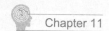

(2) Treatments for bipolar disorder.

The drug is the first choice for the treatment of bipolar disorder, on the other hand, on the basis of drug treatment, the use of psychological therapy is better than the simple drug treatment, which can improve the medication compliance, reduce the rate of re hospitalization, improve social function. Comprehensive treatment should be adopt in the treatment of bipolar disorder, including drug therapy, physical therapy, psychological and crisis intervention, aim to improve the curative effect and treatment compliance, prevent self-injury, and improve social function.

Drug therapy is the most effective treatment for bipolar disorder, and has been supported by a large number of evidence-based medical evidence. On the basis of mood stabilizer treatment, combined with other drugs according to the disease condition. Manic state: preferred a mood stabilizer treatment, combined timely with another mood stabilizer, or antipsychotic drugs, or benzodiazepines according to the different conditions. Depressive state: cautious use of antidepressants based on mood stabilizers. Mixed state: emotional stability, sodium valproate or second-generation antipsychotics.

The psychotherapy bipolar disorder includes mental health education, cognitive behavior therapy, interpersonal and social rhythm therapy, and short-term psychoanalysis. The forms of treatment include individual treatment, couple therapy, family therapy, and group therapy. Electroconvulsive therapy is one of the best choices for quick, safe and effective for severe depression, refractory bipolar disorder and rapid circulation, especially for anorexia, stupor or the risk of serious injury and suicide. The dosage of drugs should be reduced before electroconvulsive therapy.

6.3 Depression

Depressive disorder is a kind of mental disorder caused by various reasons, which is characterized by significant and persistent depression, lack of intrinsic vitality, or decreased interest. The cause of depression is very complex, which is related to many factors, such as heredity, biology, psychology, society and environment. The lifetime prevalence of depressive disorder was 12.7% and 21.3% in men and women, respectively.

(1) The main clinical symptoms of depression.

The main clinical symptoms of depression are:

1) Depression: feeling sad, depressive mood, crying, and inner pain in most of the time, this state is not affected by the external environment.

2) Lack of interest and pleasure from daily life to experience happiness, not willing to do any things.

3) Lack of energy or fatigue, the patient is also very tired even if nothing is done, work efficiency.

Depression patients evaluate lower on the self and the surrounding environment, often blame self, inferiority; often pessimistic despair, have a sense of guilt, have suicidal ideas, attempts and behavior sometimes. Patients with depression are usually associated with damage on memory, attention, thinking ability and other cognitive functions, decreased efficiency on work or learning and ability; also accompanied by sleep disorders.

(2) Treatments for depression.

The aim of treatment is to relieve depression and depressive symptoms, reduce morbidity and suicide rate, improve the quality of life, improve social function and relapse prevention. The main treatments include drug therapy, psychotherapy, modified electric convulsive therapy, music therapy, repetitive transcranial magnetic stimulation, etc. Drug therapy is the main method for the treatment of depression, which can relieve depression and anxiety and somatic symptoms. At present, the new antidepressants include: 5-HT reuptake inhibitors, such as fluoxetine, sertraline, citalopram, fluvoxamine, citalopram and colleagues; 5-HT and NE selective reuptake inhibitors such as venlafaxine; NE and DA reuptake inhibitors such as bupropion; NE and specific 5-HT antidepressants such as mirtazapine.

For depressive patients with obvious psychosocial factors, they often needed to be combined with psychotherapy. Some studies have shown that the therapeutic effects are considerable between drug and psychotherapy in mild to moderate depression. Psychotherapy includes general supportive psychotherapy, dynamic psychotherapy, cognitive-behavioral therapy, interpersonal therapy, marriage and family therapy. Psychological therapy can help patients to identify and change the cognitive distortions, correct patients with maladaptive behavior, improve interpersonal communication skills and psychological adaptation. Electroconvulsive therapy can be used in patients with severe negative suicide attempts and no effect with antidepressants. Electroconvulsive therapy is quick and effective. Generally 6-10 times are as a course of treatment. Drug therapy is needed after electroconvulsive therapy.

[Case 2]

A 19-year-old girl. One year ago, the girl had sleep disorder (drowsiness or insomnia) and poor spirit. She had a kind of unspeakable anguish and depression, which is expressed as "chest like a stone, suffocated". She feel hopeless, often want to cry and mood suppression, had no expression at the joke and had feel flat and uninteresting to see her former lover film. Nightmares, loss of appetite, depression and cannot be relieved, very anxious and pessimistic, even want to die. Two questions are raised as follows:

(A) What abnormal symptoms of psychological disorder is she showing?

(B) What mental disorders she has?

6.4 Anxiety disorder

Anxiety disorders are states of mind, characterized by excessive or problematic worrying, individuals become distressed or dysfunctional as a consequence. They are more likely to concern the ideas about illness, health or injury, and such concerns result in distress and dysfunction. The anxiety disorders include, generalized anxiety disorder, panic disorder, agoraphobia, simple phobias, social phobia. There is much overlap between these disorders, and comorbidity for depression is high. The main features of generalized anxiety disorder, panic disorder and agoraphobia will be described.

6.4.1 Generalized anxiety disorder

(1) The main clinical symptoms of generalized anxiety disorder.

The main clinical features of generalized anxiety disorder are the excessive anxiety and worry (apprehensive expectation) occurring more days than at least 6 months and occurring about a number of events or activities (such as work or school performance). Some people are anxious all the time in almost all situations. The disorder usually begins in mid-teenage years, but patients often only seek help in their late twenties and thirties. Most patients (60% to 80%) will report having been anxious or worried all their lives. This reflects a consistently high level of trait anxiety.

Other clinical features include being easily fatigued, restlessness or feeling on edge, difficulty concentrating or the mind going blank, irritability, muscle tension and sleep disturbance. Patients with generalized anxiety disorder overestimate the likelihood of unpleasant events happening to them.

(2) Treatments for generalized anxiety disorder.

The effective treatments for generalized anxiety disorder include psychotherapy and drug therapy. Cognitive-behavioral therapy and psychodynamic psychotherapy can be used in the treatment of generalized anxiety disorder. The techniques commonly used in cognitive behavior therapy include normalization, fear

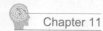

exposure, fear behavior blocking, and problem solving and time management. It is necessary to deal with the problems related to the recurrence of anxiety disorders, such as family problems and interpersonal problems. Cognitive-behavioral therapy can be operated easily, and can effectively improve the anxiety and worried of patients with generalized anxiety disorder, not only has short-term efficacy, but also has a positive effect in long-term in follow-up study. At present, the psychodynamic therapy for the treatment of generalized anxiety disorder is a short course of treatment, generally one time per week, a total of 10-20 times. Evidence based psychotherapy for the treatment of generalized anxiety disorder is less.

Anti-anxiety drugs and antidepressants in the treatment of generalized anxiety disorder. Paroxetine, sertraline, alprazolam, buspirone, doxepin and propranolol are the commonly used drugs. The generalized anxiety disorder patients with depressive symptoms should be choice the antidepressant drugs firstly. The effective drug treatment should be maintained at least 8 to 12 months.

[Case 3]

A 40-year-old woman. She always has palpitations, shortness of breath, and chronic indigestion. She feels upset, angry, restless and uncomfortable when she had some trivial things. She always been nervous and restless, worry about the things in life, always feel that some bad things would happen. Two questions are raised as follows:

(A) What's wrong with the woman?

(B) What can we do to help the woman?

6.4.2   Panic disorder

(1) Main features of panic disorder.

Panic disorder is an anxiety disorder characterized by recurrent panic attacks, which are not limited to any particular situation and with unpredictable. The lifetime prevalence rate was 0.5% to 4.7%, and the 1/3 to 1/2 patients had the symptoms of agoraphobia. The first peak of panic disorder onset appeared in late adolescence or early adulthood, the second peak appeared in 45-54 years old, after the age of 65 had rare. The patients suddenly have intense panic, with dying feeling or feeling out of control in the absence of any incentives. Patients feel that they would be die or loss of control, getting nervous, or even not realistic, often accompanied by symptoms of obviously autonomic nerve function disorder, such as palpitation, chest tightness, dyspnea, throat tightness, limbs trembling, sweating etc. Some patients worry about their heart problems, dare not to move. PD lasted a few minutes or hours, but usually no more than 1 hour. The patients can recall the symptoms because of clear awareness, and worry about the relapse after the first attack. As this reason, the patients avoid the scene of outbreak or limit their activities, which affect their work and life. Depressive symptoms are also common, and approximately half of all people with panic disorder also have depressive disorder.

(2) Treatment for panic disorder.

Treatment for panic disorder includes psychotherapy and medication. Psychotherapy includes supportive psychotherapy, cognitive behavior therapy, and psychodynamic psychotherapy. Supportive psychotherapy includes support, understanding, empathy, and so on. The commonly used techniques in cognitive behavior therapy include mental health education, cognitive correction, relaxation training, exposure, etc. According to the clinical characteristics of the patients, several techniques are applied in combination, and the patients can get good results by short-term self-training or training under the guidance of doctors. Evidence based medical evidence suggests that cognitive-behavioral therapy for panic disorder has clear short-term and long-term efficacy. Cognitive-behavioral therapy has the advantage of reducing the fear of panic disorder, and it has the advantage of improving the symptoms of panic among different groups, such as the young and the elderly. Evidence based support and dynamic psychotherapy are less.

Drug treatment for panic disorder includes anxiolytic and antidepressant drugs. The commonly used anti-anxiety drugs mainly include benzodiazepines, azaperone and β-antagonist. Antidepressants are mainly SSRIs and TCAs. The drugs commonly used for panic disorder include imipramine and SSRIs (i.e., paroxetine and escitalopram). The drug treatment is often maintained at least 8 to 12 months.

6.4.3 Agoraphobia

(1) Main features of agoraphobia.

The essential feature of agoraphobia is a fear or anxiety about being in places or situations from which escape may be difficult. Typical fears include being outside the safety of the home, traveling on public transport, being in crowded places, or having to queue. For example, people with agoraphobia fear crowded, bustling places, such as the marketplace or shopping mall; they fear enclosed spaces, such as buses, subway cars, and elevators; they also fear wide open spaces, such as open fields, particularly if they are alone. The anxiety leads to an avoidance of many social situations and the individual becomes increasingly restricted and "imprisoned" in their own home. The condition often develops as a result of panic disorder.

(2) Treatment for agoraphobia.

Psychotherapy therapy is the main treatment of agoraphobia. The commonly used psychotherapy is cognitive behavior therapy, systematic desensitization therapy, exposure or shock therapy. The cognitive and physiological models of panic control therapy (respiratory control, cognitive reconstruction, anxiety and panic education) and exposure therapy are commonly used in the treatment of agoraphobia. Current clinical studies have shown that cognitive-behavioral therapy has a definite effect on phobia, and the effect of cognitive-behavioral therapy was longer than that of drug therapy.

Anti-anxiety drugs can be used to alleviate the fear of anxiety symptoms, such as clonazepam, alprazolam, lorazepam, etc. But the anxiolytic effect is not durable, and has the shortcoming of dependence. β-antagonist (propranolol) can alleviate autonomic nervous excitement about somatic symptoms. The first-line treatment drug on agoraphobia is SSRIs such as paroxetine, sertraline, fluoxetine etc. SNRIs drugs are also effective in the treatment of agoraphobia.

6.5 Obsessive-compulsive disorder

(1) Main features of obsessive-compulsive disorder.

Obsessive-compulsive disorder is characterized by persistent, intrusive, unwanted thoughts or images that the individual finds difficult to control or put out of mind. The thoughts are usually unpleasant and are usually concerned with dirt, contamination, harm to others, sex or blasphemy. The individual recognizes that they are own thoughts and usually tries to resist them. The individual may develop behavior to try to reduce the anxiety and distress that caused by persistent thoughts. Individual's anxiety is temporarily relieved by the behavior but soon returns. The patients feel pain about their symptoms, and have insight to this disease, often see the doctors on one's own initiative.

(2) Treatments for Obsessive-compulsive disorder.

The most commonly used psychological therapy for obsessive-compulsive disorder is cognitive-behavioral therapy, and the core of cognitive-behavioral therapy is exposure, prevention and cognitive reconstruction. The patient was exposed to the symptoms of obsessive-compulsive symptoms, while encouraging patients to control their compulsive behavior (response prevention). This process of exposure often adopts the graded exposure technology, in accordance with the level of anxiety gradually from weak to strong. For patients with obsessive-compulsive disorder or compulsive behavior, stopping thought is often used. Through the imagination of the patient to imagine the symptoms of the process of thinking, combined with the means of external control, artificially suppressed and interrupted their thinking, attempts to promote patient's implicit behavior and forced thinking disappeared. But the clinical results of thought stopping are not sure.

The main therapeutic drugs for obsessive-compulsive disorder were SSRIs. The drugs commonly used are clomipramine and SSRIs drugs, such as fluoxetine, sertraline, paroxetine, citalopram, clovoxamine etc. 50%-70% patients are effective with the treatment of drugs, but the obsessive-compulsive symptoms cannot be completely eliminated. For the treatment of OCD, the dose of SSRIs was higher than that of the treatment of depression.

It is generally believed that psychotherapy combined with drug therapy is an ideal treatment for obsessive-compulsive disorder. Combination therapy can make patients more likely to accept cognitive-behavioral therapy, and cognitive-behavioral therapy can be used to maintain efficacy, reduce recurrence or relapse.

The surgical treatment can be used when drug treatment and psychological is invalid. There are mainly such as stereotactic cingulotomy, internal capsule forelimb amputation, caudate nucleus under tractotomy, and deep brain stimulation. Previous studies also have shown that the low frequency repetitive transcranial magnetic stimulation of the left orbitofrontal cortex has an independent effect on obsessive-compulsive disorder.

[Case 4]

A 46-year-old woman. She was afraid of dirt, worried about contamination with bacteria, viruses, and infectious diseases over the past five years. The woman dare not use public toilet and shake hands with people, repeated washed hand and bathed as soon as possible when she back at home. The woman cannot dismiss garbage or clean the toilet at home. She will lose her temper that his husband did not wash hands and bath repeated when back home. The relationship between husband and wife is very tense. Two questions are raised as follows:

(A) What disorder do you think the woman has?

(B) What methods can treat the disorder?

6.6 Somatoform disorders

(1) Main features of somatoform disorders.

The somatoform disorders are a group of disorders which are characterized as significant physical symptoms, but without organic cause. Usually, these symptoms are inconsistent with possible physiological processes, and there is strong reason to believe that psychological factors are involved. People with somatoform disorders usually truly experience the symptoms, do not consciously produce or control the symptoms. There are at least five types of somatoform disorders: somatization disorder, undifferentiated somatoform disorder, hypochondriacal disorder, somatoform autonomic dysfunction and somatoform pain disorder.

1) Somatization disorder. It is characterized by a variety of physical symptoms that occur repeatedly and frequently, which involve any system or organ of the body. The most common is gastrointestinal discomfort, such as pain, hiccups, acid regurgitation, vomiting, nausea, etc. Abnormal skin sensation, such as itching, sensed burning, tingling, numbness, pain, etc. Main aspects of sexual and menstrual complaints are common. Somatization disorder is often accompanied by significant symptoms of depression and anxiety.

2) Undifferentiated somatoform disorder. The characteristics of the patients with this disorder complained

with diversity and variability, which is similar to the somatization disorder, but lack of typical symptoms.

3) Hypochondriacal disorder. Patients insist that they have one or several serious body disease. The patient attention too much to his body feeling, make hypochondriac explanation to the physiological phenomenon and abnormal feeling, and show the corresponding physical symptoms. The patient repeatedly seek medical treatment everywhere, makes each kind of medical examination. Despite the negative results of various tests, doctors' interpretation and guarantee cannot dispel their doubts. Patients feel pain and often have symptoms of anxiety or depression.

4) Somatoform autonomic dysfunction. The disease is characterized by patient's clear dysfunction in autonomic nervous system of organ symptoms. The most common organ system involvement is cardiovascular system, respiratory system and gastrointestinal tract. With the symptoms of autonomic nervous excitement, such as palpitations, sweating, blushing, tremors and other symptoms on the basis, the patients also have individual characteristics and subjective symptoms, such as indefinite position of pain, burning sensation, heaviness, tightness, swelling, which cannot be find the evidence

5) Somatoform pain disorder. It is a kind of persistent severe pain which cannot be explained reasonably by physiological process or physical obstacle. The peak age of onset was from 30 to 50 years old. Emotional conflict or psychosocial factors directly lead to the occurrence of pain in patients. The patient often vividly describes the location and nature of the pain, which cannot be found in the body. Somatoform pain disorder often accompanied by anxiety, depression, insomnia, and impaired social function.

(2) Treatments for somatoform disorders.

Somatoform disorders should be treated with comprehensive therapy. Cognitive behavior therapy is effective in the treatment of somatoform disorders, including physical symptoms, psychological distress and dysfunction. Supportive psychotherapy is needed for patients with somatoform disorders, which is very important to establish a good relationship between doctors and patients. In the course of treatment, we should pay attention to the evaluation of patient's social support system, identify and reduce the daily life problems that promote or aggravate the physical symptoms of patients, reduce the secondary benefits of physical symptoms. According to the personality characteristics of patients, life history and disease characteristics, we should evaluate the relationship between emotion and somatic symptoms, test negative beliefs of patients, change the avoidant behavior can help patients with somatoform disorders.

[Case 5]

A 38-year-old woman. The woman suddenly felt his heart beating very fast, chest stuffy, worried about she suffering from heart disease one day a year ago. After that the woman went to the hospital and did a variety of tests repeatedly. The doctors said she has no problem with the heart. However, she thinks her heart disease is getting worse. Two questions are raised as follows:

(A) What disorder do you think the woman has?

(B) Which method do you think is the best to treat the woman?

6.7   Stress related disorder

For the related description, please refer to Chapter 4.

6.8   Personality disorder

For the related description, please refer to Chapter 6.

(李 平)

Chapter 12

Childhood and Senile Issues

Similar to somatic diseases, psychological problems are more easily to attack children and the senile people. Because of immaturity or senility, these people often have more specific problems and need more care. These problems are even more difficult to manage in clinics. The reasons of these problems are many and varied, some of which are related with nervous system development and change. In this chapter, we will discuss the common issues of children and senile people, their etiological factors and the optimal treatments.

1. Factors affecting the psychological problems of children

Children Mental Hygiene, a branch of Psychology, mainly studies the psychological features and personality traits of children at different ages, and it aims to offer good social impact and education training to children so as to make them optimistic, wise, reasonable, strong-willed, and possess admiring personalities as well as social adaptability. Namely, they are expected to gain all-scale healthy development in aspects such as virtue, intelligence, physical condition and aesthetic ability.

1.1 Factors affecting the psychological problems of children

1.1.1 Eugenics is the basis of children mental health

Congenital quality plays a vital role in children mental health, and is the key factor to weigh children mental health. If a child was born with the problem of cerebral agenesis, s/he would not grow into a mentally healthy people anyhow. For example, a child who was born with trisomy 21 syndrome (Down's syndrome) can hardly become a people with healthy personality. Therefore, eugenics has a significant influence on children mental health.

1.1.2 Influence on children mental health from courtship and marriage

Marriage is the perfect result of love. People should not rush to get married without deep love foundation. For the health of the next generation, close relatives and people with certain genetic diseases cannot get married as the possibility of their children suffering from developmental malformation is so high. If let them get married and give birth to babies, there would be more mentally unhealthy people in the society. After getting married, couples should further develop and deepen their love, admiring each other, respecting each other, caring about each other, which are much beneficial to the development of children's physical and mental health. If the relationship between parents is strained, namely, they keep quarreling, fighting, suspecting, abusing and even being indifferent to each other, it will lead the children to live in the sense of insecurity and pain, which will even make the children be depressed, anxious, sensitive, suspicious, self-abased, nervous, terrified and painful. Once the parents get divorced, their children are mostly psychologically hurt and easily have psychological problems.

1.1.3 Influence on children mental health from fertilization age and antenatal training

Researches hold that the best age for women to be pregnant is between 25 to 29 years old. Either too young or too old would have an adverse influence on children's physical and mental health. If the limit is set under 20 years old, it would affect offspring's physical and mental health due to the immature of reproductive organs. If over 35 years old, the rate of giving birth to children with Down's syndrome or other defects will increase accordingly as a result of the productive organ recession caused by the aging of egg cells.

During pregnancy, antenatal training is quite important to the growth and development of a fetus. Antenatal training refers to a serious of perfect measures which are carried out on purpose for the growth and development of a fetus. Mother's body is an important place for a fetus to grow and develop, thus any physical or mental changes a pregnant woman experiences will have an impact on the fetus. The mood of a pregnant woman is rather important in the antenatal training. Research has shown that change in mood of a pregnant woman would affect the fetus through the change of blood and endocrine components.

If a pregnant woman lives in a circumstance with depression, negative pessimism, anxiety, worry, fear for long, it will affect the blood supply to a fetus's fetal brain, which will cause cerebral vascular constriction and blood supply reduction, and affect brain development. Excessive fear can even cause developmental malformation of brain. Pregnant women with mood disruptions are more likely to suffer from complications during pregnancy and delivery.

For example, pregnant women who are severely anxious will have serious pregnancy response, associated with nausea and vomiting, which affects fetal development and easily causes premature delivery, abortion, dystocia and so on. It will also cause great harm to child's physical and mental health. Dystocia may keep the newborn in the birth canal too long, which causes neonatal asphyxia. With the lack of blood and oxygen to the brain, neural system will get damaged, and the same goes to mental activities. Some people think that attention deficit hyperactivity disorder is relevant to dystocia damage, so it is important for pregnant women to maintain good moods for the sake of child's mental health.

1.2 Appropriate environmental stimuli can promote children's mental health

Physiological needs and attachment to mothers are important factors for children's mental health, but appropriate environmental stimuli are also of prime important for the promotion of children's mental health. Appropriate external environmental stimuli are beneficial to mental health, and can promote the development of children's sensory organs and intelligence. To a certain extent, the level of children intellectual development is proportional to the amount of information entering the brain through the sensory organs stimulated by the external environment, that is to say, more diverse the external things children contact with, more important it is for children intellectual development. Of course, the amount of external environment stimulus must be appropriate, and excessive stimulus brings disadvantages to children's mental health.

1.3 Maternal love is an important factor for children's mental health

Nutrients supply, appropriate information stimulus and maternal love are the three main factors for children's mental health. The period from birth to 3 years old of a child is a significant stage in the process of children growth. Caresses from mothers are especially important to the development of children's mental health. At the early stage, children's main demand for maternal love is the desire of skin touching, mainly through mother's touch, hug and intimacy.

1.4　Family parenting pattern and children's mental health

During the period of babyhood, the satisfaction of babies' basic physiological needs, the external environmental stimulus and the way of maternal needs, have a great impact on children's intellectual development, emotional development and personality development. As the children grow up, the interaction between them and their parents, and other family members becomes more close and complex. In this process, family atmosphere, the status of a child at home and the educational methods parents employ play a more important role in children physical and mental health.

Foreign researches on parenting pattern mostly classify it into two categories: democratic and authoritative. In a democratic family, parents are gentle and tolerant of their children. For many things, parents give credit for what their children have done, encourage them to show themselves and cultivate their creativity. Family members discuss and decide on family affairs together. However, in an authoritative family, the rights of parents are sovereign, and children who have no right to have their voice heard are supposed to obey their parents. Children living in those different circumstances have distinct characteristics. Children who grow up in a democratic family are generally outgoing, enthusiastic, generous, lively, cheerful, confident, independent and enterprising with great interpersonal and socially adaptation abilities. On the contrary, children who grow up in an authoritative family are generally introverted, self-abased, quiet, resigned, not expressive, lack of curiosity and initiative with poor interpersonal and social adaptation abilities.

In our country, especially for the generation after 80s and 90s, most of them are the only child in a family. In the process of family upbringing, their behaviors are not properly guided, which lets them do whatever they like. Many parents mistakenly take spoiling as maternal love, which leads to the prevalence of "over-protection" phenomena. With time going on, many children develop a lot of undesirable behaviors and personality traits.

1.5　Age, personality traits and children mental health

1.5.1　Characteristics of children mental health at different ages

Psychology divides children age grades into five stages: suckling stage (0-1 year old), infancy stage (1 year old-3 years old), preschool stage (3 years old-6 or 7 years old), childhood (6 or 7 years old-11 or 12 years old), adolescence (11 or 12 years old-14 or 15 years old). The psychological development of children is a gradual process from quantitative change to qualitative change. Children have different psychological traits at different ages, which are typical and stable. Children age characteristics are the presentation of the qualitative change. Therefore, parents and educators should offer education and training on the basis of children psychological characteristics at different ages. In life there are mainly two practices which are not conducive to children's mental health: one is superior education, of which children can hardly understand the content and methods; the other one is retrogressive training and over-protection, that is, when children's psychology have already developed to a higher level, parents still follow the previous way to educate them and give excessive protection. These two wrong practices result in the consequence that children cannot do what they want and has no ability to do what they should, which seriously hinder the development of mental health and is the reason of the formation of so many bad personality traits.

1.5.2　Personality traits and children's mental health

The personality traits of Children's mental health mainly reflect in two aspects. On the one hand, for a certain child, it is imbalanced between his/her personality traits and the development at his/her age. On the other hand, for different children, individual difference exists in aspects such as ability, personality, disposition and so on. Therefore, we should offer different measures to different children according to their different personality traits in both the content and methods of education, so that it can be conducive to the development of children's mental health.

As every child is born with his/her own unique personality type, parents and teachers should provide different ways of education on the basis of children's different personality types, or it may bring unwanted harm to children's physical and mental health. Domestic and overseas studies have pointed out that since the beginning of infantile period, if children are educated in accordance with their personality types differently, they will form good personality traits and gain benefits in physical and mental health; otherwise, children would get hurt and even get mental illnesses and behavior barriers.

2. Common psychological barriers of children

2.1 Mental retardation

Mental retardation attacks human body before the maturation of the central nervous system (18 years old), the related clinical characteristics reflect in difficulties of social adaptation and mental disorders. According to the level of intelligence deficiency and the degree of social adaptability deficiency, it is divided into four levels.

2.1.1 Mild mental retardation

The score of such patient's IQ is between 50 to 69 points. The number of such patient's accounts for about 85% of all the mental retardation, who's IQ can reach the normal level of 9-12 years old. It is often difficult to be found in the early days, as there are no obvious abnormalities found in bodies and the development of nervous system. During the infantile period, those kinds of patients are found backward in language and motor development. Some children even do not start to speak and walk until the age of 2-3 years old. After entering primary school, those children show poor learning ability gradually, especially in maths. They would often fail the exams or have to repeat a year to catch up with others. Their performance in the course of Chinese would not be prominent. As growing up, their learning abilities in all aspects are not good; besides, they usually have poor communication abilities. However, they can still take care of themselves, and can do some simple labor and non-technical work. They have poor abilities in aspects such as computing, literacy, or abstract thinking. They are rigid and do not rely on others. Their body development is normal with the same average life expectancy as normal people.

2.1.2 Moderate mental retardation

The score of such patient's IQ is between 35 to 49 points. The number of them accounts for about 10% of all the patients suffering from mental retardation. Compared with normal children, they are generally found backward in language and motor development, especially shown in expression, comprehension and application of language. These children can learn to speak, but with unclear pronunciation and impoverished vocabularies. Their words are simple as they usually lack abstract thinking ability, which makes their words fail to express what they what to say. Their cognitive competence is superficial and one-sided, and their discernment of the surrounding environment is poor with low adaptability. After the patients grow into adults, their level of IQ equals to that of normal children at the age of 6 to 9 years old, and they still do things inefficiently. All aspects of the development of patient's bodies are not good, namely, most of them would suffer from organic diseases. Their life length can reach the level of an adult, and under guidance they can handle simple self-care.

2.1.3   Severe mental retardation

The score of such patient's IQ is between 20 to 34 points, the number of whom accounts for about 10% of all the patients suffering from mental retardation. The IQ level of these patients equals to that of normal children at the age of 3 to 6 years old. They are born backward in growth and development, and usually accompanied by organic diseases. Besides, the morbidity of diseases such as epilepsy of central nervous system, cerebral palsy or somatic malformation is rather high. Usually, parents would find their children who suffer from severe mental retardation fall behind in growth and motor level compared with children of the same age. The development of language is particularly backward with unclear pronunciation, and some serious patients cannot even speak. After specialized training, the patients can speak simple words, but can neither establish effective communication, nor calculate, learn or work. They lack the ability of abstract thinking and have no concept of numbers. They have problems of emotional response and are usually impulsive. After the patients grow into adults, they can do very simple manual labor with the care of someone else.

2.1.4   Extreme severe mental retardation

The score of such patient's IQ is between 0 to 20 points, it accounts for about 10% of all the patients suffering from mental retardation. Their actual IQ level is close to that of children under 3 years old. They usually suffer from physical abnormalities and severe central nervous system developmental barriers. They can hardly express themselves and understand what others said. They usually express themselves through the primitive ways of screaming or crying. It is hard for them to tell well from bad and avoid danger. They do not have the ability to defend and protect themselves. They completely lose the ability to take care of themselves and need to be cared by others.

2.1.5   Treatment

The etiology of mental retardation is complex, most of which are still undefined so far, so there are still difficulties in finding proper treatments. The principle of the treatment is "three earliest", namely, early detection, early diagnosis and early treatment. In fetal period, it is necessary to take antenatal inspection timely, and to take early screening of chromosomes or genetic diseases. It is vital to provide early intervention while pregnancy, and offer treatments according to the etiologies to reduce the birth of babies with such imperfections. During the infantile period, early detection and treatments are necessary to reduce the damage to brain as much as possible, so as to delay the brain function impairment. For elderly children, the treatments focus on caring, education and training of basic living skills. For children with mild mental retardation, they can receive special school education. For children with moderate mental retardation, we can strengthen the training for them properly. For children with severe and extreme severe mental retardation, nursing and caring are the main methods, and among them, for people with mental or neurological symptoms, proper drug symptomatic treatments should be given.

2.2   Specific and pervasive developmental disorders

Children autism

Childhood autism is caused by a kind of serious pervasive developmental disorder, mainly reflecting in varying degrees of speech developmental disorder, interpersonal disorder, and narrow range of interest and stiff behaviors. Most of the patients also suffer from mental retardation and poor prognosis. The main features of Children Autism are interpersonal disorder and communication disorder. Most of the children with autism are backward in language development compared with normal children, or retrograde in language development after normal language development. As growing up, they speak less and less, sometimes keep silent and even lose the ability to speak. Patients have barriers in expressing themselves and the application of language. With the retrogression of social function, they cannot establish normal interpersonal relationship with others. They lower heads often, get used to be alone and lack attachment to their loved ones. They cannot make friends with children of the same age. For instance, they do not take an active part in activities in school, and show little interest in recreational activities and games. Instead, they usually stay alone, and once their daily living patterns are interrupted, they will be disturbed, emotional, scream, attack and so on. Intelligence levels differ among children with autistic, and the majority of them are influenced in intelligence while some others still have normal intelligence.

The methods of treatments for autism are mainly education, training, psychological treatment, drug treatment and so on. Among them, the most effective way is education and training. Education, training and psychological treatments mainly include: discrete unit teaching, language communication training, interpersonal development intervention, structured teaching method, sensory integration training, game training and other comprehensive intervention measures. All of them aim to correct some misconducts of patients, such as stiff behaviors and self-injury, to improve their perception and motor activities and enhance their cognitive ability as well as communication and social interaction competence. Children with neuropsychiatric symptoms are advised to be given proper drug treatments such as risperidone, methylphenidate, valproate, carbamazepine, diazepam stability and other drugs.

2.3   Behavior and emotional disorder in childhood and adolescence

2.3.1   Attention deficit and hyperactive disorder

Attention deficit and hyperactive disorder (ADHD) is featured as various petty actions and activities, impulsive behavior, egocentrism, bad temper, poor self-control ability and inattention that should not be shown at their age. ADHD will seriously affect the normal study, but the intelligence of children will not be affected. ADHD has two main symptoms, including inattention and excessive activities, associated with impulse, caprice and learning disability. Children generally fall ill at the age of six and the symptoms are apparent at school age. As the children grow up, they will get better. A few children may show the symptoms even when they become adults. Inattention is one of the main symptoms of ADHD. The patients cannot concentrate on their own things and they may be influenced by the surroundings. They have excessive petty actions in class and cannot listen attentively to the teacher, often attracted by the surroundings. They cannot focus on one thing and distract their attention frequently. Their inattention leads to carelessness, negligence and lack of perseverance. They are always dilatory in doing things and constantly look for excuses to stop halfway. Some children stare blankly, fascinatedly and absent-mindedly, utterly ignorant to course content and questions raised by teachers. The patients have more actions than other children, such as running wildly, making noise, fiddling with what they see, swinging around when sitting on the chair and running wildly after leaving the chair. They like to speak and make noise without regard to the occasions. They like to interrupt others and do not conform to the class discipline. ADHD has two kinds of symptoms. One is sustained hyperactivity. The hyperactive behaviors of patients are tested to be the same on different occasions. The other one is situational hyperactivity. Patients show the symptoms on certain occasions and it will be less harmful to the children. Patients have the normal intelligence and their poor grades are due to the inattention in class. A few patients' nervous system examination shows positive signs.

Treatment for ADHD mainly includes psychotherapy, special education, drug therapy (methylphenidate

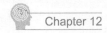

amphetamine atomoxetine) and parents' education and training. Patients should eat more food rich in zinc and selenium, such as fish, eggs, and lean meat, peanut and dairy products. In school and family, teachers and parents should care, encourage, help and forgive the children, helping them build up self-confidence and overcome difficulties. The children should take part in some cognitive activities that can improve their concentration. The excessive and bad behaviors can be corrected by specific training program, reward and punishment training and behavior training. The improvement of children's behavior should be recognized and encouraged in order to boost their confidence and make for the treatment. Vulgar and violent words and behaviors should be avoided in the process of education for not hurting children's self-esteem.

2.3.2 Tourette syndrome

Tourette syndrome (TS) is mainly diagnosed in childhood, featured as motor or phonic tics. According to the age, duration, clinical features and phonic tics, the Tourette Syndrome can be divided into three clinical types, including transient tic disorder, chronic motor or vocal disorder and Tourette syndrome. Common symptoms are blinking, squeezing eyebrow, wrinkling forehead, sniffling, canthus and lips tics to one side, stretching out the neck, shaking head, crooking neck, shrugging shoulders, biting lips, opening mouth, clearing throat, roaring, imitating and repeating the same words. Tourette syndrome mainly includes motor tics and phonic tics or both as well as simple motor tics and multiple motor tics according to the complexity. Tics occur in one or more parts of the body. Simple tics are characterized by tics of one group of muscles while multiple tics are bouncing, spinning, buckling body, beating body or indecency. The symptoms of simple phonic tics are clearing throat, coughing, roaring, sniffling, imitating monosyllabic sounds like animal sounds and the symptoms of multiple phonic tics are repeating the same words, imitating others" language and talking billingsgate. The symptoms of Tourette syndrome are involuntary, paroxysmal, rapid, repeated and non-rhythmic. Tourette syndrome can be controlled by will power in a short period of time, but it cannot be controlled in a long time. When suffering from psychological stimulation, emotional stress, learning pressure, body disease or other stressful situations, children will show the symptoms more frequently. The symptoms will relieve or disappear when they fall asleep. According to the different types of tics, the ages and duration of the disease are different as well. Children may suffer from Tourette syndrome from pre-school age. Simple tics may occur repeatedly in one day, no more than two weeks and the duration is less than one year. Multiple tics occur frequently and the duration is more than one year. The longer the duration lasts, the greater the influence of patient's social functions will be.

Treatment for TS plans should be taken according to different clinical manifestation and condition. Those who show transient or light symptoms can be simply treated by psychotherapy, mainly including cognitive therapy, behavioral therapy, family therapy and habit reversal training. The patients and their relatives should have a correct understanding of the disease, helping the children to relieve tension, remove psychological factors and actively cooperate with doctors during the treatment. As for the multiple tics, psychotherapy combined with drug therapy is recommended and common drugs include haloperidol, tiapride, clonidine, risperidone and clomipramine.

2.3.3 Conduct disorder

Conduct disorder refers to persistent oppositional defiant behavior of teenagers and the main characteristics are anti-social behavior, steal, fight, disrupting public order and aggressive behaviors. These abnormal behaviors seriously violate social norms at their age and exceed naughty and antagonistic behaviors of children and adolescents.

The treatment for conduct disorder is a difficult problem, there is a lack of specific treatment methods, the effect of a single therapy is poor, more individualized education, drug therapy, psychotherapy and behavioral therapy were used.

2.3.4　Emotional disorder

Emotional disorder in childhood and adolescence. Children suffer from emotional disorder mainly in childhood and adolescence with psychosocial factors as the main causes and mental disorders of anxiety or fear as the main symptoms. Emotional disorder mainly includes separation anxiety disorder, specific phobia and social anxiety disorder, such as school phobia. Some children influenced by psychological factors are afraid of going to school. They may show the symptoms of palpitation, headache, abdominal pain, vomiting and frequent urination before school and at school. Some children even refuse to go to school (mainly quoted from Psychiatry textbook version 6).

Treatment: The treatment of emotional disorders in children and adolescents mainly include family therapy, drug therapy, benzodiazepines such as alprazolam, Moxa, antidepressants such as doxepin, imipramine, fluoxetine, etc.

3.　Senile Psychological problems

According to the new age standard established by World Health Organization, people more than 80 years old enter into senile stage. The function of various body organs gradually degenerate with age and their mental health will be influenced as well:

3.1　Loneliness

Retirement and change in role will lead to loneliness in senile people. They leave the former company they worked in, especially those who retire from leadership positions having great psychological gap and obvious sense of loss. From their perspective of view, they are valueless, helpless and hopeless. They sit around all day so they are prone to feel lonely. Their children are busy with their own family and careers, negligent of communicating with parents. The elderly have little friends and lack of social activities. The empty nest elderly without families around are prone to feel abandoned by the world, thus feeling sad and questioning their personal values. They consider themselves to be valueless for the society and family and remain negative, pessimistic, depressed and hopeless. Some people even have negative behaviors.

3.2　Sense of emptiness

It is common in the elderly who are unprepared to retirement life. They cannot adapt to the change from orderly, regular and intense work state to aimless, irregular and relaxed life state. They may feel incompatible with their surroundings and sit around all day with no arrangements for life. They become lazy and spiritless, unaware of how to spend their time and live their lives. They will be depressed, anxious, frightened, worry and puzzled. Some people will have negative thoughts and behaviors and age quickly, greatly influencing their body and mind.

3.3　Personality changes

When people enter into senile stage, their life journey is drawing to an end. During this period, there will be various "loss", such as death of relatives, retirement, and loss of money, status, right and reputation. With physical aging, disease and body hypofunction, the personality of the elderly will change to be suspicious, sensitive, solitary, obstinate, selfish, garrulous, emotional, hard to communicate, sick of new things, hard to accept new things, afraid to change and adapt to new things, recalling past repeatedly and resistible of the reality. The gap between parents and children widens, forming a sense of distance imperceptibly. The changes lead to decreased interpersonal skills and social adaptability.

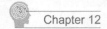

3.4　Cognitive change

When people get old, their memory will get worse. Many elderly people become absent-minded and increasingly forgetful. They forget to bring keys when they leave home and forget to turn off the gas after cooking. Sometimes they call their children for the missing of belongings and doubt if others take them away. They are often anxious, distressed, guilty, helpless and depressed for their memory loss. Memory loss is a physiological process and normal phenomenon that brain cells gradually get old and degenerate. It is worth noting that the brain cells decrease rapidly and degenerate obviously, especially accompanied with mental symptoms of depression, anxiety, delusion and hallucination, which will lead to organic disease including senile dementia.

3.5　Sleep change

When people enter into senile stage, they will need less sleep. The duration, rhythm and cycle of sleep will also change with age. Elderly people will sleep less and lightly and they are easy to wake, early to wake and difficult to fall asleep after waking up. Some elderly people cannot fall asleep after they lie down for more than one hour, which leads to anxiety. Some sleep too much, feeling drowsy all day. They doze and yawn, feeling lazy to move, tired after waking up and depressed all day. Some fall asleep at daytime and wake up at night. The reverse sleep time severely influences life quality. All of the physiological changes show brain dysfunction.

4. Senile mental disorders

4.1　Neurocognitive disorders

4.1.1　Senile neurocognitive disorders

Senile neurocognitive disorders also known as Senile Dementia of Alzheimer Type (SDAT). SDAT is a series of primary retrogressive cerebral degeneration diseases and a progressive and irreversible development process, which is diagnosed in senile stage and has long incidence period. SDAT is caused by cerebral cortex atrophy, neuronal degeneration and change of neurotransmitter of the brain, mainly manifested as hypomnesis and amnesia at first. The symptoms are mild and easy to be neglected. The personality of patients will change to be sensitive, suspicious, sluggish, garrulous, stubborn, indifferent and selfish at first. Emotional changes will occur in patients gradually and they will be anxious, depressed, excited and indifferent. Severe cases may be accompanied by hallucinations delusion. Hallucination is featured as auditory hallucination and delusion includes jealousy, persecution and reference delusion, mostly in jealousy delusion in early stage. Progressive decline in memory and intelligence will lead to a vague idea of what happened to the patients. Patients find difficulty with organizing and planning and it will soon develop into a complete dementia. Patient's ability of calculation, judgment and comprehension all decreased progressively. They are unable to speak clearly and behave themselves. They have emotional disorder and special addition. The patients always get lost and cannot find the way home. People with late-stage dementia are unable to take care of themselves and they need to lie on bed for a long time. The mental symptoms of delusion and hallucination aggravate. They may mutter to themselves, laugh and behave strangely. When the patients get worse, they are unable to control their bladder or bowels, which lead to the death of systemic infection or multisystem organ failure. The disease will develop progressively. The average mortality was 4 to 5 years after onset; some people will live shorter and some will live up to 10 years.

Treatment: Treatment includes drug therapy and non-drug therapy. Firstly, treatment aimed at the cause of the disease will be conducive to finding the possible cause. Secondly, treatment measures should be taken according to the influence of social functions and decline of memory and intelligence. The families should strengthen nursing. The patients with poor memory should carry ID card with patient information in order to contact the families freely when accidents happen. It is inadvisable to change the rooms of the patients so as to provide comfortable living environment and adequate nutrition for them. Patients who have physical disease should be treated as well. Patients with lower intelligence should be treated by nutritional cranial nerve drugs. Patients with mental symptoms should be treated by antipsychotic drugs, beginning with small-dose and gradually reducing and stopping the drugs according to the symptoms. Drugs used for improving cognitive function include donepezil, huperzine A, rivastigmine and memantine, which can improve cognitive function and slow the progression of the disease.

4.1.2　Vascular dementia

Vascular dementia refers to the dementia caused by vascular disease, with the symptoms of acuteness, rapid progress and fluctuations. Patients have the medical history of cerebrovascular disease, such as cerebral hemorrhage, transient ischemic attack and cerebral infarction. Neurologic examination may show corresponding symptoms and signs. Common mental disorders are talking nonsense and hallucinating at night. Patient's personality will not be influenced obviously and they have self-insight at early stage. Vascular dementia is accompanied with the symptoms of depression, anxiety, hallucination, delusion, excitement and emotional instability.

During the treatment of vascular dementia, the treatment for primary disease should be the first step, including controlling blood pressure and reducing blood sugar and blood fat, which can effectively prevent vascular dementia. Vitamin E, vitamin C, Ginkgo Bi loba Leaf, donepezil, piracetam and cerebroprotein hydrolysate can improve cognitive symptoms, nourish cranial nerves and promote catabolism of brain cells. Patients with mental symptoms, insomnia, behavior and emotional disorders can be treated by antipsychotics.

4.2　Senile depression

Senile depression is the emotional and mental disease in senile stage, including patients with depression above the age of 55 or 60 as well as the patients first diagnosed above the age of 55 or 60. The two kinds of patients both have the characteristics of senile stage. The clinical symptom is mild depression, but its harmfulness cannot be neglected. If the patients are not treated timely, it will lead to serious consequences, including decreased life quality, increased risk of physical and mental disease (cardio-cerebrovascular diseases) and risk of mortality. Typical symptoms of depression are low spirits, decreased interests and decreased activities of volitional behaviors while the main symptoms of senile depression are physical discomforts including dizziness, chest distress, shortness of breath, irritability, impatience, chills and fever of the body, anorexia, stomach problems, sleep disorders, sensitivity, memory loss, inattention, low self-evaluation, bad self-feeling, silence, laziness and excessive attention to their physical discomfort. Without prompt treatment, the life quality of the patients will be greatly influenced and the risks of physical disease will be increased.

Treatment for senile depression is divided into psychotherapy and drug therapy. Psychotherapy mainly includes supportive psychotherapy, listening, rational emotive therapy, cognitive behavior therapy, interpersonal psychotherapy, individual psychotherapy, marriage and family psychotherapy and group psychotherapy. The patients who have not improved by psychotherapy only can be treated by drug therapy and the common antidepressant drugs are paroxetine, duloxetine, sertraline, venlafaxine and citalopram.

（张　兰　朱菊红）

Chapter 13

Crisis Intervention and Psychiatric Rehabilitation

Crisis intervention services are now widely recognized as an efficacious treatment modality for the provision of emergency mental health care to individuals and groups. During the course of a lifetime, all people experience a variety of personal traumas, such as divorce or illness, while many others will also live through cataclysmic events, such as natural disasters or acts of violence, that result in a state of crisis. Although exposure to traumatic stressors can trigger adverse, long-term effects that can become extremely difficult to resolve without the timely delivery of effective, psychological intervention, crisis states can also provide an avenue for personal growth. This chapter presents a summary of common crisis forms and modem crisis intervention theory.

1. Crisis intervention

Crisis refers to an unanticipated event that actually or potentially disrupts or undermines the normal functioning of a significant segment of the body or the community. Clinical and empirical writings often distinguish group-level crises from individual-level crises and emergencies, for example suicidal behavior or intent, homicidal behavior or intent, physical maltreatment, sexual assault, and treatment goals for groups and individuals who experiencing crises are similar. And in crisis work the possibility of dealing with suicidal and homicidal patients or both is always present.

1.1 Suicide and crisis intervention

Suicide is a global public health problem, about 1 million people kill themselves each year, or about one every 40 seconds. Worldwide suicide rates have increased about 60 percent in the last 45 years. Eastern European countries, particularly in the Baltic Sea area, are the leaders along with Hungary (World Health Organization, 2011). In the United States, 30,000 to 35,000 people kill themselves every year (Centers for Disease Control and Prevention, 2008; U.S. Department of Health and Human Services, 2003), which translates into about 85 people a day. That number is probably very conservative because many suicides are ruled accidental either due to political, religious, and emotional considerations or because medical examiners just cannot say for sure). Most official reports indicate that the real numbers of suicide attempts as well as injury caused by suicide attempts are grossly underreported. Experts claim that upward of 60,000 Americans die annually by suicide (Ross, 1999). Between 300,000 and 600,000 U.S. citizens a year survive a suicide attempt, and about 19,000 of those survivors are permanently disabled as a result of the attempted suicide (Stone, 1999, p. 1; U.S. Department of Health and Human Services, 2003). Suicide ranges from the 10th to 11th leading cause of death in the United States (Centers for Disease Control and Prevention, 2011; National Institute of Mental Health, 2011). Despite this, suicide has received relatively less attention. In this chapter strategies are presented to help crisis workers strengthen their skills in assessing, counseling for, intervening in, and preventing lethal behavior, with the major emphasis on suicide.

We effort to address the problem have been increasing recognition by governments, community members, and professional groups of the need to do more. So, some nongovernmental organizations have been developed, which implements, and funds suicide prevention projects in worldwide. Those organizations utilize the international network of experts to decide what projects are most likely to prevent suicide, and select the investigators to work on them, and they are an active partner in conducting the projects from the beginning to the end.

The primary purpose of this book is to present applied therapeutic counseling in general, and crisis intervention in particular, in a way that effectively describes actual strategies to alleviate the crisis. In our experience, most patients who enter counseling or psychotherapy do so because of some sort of crisis in their lives although "preventive" counseling is the ideal, personal crisis generally provides the impetus that impels real patients into contact with a helping person. And, rather than assume that individuals in need seek services independently, crisis intervention appropriately takes services to victims. Crisis intervention seeks to mitigate the social and psychological effects of the stressful event. The primary therapeutic goal of crisis intervention is to restore a sense of equilibrium, characterized by the ability to creatively problem-solve and feel efficacious, as when coping resources are not taxed. Crisis intervention may mainly include activities associated with traditional mental health care.

1.2   Suicide prevention

1.2.1   Why focus on suicide?

We pay attention to suicide because it is there, and is an unavoidable, sometimes devastating, life issue. Whether one can live or chooses to live is the only truly serious philosophical problem. Camus claims that man invented God in order to be able to live without killing themselves and that the only human liberty is to come to terms with death. And he claims suicide is prepared within the silence of the heart, as is a great work of art.

Sigmund Freud argued, "Life is impoverished, it loses its interest, when the highest stake in the game of living, life itself, cannot be risked" (1970). Early on Freud saw aggression as a product of frustration of sexual impulses and, indeed, tended to see all life energy as sexual energy. However, after World War I Freud decided there were two opposing basic instincts: life (eros) and death (thanatos) drives. All instincts sought tension reduction. To illustrate, libido sought to reduce sexual tensions, whereas the death instinct sought the elimination of the tension of life itself. Freud contended that much external aggression against others was necessary to avoid self-destruction. In discussing depression Freud felt that people did not find the energy to kill themselves unless they were first killing an internalized object previously identified with and then turned this prior external death wish against a fragment of their own ego. Freud also believed that suicide is more likely in advanced civilizations requiring greater repression of sexual and aggressive energy.

Second, one studies suicide and death in order to live better. One could argue that the cloud of a shortish, finite lifespan tends to cast a pall over all of our lives, and this can lead to a pervasive underlying mild functional depression, a lack of hope about life's ultimate worthwhileness, or even despair (Becker, 1973). One could argue convincingly that suicides more often than not have failed troubled lives and relative biological unfitness and usually find a premature, perhaps unnecessary resolution to their life problems. That is, suicide is often a kind of Darwinian inability to live at all or to live well enough to survive.

Third, what is it that we are proposing to study? Suicide is unlike the other behavioral sciences in that it has usually included not just the study of suicide but also its prevention. In a sense suicide is like internal medicine. Suicide includes not only completed suicide and nonfatal attempted suicide but also partial self-destruction, suicidal gestures and ideation, parasuicide (Kreitman, 1977), deliberate self-harm, self-mutilation, and a panorama of related self-destructive behaviors and attitudes (Maris, 1992d). As we shall see shortly, completed suicide is a relatively rare behavior-occurring at a rate of 1 to 3 per 10,000 per year in the general population. However, completed suicide is just the tip of the proverbial self-destructive iceberg. One must always consider the full range of a subject's dependent variable. Of course, we also have to be careful not to make our dependent variable overly broad. Because suicide is not one thing but many related overlapping phenomena, it follows that neither does it have one cause or etiology.

Not only is the focus here be on completed suicide, it is on the treatment of suicidal individuals, as well. We should not forget that suicides tend to die one at a time and have their own unique life histories. High-risk groups, profiles according to the Minnesota Multiphasic Personality Inventory depressives, alcoholics, and so on, never kill themselves—individual people do. This should suggest to clinicians that suicide treatment plans and suicide prevention and intervention strategies need to be tailored to fit the special needs, pain, situations, and biology of a particular individual.

Finally, the study and prevention of suicide are interdependent. Understanding logically precedes intervention and control. Without a solid scientific foundation suicide prevention is doomed to be ineffective. Thus, another reason why we study suicide is to be able to intervene effectively in self-destructive behaviors. Individuals, who are in pain, hopeless, depressed, anxious, psychotic, and so on, have a right to relief short of irreversible cessation of their consciousness.

1.2.2   Epidemiology and problem

(1) Epidemiology

Suicide is not one thing or problem but is in fact many different overlapping yet somewhat distinct problems. And the success or failure of suicide science depends in large measure on how carefully we specify and operationally define our dependent variables. Also, broad epidemiological or socio-demographic problems of suicide are quite different from individual suicide case treatment problems.

Each year worldwide approximately one million individuals die of suicide, 10-20 million attempt suicide, and 50-120 million are profoundly affected by the suicide or attempted suicide of a close relative or associate. Asia accounts for 60 percent of world's suicides, so at least 60 million people are affected by suicide or attempted suicide in Asia each year (Beautrais, 2006). Even though suicide is rare we have to take it seriously, because it is a premature, fatal outcome—often with devastating interpersonal and economic consequences.

Age is a powerful factor in increased suicide rates. The highest suicide rates in the United States are and always have been found among older and middle white males, where the loss of a spouse, years of heavy drinking, job stagnation or loss, increased risk of depressive illness, and negative events were all noted as suicide forces. In China, the suicide rate for women is higher than that for men, too. There is over 40 percent were young rural women 15-34 years of age. The high suicide rate of women is in rural China, which has been attributed to the situation of women in the traditional patriarchal structure of Chinese society which causes woman's social and economic status to be problematic in and out of marriage (Lee et al., 2000). Children have remarkably low suicide rates, which are related to child's conceptual inability to comprehend the concepts of death and suicide, and lack of access to lethal means to attempt suicide.

On the other hand, gender plays a complex and important role in suicidal behavior, too. By early adolescence, males behave more lethally than females and differences in mortality rates continue across the entire lifespan and across cultures. Male suicide appears most significantly tied to an all greater frequency and level of violence and aggression and the relative lack of social sanction for accepting a helpless-dependent position in a help-giving relationship. In addition, the significance of relatedness to others and the importance of social supports appear to serve women most profoundly both as a protection against suicidal urges and as a precipitant for nonfatal suicidal behavior. There is in fact a growing divergence of rates, with male rates increasing and female rates decreasing. At the same time, there is an increasing trend for females to behave like males in their selection of firearms as the modal method of choice to complete suicide.

Suicide is not only a problem for Europe and North America, but also for Asia. In Asia, suicide has received relatively less attention for lack of resources and competing priorities. Generally as we age our suicide potential also rises. Especially for white males, suicide rates are highest in the oldest age groups (Richman, 1992). Female suicide rates usually peak in the 45-54 age group, then, drop slightly in older age groups. The relationships of suicide rates to other important predictor variables (marital status, occupation, mental disorder diagnosis, alcohol and substance abuse, methods of attempting suicide, etc.) are elaborated on in subsequent chapters.

(2) Problem

Are suicide, self-destructive behavior, and suicide ideation common treatment problems? We know suicide and self-destruction are fairly common problems among psychological or psychiatric patients, it may lead to malpractice litigation. The most common psychiatric diagnoses associated with suicide outcome of patients are the affective or mood disorders (especially, major depressive episode), the schizophrenias, substance abuse, and so on. So some critical questions facing suicide prevention workers are: which individuals are at risk of suicide? How high is their risk? When and under what circumstances is the suicide event likely to occur? Even in depressed psychiatric hospital patient populations, completed suicide is still relatively rare. As with any rare event, when one attempts to predict the outcome the tendency is to get false positives—here the misidentification of patients as suicides when they are not.

Some psychiatrists (e.g., Motto, 1992) argue that suicide prediction is an impossible task if we mean a high suicide probability of a particular individual suicide within a short time frame. Several helpful standardized suicide assessment and prediction scales have been reviewed in detail elsewhere (Rothbe and Geer-Williams, 1992). Therapists need to use subjective clinical judgment as well as objective tests and measurements when attempting to assess the suicide potential of individuals.

Another therapy or treatment problem concerns how does one become a competent suicide interventionist? How can patients and their families locate qualified physicians, psychologists, nurses, social workers, and pastoral counselors, for example, specializing in suicide prevention and treatment?

1.3   Varieties of self-destructive behaviors

At first blush suicide seems simple and clear, which is some pained individual ends their own life-period. However, suicide is not one thing but many, and it can be divided at least into completed suicides, nonfatal suicide attempts, suicidal ideation, and indirect self-destructive behavior.

1.3.1   Completed suicides

Suicides are individuals who have actually died by their own hand, have been sent to a morgue, funeral home, burial plot, or crematory, and are beyond any therapy. The typical suicide is an older male who is depressed, maybe alcoholic; lives alone or is socially isolated; uses a highly lethal irreversible method; dies after his first suicide attempt; has grown increasingly hopeless and cognitively rigid, may have some debilitating, nagging physical illnesses; has recurring work, sexual, and marital problems; has experienced a series of stressful, negative life events; in some cases has had a prior suicide in his family; and often sees suicide as the only permanent resolution to his persistent life problems (Maris, 1981) concept of a "suicidal career." The rates

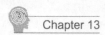

and prevalence of completed suicides were reviewed previously and need not be repeated here. Of course, not all suicides have all of the traits in the typical completed suicide profile, and it is different for patient suicides from suicides in the general population that have never been treated.

1.3.2 Nonfatal suicide attempters

A nonfatal suicide attempter is someone who intentionally injures him or her but does not die, and who is available for treatment. A typical nonfatal suicide attempter is a younger female who uses less "lethal" methods to attempt suicide (such as an overdose, other "poisoning" or cutting), is perhaps more ambivalent about dying, is often motivated by interpersonal dynamics including revenge or change in an important relationship, may be more impulsive, and whose problems can be related to anxiety or panic disorders and other Axis II personality disorders.

It is well known that nonfatal suicide attempts outnumber completed suicides but the exact ratio is speculative. Stengel (1964) first estimated that nonfatal suicide attempters outnumbered completers by a ratio of 6-8:1. Stengel (1964) contended that only about 10-15% of suicide attempters ever completed suicide. Linehan (1986) also gets the same conclusion.

But at the same time, we must realize that a very large percentage of completed suicides never make nonfatal attempts, are never treated, never present at a clinic or hospital.

1.3.3 Suicide idea

Suicide ideas are individuals who think about or form an intent to commit suicide of varying degrees of seriousness but do not make an explicit suicide attempt or complete suicide, which can vary from nonspecific. Suicide ideation is probably most closely associated with depressive disorders, and 67 and 84% of them maybe have suicidal ideation. Two of the more common suicidal ideas or motivations are to escape from one's life problems and to get revenge on others, not necessarily a wish to die.

Intention to suicide is a crucial component in suicidal ideas; however, it is also one of the most difficult to measure-especially after the fact of completed suicide. Most suicides are expected to have both motive and intent to suicide before they can be properly classified as a suicide.

Finally, suicidal ideas may come from imitation or contagion. This is an area of suicide research deserving of special consideration.

1.3.4 Indirect Self-Destructive Behaviors and Parasuicides

Not all self-destructive behaviors are overt, explicit, or intentional. In fact, probably the majority of self-destructive actions are partial, chronic, long-term, and even unconscious. Of course, we do not need to see all human behaviors as self-destructive. On the other hand, neither can we afford to neglect the chronic, cumulative, partially self-destructive behaviors in which many of us seem to engage. It is as if we were chronically depressed and felt that we deserved punishment or pain for our real or imagined transgressions. Kreitman (1977) observed that there can be self-harm even though there is not a clear intent to suicide. In many cases suicide intent cannot be documented and may not even be present.

1.4 The theory of suicide

Emile Durkheim saw suicide as an external and constraining social fact independent of individual psychopathology. Sigmund Freud and Karl Menninger considered suicide a murderous death wish that was turned back upon one's own self. Edwin Shneidman conceives suicide as "psychache" or intolerable psychological pain. Psychiatrist John Mann tends to think of suicide as reflecting brain neurotransmitter abnormalities or deficiencies.

Theory is usually contrasted with practice. The suspicion often is that theory is secondary to practice and at worst that theoreticians are only web spinning, impractical dilettantes who really lack the skills to be able to do much of anything. However, this is only the beginning theoretically, not the stopping point. Unlike Shneidman, Mann (1991) tends to see the etiology of suicide in the brain, most likely in dysfunctions of the serotonergic system (especially low 5-HIAA levels, postsynaptic receptors, and related biological markers).

Now we turn to a description of the basic building blocks or elements of a systematic theory of suicide to definitions, major concepts, hypotheses, and so on. After discussing each theoretical element in some detail and reviewing commonalities and differences among suicides, the chapter closes with an example of systematic suicide theory construction.

1.4.1 Definitions

Suicide is intentional self-murder (Maris, 1991, 1993), or as Rosenberg and colleagues (1988) put it, suicide is "death arising from an act inflicted upon oneself with the intention to kill oneself." The first point to note about the definition of suicide is that it is a death. It is amazing how many scientific papers and books have been written about "suicide ..." but have samples with not a single completed suicide in them!

Second, suicide is intended. Suicide is not unintentional and it is usually intentional. However, many suicides seem to be ambivalent about suiciding, and their intention to die is not constant. An important question here is, how high does one's suicide or death wish make one get a death outcome?

Third, suicide is done by oneself and to oneself, not someone else kills you, even if you want them to, it is usually defined as murder.

Fourth, suicide can be indirect or passive. For example, not taking life-preserving medicine or intentionally not moving from the path of an oncoming train is often suicidal.

1.4.2 Commonalities and similarities

Do all suicides have some traits in common? Are these suicidal commonalities not present among nonsuicides? Shneidman argues that all suicides tend to share the 10 commonalities of suicide (Shneidman, 1985; 1993). The 10 commonalities of suicide are:

(1) To seek a solution.

(2) Cessation of consciousness.

(3) Intolerable psychological pain.

(4) Frustrated psychological needs.

(5) Hopelessness-helplessness.

(6) Ambivalence.

(7) Constriction.

(8) Egression.

(9) Communication of intent.

(10) Lifelong coping patterns.

Let us elaborate some on these common traits of suicide seriatim, in passing making a few brief asides about their possible implications for suicide prevention, for instance:

(1) Suicide can be seen as life-problem solving. Most suicides are in life situations or suicidal careers that seem to demand resolution. Suicides lives are experienced as painful, intolerable, absurd, and meaningless, so much so that suicidal death may seem to be the only way out (Maris, 1982a). Of course, the key response to this commonality is that there usually are other resolutions short of suicide.

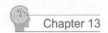

(2) Suicides want to interrupt their tortured self-consciousness, to stop the mental pain and anguish. Thus, it is understandable that analogues of suicide, sleep, anesthesia, psychosis, drug abuse, alcoholic stupor, etc. all involve alteration or cessation of consciousness. The challenge to suicide prevention here is to facilitate a meaningful change short of death through neurochemistry, psychotherapy, and so on.

(3) Psychological pain is the key commonality in all suicides. One absolutely central question for therapists to ask their suicidal patients is, "Tell me where you hurt". Often to prevent a suicide one just has to take the edge off the pain, not eliminate the pain.

(4) Most suicides have been frustrated in meeting some of their basic psychological needs. These include the 20 to 30 needs originally listed by Harvard psychologist Henry Murray (1938). Often meeting psychological needs entails resocialization, regression, and reparenting.

(5) Suicides are not just depressed. As Beck (1986) has demonstrated, suicides tend to have become hopeless that their life quality will ever improve sufficiently, and they feel helpless to do anything about it. Therapists need to convince the suicidal patient, "You can be helped". Suicidal patients need at least one significant udder.

(6) Suicides both want to die and want to live. It is common for soon-to-be suicides to make appointments for after their death. Freud claimed that we all have both life (eros) and death (thanatos) wishes. Treatment and intervention are often justified on the grounds that the therapist is after all just supporting or responding to the life-affirming pole of the would-be suicide's own ambivalence.

(7) Attempt suicide was the only thing they could do! |One of the salient mental traits of depressed suicidal individuals is the narrowing of their perceived viable alternatives, often to the extreme of dichotomous thinking (Weishaar and Beck, 1992). For example, suicides commonly think to themselves, "I must be either miserable or dead."

(8) Most of them probably just want the pain to stop. Many have tried alternatives snort of suicide but are now faced with the ultimate egression. All experience for many suicidal individuals is seen as preferable to continued existence in this world.

(9) A lot of suicides will tell you that they are contemplating suicide, if you listen carefully, are sensitive to indirect behavioral or verbal clues, and generally just pay attention. These may not be clear, but they will be at least ambiguous signs. These may include expressions of hopelessness, preparations for death, serious depression, partially self-destructive behaviors, alcoholism and exacerbation of drinking or drug use/abuse, acquiring the method of suicide, open declarations of suicidal intent or saying farewell, being placed in situations of great stress or loss, and isolation and precautions to avoid rescue. Of course, all these signs are ambiguous and most of the time they identify "false-positive" suicides, that is people who never in fact kill themselves.

(10) Suicides tend to have what we earlier called suicidal careers. They tend to be chronically self-destructive, with a repeated exhaustion of their adaptive repertoire most suicidal crises are only crises because of the long history of partially self-destructive coping.

Not only do suicides share common traits, they also are (of course) different, comprise somewhat separate and distinct types, and can be classified by their salient characteristics. For example, we reviewed Durkheim's four basic types of suicide: 1) anomic; 2) egoistic; 3) altruistic, and 4) fatalistic.

1.5 Treatment and prevention of suicide

By virtue of a symptom, set of symptoms, a complaint(s), or problem(s), an individual seeks or is referred, taken, or commanded to seek help from a person with specialized skills, licensed to observe and evaluate, refer to or offer treatment, and then treat, successfully it is hoped, the presenting issues. This is the clinical paradigm. It defines roles of patient and caregiver and simply outlines the patient-caregiver relationship and the help-giving process. But, with the suicidal patient, these are anything but simple.

The distinction between treatment and prevention is essentially one of timing: in prevention we attempt to intervene before the onset of a problem; clinical treatment begins once a problem has developed and, too often, well after optimal points of intervention have passed.

Moreover, certain features, typically present with the suicidal patient, are incongruous with a good patient's role and obligations. For example, the patient who intentionally has injured him- or herself is both the perpetrator and victim of his or her action, in contrast to being the innocent victim of an undesirable disease or injury. Moreover, not all suicidal patients share their caregiver's belief that they should be provided with life-sustaining treatment; some may maintain a persistent wish to die. Treatment compliance and the attainment of a reciprocal, collaborative relationship are often difficult.

High-risk patients have a number of character traits, skill deficits, and attachment difficulties that both explain their suicidality and negatively affect treatment alliance. Among these are significant psychopathology, limited impulse control (act first, think later), alcohol and drug abuse or both, and poor relational, communication, emotional regulation, and problem-solving skills. Among suicidal adolescents, in particular (but, perhaps, common to all life stages), stage-specific developmental characteristics further make the forming of a therapeutic alliance difficult for example, idealism and absolutism (black and white thinking), externalizing attributions, and so on. Attachment patterns common to suicidal adolescents have been described as unresolved/disorganized. So treatment drops out rates high. As the quality of the therapeutic alliance is the greatest single factor affecting treatment outcome, recognizing these issues is critical to developing a treatment plan with chance of successful implementation.

Compliance with treatment, both medication and psychotherapy, is a significant treatment problem when dealing with suicidal patients. People, even after treatment in a hospital emergency room for a suicide attempt, have low rates of compliance.

1.5.1 Counter transference

Suicidal communications, in the form of behaviors, threats, and verbalized ideation, are common to a number of mental disorders (e.g., schizophrenia and alcohol abuse). Conversely, a number of mental disorders have suicidal behavior as one of several symptom criteria, a proportion of which define the disorder (e.g., major depression and borderline personality disorder). Thus, suicidal behaviors are commonly observed in the clinical paradigm.

In fact, suicidal behaviors are the most frequent mental health, problems presenting to hospital emergency departments and that result in inpatient admissions. This is particularly true among children and adolescent inpatient psychiatric admissions.

Given our difficulty in accurately predicting when and if any at-risk patient might attempt suicide, the potential for a patient acting on suicidal urges (and consequently causing lethal medical damage) is constancy in the clinical situation and is anxiety provoking to the clinician.

Berman (1986a) estimated that one in six individuals who complete suicide is actively engaged in psychotherapy at the time of their deaths and that one-half of completers have had experience with the mental health system at some time. It is of interest, then, to consider whether these suicides might be considered prima facie evidence of treatment failures. Moreover, it is of interest to consider whether these suicides were consequent to some iatrogenic effect. Iatrogenesis is defined as a caregiver-induced negative effect (or illness caused by health care), such as hopelessness engendered by a lack of response to sequentially prescribed antidepressants or the anger and distrust induced and reinforced by involuntary hospitalization.

Perhaps, the most significant contributor to iatrogenesis is negative counter transference. In its most

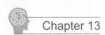

contemporary usage, negative counter transference is defined by a range of aversive reactions (thoughts, feelings, behaviors) that are manifested in clinicians in reaction to working with their psychotherapy patients. These reactions range from anger to hopelessness to dislike. In the traditional meaning of the term, these reactions are unconscious and stem from the therapists relationships in childhood (e.g., to parents). Often, however, these responses are conscious and directly related to a difficult-to-treat patient.

As noted previously, suicidal patients readily engender fears and anxieties in clinicians. They present complicated and often chronic histories, maintain a high level of threat, impose strong feelings and behaviors stemming from poor relationships with their primary caregivers (parents), pose potential emergency situations and potential malpractice litigation, should they complete suicide during the therapist watch. Each and every one of these anxieties must be successfully managed by the clinician in order to maintain an effective and helpful therapeutic position. This is no small task.

There is little doubt that suicidal patients harbor much rage, can be manipulative or help rejecting, and engage in a number of interpersonally alienating behaviors. Suicidal patients who have diagnoses of schizophrenia, schizophrenic spectrum disorders, or borderline personality disorder are, indeed, difficult to treat. These patients may experience extreme distress at having to tolerate aloneness, may be terrified at anticipated abandonments, and may have diffuse boundaries—any or all of which test the most experienced of therapists" skills at maintaining appropriate therapeutic positions. Moreover, a patient who threatens suicide is, at once, rejecting the offered help and efforts of the therapist.

Negative therapist attitudes toward suicidal patients are also observable in the pejorative labeling attributed to difficult-to-treat patients. Suicidal patients are often seen suggesting that they are devious and indirect in attempting to control others and outcomes or both, rather than more simply deficient in skills to be in better control. As few people like to be manipulated, perhaps especially therapists whose job it is to manipulate, protective distancing is likely to result from perceived manipulators. This is the antithesis of what is needed to change a patient's interpersonal behavior and to teach more effective skills.

Similarly, therapists are wont to label help-rejecting patients resistive. Rather than seeing this as an obstacle of therapy, resistance needs to be reframed as one of the reasons this patient needs therapy; that is resistance, is a protective device, probably learned in childhood, which has gained functional autonomy with age. Patients need to be helped to analyze the defense and to learn to risk trusting behaviors in the context of the therapeutic relationship.

Finally, suicidal persons challenge caregivers to examine their own issues regarding life and death, to keep clear the boundary between personal beliefs and professional ethics, and to examine carefully their attitudes toward involuntary detention and treatment.

1.5.2 From assessment to disposition

Risk assessment initiates treatment by first addressing the appropriate setting. If a patient is evaluated as at high risk for imminent suicidal behavior, immediate action is called for to protect the patient from him- or herself. Psychiatric hospitalization is generally thought to provide the most secure environment and best opportunity to provide sanctuary, to manage and observe behavior, and to initiate treatments. Thus a rationale or cost-benefit analysis for inpatient hospitalization is the first consideration for an acutely suicidal patient.

The decision to hospitalize is based on a number of criteria reflective of patient's acute psychopathology, observed ability to regulate self, alternative sources of support and monitoring, and so on. Among the variables to consider are the following:

(1) Psychopathology that describes symptoms of decontrol or impending decompensation such as disorientation, dissociation, and impulsive behavior; high levels of perturbation (agitation); thought disorder (e.g.,

hallucinations and delusions), and high levels of rage, panic, or uncontrolled violent behavior.

(2) Medical problems consequent to a suicide attempt placing the patient in danger of losing life, if untreated.

(3) Stress at high and unresolvable levels.

(4) Attachment problems such as the absence of a supportive family or surrogate system to monitor and prevent isolation or the presence of an abusive, rejecting, or psychiatrically impaired interpersonal system; the absence of a therapeutic alliance; or the absence of other attachments of personal value and efficacy, such as employment, function and so on.

(5) Highly death intentioned suicidal thinking or behavior indirectly suggesting high intent.

(6) Evaluated acute risk in the context of a family history of suicide.

There are clear benefits to the stabilization and sanctuary that hospitalization provides: The patient is removed from sources of stress; an immediate change in (pathological) system dynamics is effected; 24-hour support and monitoring are available that counteract isolation and loneliness and encourage activity and interpersonal involvement; maximum control over suicidal and aggressive urges is available; hope and mastery are instilled through stepwise goal attainment programs; medical consequences and complications from self-injurious behavior can be treated and monitored; and medications may be reconsidered arid titrated to therapeutic levels. For some, hospitalization is an aversive experience and is, thus, a contingent reinforce to sufficient self-regulation to deter future rehospitalization.

There also are clear costs: hospitalization interrupts the consistency and alliance building of an outpatient contract; reinforces regression and, for some, fosters an institutional dependency; and removes the patient from the in vivo context in which coping and mastery skills need to be applied and reinforced. Furthermore, the hospitalized patient loses some degree of autonomy and may feel stigmatized. These pose significant problems to outpatient alliances (problems of trust, for example) and reentry, for example, for an adolescent who must now return to school and peers.

One point should be made eminently clear: Hospitalization does not necessarily prevent suicide. Suicides can occur in hospitals, although policy and procedural safeguards typically deter such outcomes, on passes and via elopement from an inpatient unit, and quite soon after discharge, suggesting that this is a particularly crucial treatment decision point. Also, the decision to hospitalize is best considered when the patient voluntarily consents to this treatment setting. Involuntary hospitalization is mandated by state statute under conditions (with regard to suicide) of evaluated imminent danger to self.

1.5.3　Inpatient and outpatient treatment

The immediate treatment goal of inpatient hospitalization is the absence of current suicidal ideation and intent. Within the typical parameters of managed care, this goal must be met rapidly; economic pressures are now added to the matrix of considerations in determining discharge decisions. Clearly, when the patient is still considered to be unsafe from his or her own self-destructive urges, a well-documented appeal for extended treatment should allow sufficient additional time to stabilize most patients.

At the most acute phase of risk, an imminently suicidal patient is immediately confronted with a treatment environment in most psychiatric inpatient units that promotes protection, safety, and connectedness. The patient is denied access to immediately accessible means to suicide—for example, sharp objects are confiscated at admission—and units are reasonably suicide-proofed in their design; for example, breakaway shower rods are used and windows are barred or effectively screened internally. Watch procedures and monitoring protocols are established ranging from one-to-one constant observation to various levels (e.g., 15 minutes) of logged checks. No unit, however, can be totally suicide proofed and in-hospital suicides do occur. In addition, it should be kept in mind that a suicidal act can lead to death in less than 5 minutes; thus, any level

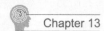

of surveillance other than that of close observation, one-to-one or group, is insufficient to prevent suicide. A typical initial treatment plan will evolve at admission or after a few days' observation. Secondary treatment goals, of course, would be established for assessed underlying problems (for depressed mood, social skills, self-esteem, etc.).

Inpatient care usually involves a screening evaluation and team-developed treatment plan, treatment according to that plan, followed by discharge planning and implementation. As indicated by the initial and follow-up evaluations of suicide risk, affirmative precautions are instituted—with an ever present awareness that suicides can occur in the best of inpatient units. Unit policies and procedures should define steps to safeguard the environment and protect the patient, in addition to staff responsibilities, roles, and so on.

The hospital promises to provide the patient safety, a responsibility it already has, while the patient commits to not act in a suicidal manner and to inform the staff should suicidal urges become overwhelming. The no-suicide contract actually is a clinical tool used to assess the therapeutic alliance and to identify explicitly a treatment goal.

The frequency of suicides that occur shortly after hospitalization is disturbing. Several implications need to be considered: Did the assessment of suicide risk at the time of discharge inadequately consider the toxic effect of the external social milieu or the loss of constant support provided by hospital care? Was the patient sufficiently advised of the need for continued compliance with the treatment plan and referral for outpatient care? Did the patient intentionally deceive/mislead the treatment team in appearing well-enough for discharge? Was follow-up outpatient care not sufficiently accessed? Was patient's family or significant other insufficiently aligned with follow-up care needs or with the continued need for surveillance and reporting?

Outpatient treatment begins with the assessment of suicide risk and the decision not to hospitalize. If the risk for suicidal behavior is high but not sufficiently imminent to demand hospitalization, the need for monitoring may still be present through the period of perturbation or crisis. A person close to the patient and capable of providing both vigilance and relief from aloneness should be considered and may be necessary. Home environments should be suicide proofed, as much as possible, particularly as they pertain to available and accessible firearms and medications. Frequent contact with the primary caregiver is important through either increased session visits or telephone communication. Pharmacological interventions should be considered for assessed diagnoses. With these immediate supports established, treatment planning ensues.

1.5.4   Treatment planning

Treatment planning involves designing interventions that aim first at reducing the risk of suicidal behavior and second at reducing the predisposition to being suicidal. It is a truism that the better the assessment, particularly in understanding the suicidal person5s vulnerabilities and pathologies, aims or goals of suicidal behavior, and resources (protective factors), the easier the treatment planning. In addition to deciding structural issues such as the site of treatment (inpatient vs. outpatient), treatment planning speaks to the sequencing of treatment, for example, with dual-diagnosis patients; the particular type(s) of psychosocial intervention; the need for biological interventions, such as medication or electroconvulsive therapy; the frequency and duration of interventions; the measurable goals of interventions, the accomplishment of which leads to termination from treatment and follow-up planning; and environmental manipulations and enhancements to support treatment goals.

Treatment planning further specifies particular symptom remission related goals (the reduction in frequency, intensity, duration, or specificity of suicidal ideation; decreased hopelessness; improved access to supports, etc.). Specific throughout the treatment planning should be considerations of ongoing risk assessment and the need for collateral consultations.

1.5.5　Treatment approaches

(1) Crisis intervention

Crisis intervention and management approaches to the suicidal patient are designed to ensure patient's safety and life until the precipitant crisis situation can be resolved and a precrisis equilibrium restored. The steps of crisis intervention might involve 1) restricting access to lethal means (e.g., removal of available and accessible weapons); 2) decreasing personal isolation (e.g., monitoring activities and behavior through constant interpersonal watch); 3) decreasing anxiety, agitation, or insomnia (e.g., through medication or relaxation training procedures); 4) increasing accessibility (e.g., through telephone availability) and frequency of contact; 5) establishing a collaborative, problem-solving focus to treatment and fostering patient's problem-solving skills; 6) removal from stressful or toxic environments (e.g., through hospitalization); 7) system interventions to shift immediate (e.g., family) dynamics; and 8) negotiating safety considerations and developing contingency plans.

(2) Brief therapy

Brief therapy is a time-limited intervention that, especially in the era of managed care, attempts to focus on maximizing change, accomplishing goals and need fulfillment, and problem-solving. One example of this intervention approach is solution-focused brief therapy. As described by Fiske (1997), solution-focused brief therapy transfers the treatment focus from problems and pathology to solutions and competencies. This shift in focus is toward the future doing more of what works and something different if something is not working. The model emphasizes exceptions to the problem ("nothing occurs always!"), using patient's strength, competencies, resources, and successes; helping patients define their goals; and effecting small changes that generate yet larger, more profound, and pervasive changes.

(3) Cognitive-behavioral therapy

Cognitive-behavioral therapy is also structured and problem focused. In a time- limited approach, CBT aims to identify and change dysfunctional cognitions (thoughts, beliefs, schemas, etc.) and behaviors. Problems are conceptualized as having interacting dysfunctional thoughts, moods, and behaviors. By identifying and changing any one component, problem solving can occur.

The basis for a cognitive approach is rooted in a substantial body of research linking cognition and suicide (cf. Ellis and Newman, 1996). Hopelessness, problem-solving deficits, perfectionism, and a variety of dysfunctional attitudes and irrational beliefs have been found to be characteristic of suicidal individuals. Teaching problem-solving thinking, reattaching to reasons for living, and defusing black-and-white thinking, then, become tools for correcting maladaptive thinking.

For adults, the typical point of attack is on patient's cognitive distortions and automatic negative thoughts that underlie a depressive mood state, or even more malignant states of hopelessness (Berchick and Wright, 1992). For children and adolescents, behaviors are easier to observe and monitor, therefore modify (Trautman, 1995). For both adult and adolescent patients, the CBT therapist is active and assertive, providing explanations and positive feedback with frequency.

Above all, the CBT model is collaborative. Therapist and patient (patient's family), identify patient's problems, strengths, and previous attempts at problem solving. By viewing the world through patient's eyes, the therapist is able to identify and label patient's errors in thinking, automatic thoughts such as overgeneralization, jumping to conclusions, and dysfunctional attributions, and to help the patient develop alternative explanations, interpretations, and beliefs. In particular, a primary target of treatment is to change patient's view of suicide as the most desirable (or only) alternative to the present, pained experience of living.

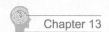

Problem-solving thinking and skills are developed and practiced. A significant goal of treatment is to increase the frequency of pleasant and rewarding thoughts and experiences (activities).

(4) Dialectical behavior therapy

Dialectical behavior therapy (DBT) was developed by Linehan (1993) specifically to treat the chronic suicidal patient who lives a suicidal career high in suicidal ideation, frequent in suicide talk and threat or both, and high in repetitive suicide attempts of varying degrees of lethality. DBT differs from traditional cognitive-behavioral approaches to treatment in that it is based on making behavioral techniques more compatible with psychodynamic models (see below). The model posits that the chronic suicidal individual 1) lacks and must acquire self-regulation (of emotion and behavior) and distress tolerance skills and 2) must be motivated to strengthen and generalize skills to out-of-therapy situations.

DBT utilizes a problem-solving strategy, addressing patient behaviors through a collaborative behavioral analysis and hypothesis formulation. Possible changes (behavioral solutions) are then generated to be tested and evaluated. Dialectical strategies balance and at- tempt to synthesize coexisting opposites and tensions, helping the patient accept reality as ambiguous and constantly changing. The therapist validates patient's view of life (and death) while implementing alternative problem-solving analyses and responses. Detailed chain analyses of environmental and behavioral events linked to suicidal behavior are conducted to elicit patterns and to identify alternative solutions. Patient's capacity (skills) to modify problematic precipitating events or conditions that inhibit or interfere with the use of existing skills must then be understood. Skills, then, are either taught or inhibiting forces reduced. A commitment to learning nonsuicidal behavioral responses while tolerating negative affect is a significant target of DBT treatment.

(5) Psychoanalytic/psychodynamic approaches

Psychoanalytic/psychodynamic approaches to treating the suicidal patient assume that suicidal behavior is an expression of unconscious conflict. The goal of treatment is to gain insight in order to resolve the intrapsychic pain, self-hatred, and so on. The classic psychoanalytic approach, or Freudian model, theorized that suicidal urges expressions of a turning inward of aggressive/hostile impulses—an attack against the ambivalently held internalized love object. Freud (1917/1963) noted that self-reproaches are reproaches against a loved object which have been shifted away from it onto patient's own ego, Libido invested in another ("object libido") is withdrawn and directed back into the self and an identification takes place between the ego and the lost object. The ego could only kill itself, Freud argued, it can treat itself as an object.

More modern analytical approaches define the core conflict in different terms, each then posing a different cause for suicide to be understood and resolved. Object relations theory emphasizes that suicide represents a failure in the task of separation-individuation. The suicide act is an attempt to rid the self of the bad internal objects and to reunite with idealized omnipotent love objects. Research on attachment styles among suicidal teens and adults supports this, model, finding many more "insecure" styles of attachment, ranging from avoidant to clinging. Alternatively, suicide is seen as a resolution to problems of separation and individuation through a regressive wish to return to a state of symbiosis.

Self-psychology theorists argue that suicide vulnerability arises from threats of being overwhelmed by negative self-judgments (e.g., worthlessness and guilt) in the context of an intolerably intense experience of aloneness isolation. Soothing security can be derived from having soothing self-objects and from having available external holding resources. Lacking these internal resources and absent external resources for soothing, there is a profound and intolerable state of aloneness. Suicide avoids the experience of a crumbling self.

Suicide, in turn, may avoid having to accept a changed sense of self (Smith, 1985). Individuals maintain an internalized view of self—an unconscious, life-guiding abstraction that is rigidly held.

These psychodynamic formulations inform psychodynamic interventions, such as the analysis of transference, exploration of intrapsychic pain and negative early life events, identification of painful affect states, interpretation of defenses and the motives that maintain self-devaluation, attention to issues of individuation and self-soothing, and so on. Central to the treatment is the role of the therapeutic relationship. The psychodynamic therapist plays the role of good enough parent's establishes self-object transferences that convey acceptance and confirmation, protects against feared disintegration from painful affect, models soothing and nurturing, interprets transferential impulses that seek to punish a hated parent or seek rescue while supporting ego functioning, perseveres in the face of suicide ideation or through assaults on his or her competence, and so on.

(6) Psychpharmacotherapy

Psychopharmacotherapy does not target suicidal behavior. There simply is no antisuicide pill. Rather, pharmacological strategies are diagnosis-specific treatments that aim to regulate the biochemistry associated with predisposing, suicidogenic pathologies. There is evidence which is linking diminished serotonin (5-HT) metabolism and depression, thus suggesting that the administration of selective serotonin reuptake inhibitors should effect a reduction in suicidality.

Antidepressant medications, particularly the less toxic selective serotonin reuptake inhibitors, and lithium and carbamazepine for bipolar disorders are core considerations for pharmacological intervention in suicidal patients. These medications also may reduce episodic impulsive and aggressive behavior. Neuroleptics and antipsychotics are to be considered to manage chronic schizophrenia, as might the short-term use of a benzodiazepine for acute anxiety states. But the effectiveness of psychopharmacological interventions has been widely debated in the literature.

(7) Electroconvulsive therapy

Electroconvulsive therapy, in its modern form, is generally considered safe and effective in the treatment of major depression and mania and should be considered for suicidal patients whose disorders are refractory to psychopharmacological interventions. However, perhaps because there is a paucity of randomized controlled studies to document its effectiveness—or because of negative public perceptions, it has not gained widespread use or acceptance.

1.5.6   Social system intervention

(1) Family therapy

Family therapy seeks to alter system dynamics when suicidal behavior is viewed as an expression of family dysfunction and transactional difficulties. For suicidal children and adolescents, in particular, it is considered a most significant intervention, paralleling the child need for individual therapy, as family problems often precipitate suicidal behavior among youth. Among early trauma frequently linked to later suicidal behaviors are early family loss, physical, sexual abuse, and so on.

The goal of family therapy is to improve family functioning. This may be accomplished in a number of ways designed to reduce enmeshment and support greater individuation, increase tolerance and flexibility, identify and resolve communication problems, clarify dysfunctional alliances, reveal and accept previously held secrets, increase mutually rewarding behaviors among family members, decrease punitive interactions among family members, and so on. Moreover, family members might be educated about and to monitor suicide risk in a suicidal member.

(2) Group therapy

Group therapy seeks to help suicidal patients acquire and maintain a social support network. Concurrently

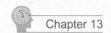

it affords a safe haven in which social skill deficits may be observed and social skill development may occur. Interpersonal learning and support are developed through the sharing of problems, perceived commonalities among group members, and reinforcing feedback among members and by therapists. In particular, the impact of one^ behavior on others can be observed and understood. Among the skills that may develop in group are those of listening and empathy, an understanding of group qua family dynamics, and the containment and regulation of impulses. Group leaders/therapists model good parents and teaching specific skills while exploring pathological defenses, cognitive distortions, and so on.

To sum up, the effective prevention of suicide and suicidal behaviors is in the best interest of all communities. Prevention efforts communicate that life is valued. It should make no difference whether that message is given to those suffering with cancer, with AIDS, with alcoholism or with suicidal despair. Prevention efforts might actually save lives, provide years of productive life, and enhance protective factors that generalize across the potential mental and public health problems.

However, even if we accomplish a more scientific basis for these efforts, we are not naive enough to believe that we can prevent all suicides. And with each of these suicides, there will be many survivors.

2. The concept of psychiatric rehabilitation

Psychiatric rehabilitation, also known as psychosocial rehabilitation, is the process of restoration of community functioning and well-being of an individual diagnosed in mental health or mental or emotional disorder and who may be considered to have a psychiatric disability.

2.1　The origin of psychiatric rehabilitation

Psychiatric rehabilitation emerged as a significant field of practice and study during the 1970s and 1980s, in part as a response to the tragedies of the deinstitutionalization movement, which beginning in the 1950s, discharged large numbers of state hospital patients to a psycho-social community. In essence, deinstitutionalization accomplished a single outcome: transferring patients with severe mental illnesses to the community, a relatively easy task in comparison to the goals of rehabilitation. Said another way, deinstitutionalization opened the doors of the institutions and literally gave people a prescription for their medicine when they left. Rehabilitation attempts to open the doors of the community and help people figuratively develop a prescription for their lives.

2.2　The definition of psychiatric rehabilitation

Psychiatric rehabilitation is not a practice but a field of academic study or discipline, similar to social work or political science; other definitions may place it as a specialty of community rehabilitation or physical medicine and rehabilitation. As psychiatric rehabilitation services and concepts have become more common in helping people with severe mental illnesses to regain their valued roles, the necessity of developing a standard definition of psychiatric rehabilitation has become apparent. On September 29, 2007, the following definition was approved and adopted by the Board of Directors of United States Psychiatric Rehabilitation Association, the major professional association of the field of psychiatric rehabilitation.

Psychiatric rehabilitation promotes recovery, full community integration, and improves the quality of life for persons who have been diagnosed with any mental health condition that impairs their ability to lead meaningful lives seriously. Psychiatric rehabilitation services are collaborative, person-directed, and individualized. These services are an essential element of the health care and human services spectrum, and should be evidence-based. They focus on helping individuals develop skills and access resources needed to increase their capacity to be successful and satisfied in the living, working, learning, and social environments of their choice.

The term was added to the U.S. National Library of Medicine's Medical Subject Headings in 2016.

There, psychiatric rehabilitation is defined as: specialty field that promotes recovery, community functioning, and increased well-being of individuals diagnosed with mental disorders that impair their ability to live meaningful lives.

2.3   The common methods of psychiatric rehabilitation

The mission of psychiatric rehabilitation is to enable with best practices of illness management, psycho-social functioning, and personal satisfaction. Treatments and practices towards this are guided by principles. There are seven strategic principles:

(1) Enabling a normal life.

(2) Advocating structural changes for improved accessibility to pharmacological services and availability of psycho-social services.

(3) Person-centered treatment.

(4) Actively involving support systems.

(5) Coordination of efficient services.

(6) Strength-based approach.

(7) Rehabilitation is not time specific but goal specific in succeeding.

Principles guide psycho-social rehabilitation practices to be better.

Recovery through rehabilitation is defined possible without complete remission of their illness, and it is geared towards aiding the individual in attaining optimum mental health and wellbeing.

The common methods of psychiatric rehabilitation mainly include two parts:

(1) Psychotherapy and psycho-social treatments, which include:

1) Individual psychoanalytic psychotherapy

2) Interpersonal psychotherapy

3) Brief psychotherapy

4) Group psychotherapy

5) Cognitive and behavioral therapy

6) Family therapy

7) Couples therapy

8) Hypnosis

9) Behavioral medicine

10) Psycho-social rehabilitation

(2) Pharmacological and brain stimulation treatments, which include:

1) Antidepressants

2) Antipsychotic drugs

3) Mood stabilizers

4) Anxiolytic drugs

5) Pharmacological treatment of insomnia

6) Stimulants

7) Cognitive enhancers

8) Complementary and alternative treatments in psychiatry

9) Brain stimulation in psychiatry

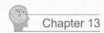

Relative studies underscore the significance of symptomatic remission, social skills building, and strengthening cognitive functioning to prepare patients for rehabilitation services and community integration. Many pharmacological interventions are necessary to reduce or extinguish positive symptoms (i.e., hallucination and delusions) and provide opportunities for the patient to develop and attain social and mental health rehabilitation, which are the optimal levels of functioning and quality of life.

2.4　People who need psychiatric rehabilitation

Psychiatric rehabilitation is not a practice but a field of academic study or discipline, similar to social work or political science. It is aligned with the community support development of the National Institute on Mental Health begun in the 1970s, and is marked by a rigorous tradition of research, training and technical assistance, and information dissemination regarding a critical population group (e.g., psychiatric disability) in the US and worldwide.

As a result of deinstitutionalization, most adults diagnosed with severe mental illnesses, such as schizophrenia, bipolar disorder, major depression, and the like, are now residing in the community. These individuals are the primary recipients of psychiatric rehabilitation services. Psychiatric rehabilitation helps persons who have experienced severe psychiatric disabilities, rather than concentrating on individuals who are simply dissatisfied, unhappy, or "socially disadvantaged". Persons with psychiatric disabilities have diagnosed mental illnesses that limit their capacity to perform certain tasks and functions (e.g., interacting with family and friends, interviewing for a job, studying for tests) and their ability to perform in various community roles (e.g., worker, resident, spouse, friend, student).

（杨世昌　马现仓）

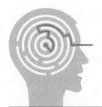

References

[1] American Psychiatric Association. Diagnostic and Statistical Manual of Mental Disorders. 5th ed. Arlington: American Psychiatric Association, 2013.

[2] Barlow DH, Gorman JM, Shear MK, et al. Cognitive-behavioral therapy, imipramine, or their combination for panic disorder: A randomized controlled trial. J Am Med Assoc, 2000, 283 (19): 2529-2536.

[3] Bateman A, Fonagy P. Effectiveness of partial hospitalization in the treatment of borderline personality disorder: a randomized controlled trial. Am J Psychiatry, 1999, 156 (10): 1563-1569.

[4] Bracha HS, Ralston TC, Matsukawa JM, et al. Does "fight or flight" need updating? Psychosomatics, 2004, 45 (5): 448-449.

[5] Brown GK, Ten Have T, Henriques GR, et al. Cognitive therapy for the prevention of suicide attempts: a randomized controlled trial. J Am Med Assoc, 2005, 294 (5): 563-570.

[6] Butle AC, Chapman JE, Forman EM, et al. The empirical status of cognitive-behavioral therapy: a review of meta-analyses. Clin Psychol Rev, 2006, 26 (1): 17-31.

[7] Chen W, Qin K, Su W, et al. Development of a structure-validated Sexual Dream Experience Questionnaire (SDEQ) in Chinese university students. Compr Psychiatry, 2015, 56: 245-251.

[8] Chen W, Xu Y, Zhu M, et al. Development of a structure-validated Nightmare Experience Questionnaire in Chinese university students. J Psychiatry: Open Access, 2014, 17: 1000147.

[9] Craske MG, Golinelli D, Stein MB, et al. Does the addition of cognitive-behavioral therapy improve panic disorder treatment outcome relative to medication alone in the primary-care setting? Psychol Med, 2005, 35 (11): 1-10.

[10] Ehlers A, Clark, DM. A cognitive model of posttraumatic stress disorder. Behav Res Ther, 2000, 38 (4): 319-345.

[11] Eng W, Roth DA, Heimberg RG. Cognitive-behavioral therapy for social anxiety. J Cogn Psychother, 2001, 15 (4): 311-319.

[12] Foa EB, Hembree EA, Cahill SP, et al. Randomized trial of prolonged exposure for posttraumatic stress disorder with and without cognitive restructuring: outcome at academic and community clinics. J Consult Clin Psychol, 2005, 73 (5): 953-964.

[13] Frank MG, Issa NP, Stryker MP. Sleep enhances plasticity in the developing visual cortex. Neuron, 2001, 30 (1): 275-287.

[14] Gabbard GO. Long-Term Psychodynamic Psychotherapy: A Basic Text. Arlington, VA: American Psychiatric Association, 2017.

[15] Gillespie K, Duffy M, Hackmann A, et al. Community-based cognitive therapy in the treatment of posttraumatic stress disorder following the Omagh bomb. Behav Res Ther, 2002, 40 (4): 345-357.

[16] Hayes SC, Follette VM, Linehan M. Mindfulness and acceptance: Expanding the cognitive-behavioral tradition. New York: Guilford, 2004.

[17] Lepage M, Ghaffar O, Nyberg L, et al. Prefrontal cortex and episodic memory retrieval mode. Proc Nation Acad Sci, 2000, 97 (1): 506-511.

[18] Loeb KL, Wilson GT, Labouvie E, et al. Therapeutic alliance and treatment adherence in two interventions for bulimia nervosa: A study of process and outcome. J Consult Clin Psychol, 2005, 73 (6): 1097-1107.

[19] Lowery D, Fillingim RB, Wright RA. Sex differences and incentive effects on perceptual and cardiovascular responses to cold pressor pain. Psychosom Med, 2003, 65 (2): 284-291.

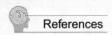
[20] Pike KM, Walsh BT, Vitousek K, et al. Cognitive behavior therapy in the posthospitalization treatment of anorexia nervosa. Am J Psychiatry, 2003, 160 (11): 2046-2049.

[21] Revonsuo A. The reinterpretation of dreams: An evolutionary hypothesis of the function of dreaming. Behav Brain Sci, 2000, 23 (6): 877-901.

[22] Rizzolatti G, Craighero L. The mirror-neuron system. Annu Rev Neurosci, 2004, 27: 169-192.

[23] Stirman SW, Derubeis R J, Crits-Christoph P, et al. Can the randomized controlled trial literature generalize to nonrandomized patients? J Consult Clin Psychol, 2005, 73 (1): 127-135.

[24] Strunk DR, DeRubeis RJ. Cognitive therapy for depression: A review of its efficacy. J Cogn Psychother, 2001, 15 (4): 289-297.

[25] Svartberg M, Stiles TC, Seltzer MH. Randomized, controlled trial of the effectiveness of short-term dynamic psychotherapy and cognitive therapy for cluster C personality disorders. Am J Psychiatry, 2004, 161 (5): 810-817.

[26] Tarrier N, Wykes T. Is there evidence that cognitive behaviour therapy is an effective treatment for schizophrenia? A cautious or cautionary tale? Behav Res Ther, 2004, 42 (12): 1377-1401.

[27] Taylor SE, Klein LC, Lewis, BP, et al. Biobehavioral Responses to Stress in Females: Tend-and-Befriend, not Fight-or-Flight. Psychol Rev, 2000, 107 (3): 411-429.

[28] Walker MP, Stickgold R. Sleep-dependent learning and memory consolidation. Neuron, 2004, 44 (1): 121-133.

[29] Wang W, Du W, Wang Y, et al. The relationship between the Zuckerman-Kuhlman Personality Questionnaire and traits delineating personality pathology. Person Indiv Diff, 2004, 36 (1): 155-162.

[30] Wang Y, Zhu M, Huang J, et al. Family Behavior Therapy for Antisocial and Narcissistic Personality Disorders in China: An Open Study. Germ J Psychiatry, 2008, 11 (1): 91-97.

12检